Laboratory/Pathology Words and Phrases

Laboratory Medicine
Anatomic Pathology
Clinical Pathology
Hematology
Dermatopathology

Health Professions Institute • Modesto, California • 1996

Laboratory/Pathology Words and Phrases

Laboratory Medicine, Anatomic Pathology, Clinical Pathology, Hematology, Dermatopathology

Sally Crenshaw Pitman
Editor & Publisher
Health Professions Institute
P. O. Box 801
Modesto, CA 95353-0801
Phone 209-551-2112
Fax 209-551-0404
E-mail: hpi@ainet.com
Web site: http://www.hpisum.com

Printed by
Parks Printing & Lithograph
Modesto, California

ISBN 0-934385-66-1

Last digit is the print number: 9 8 7 6 5

To

Leon Sidney Pitman

Contents

Preface

Laboratory/Pathology Words and Phrases is more than an update of the classic *Pathology Words and Phrases* published in 1988. It has been greatly expanded to include over 45,000 entries from laboratory medicine, anatomic and clinical pathology, hematology, and dermatopathology. (In the fall 1996 second printing, the title was changed from *Pathology/Laboratory* to *Laboratory/Pathology* to more accurately reflect the book's emphasis on laboratory terminology, lab values, lab tests, pathogens, and anatomy.)

A special feature includes 80 pages of tables of arteries, bones, muscles, nerves, and veins, listing both English and Latin forms in tabular form for quick reference. The appendix also includes an extensive table of normal laboratory values of blood, urine, and miscellaneous body fluids.

Another useful feature is an extensive list of bacteria, fungi, parasites, and viruses under the broad term *pathogen.* This should make it easier for students and others new to the field of medicine to find the name of a "bug" used in medical reports when it is not known what kind of organism it is.

Much terminology in pathology, laboratory medicine, hematology, and dermatopathology is related to neoplastic disease entities and conditions involving the cellular level, and this book necessarily includes thousands of carcinogen-related terms. A list of over 1200 laboratory tests is provided in the text.

This book is by no means an exhaustive list of words and phrases in the laboratory/pathology specialties, but we are confident that we have gathered the most relevant and useful words and phrases in those specialties. We've culled words and phrases from hundreds of transcripts of medical dictation, as well as laboratory medicine references, anatomy textbooks, scholarly journals in all specialties, and other printed and electronic references.

We hope that this book will be useful for medical transcriptionists in all specialties, not just those who work exclusively in the pathology department or laboratory. Physicians and other healthcare professionals who dictate patient health records refer to laboratory medicine and pathology in almost every report, and use anatomical terms extensively in operative reports, autopsies, and cellular pathology studies. The difficulty in compiling this quick-reference book of laboratory/pathology words and phrases was not in *finding* sufficient terms, but in *limiting* the terms to the ones most likely to be found in dictation of medical reports.

The research, editing, and proofreading of this book were done primarily by Kathy Cameron, Linda Campbell, Catherine Baxter, Dr. John H. Dirckx, and Bron Taylor. My warmest gratitude to all.

Sally Crenshaw Pitman
Editor & Publisher

How to Use This Book

The words and phrases in this book are alphabetized letter by letter of all words in the entry, ignoring punctuation marks and words or letters in parentheses. The possessive form ('s) is omitted from eponyms for ease in alphabetizing. Numbers are alphabetized as if written out, with the exception of subscripts and superscripts which are ignored.

Eponyms may be located alphabetically as well as under the nouns they modify. For example, *acid-fast bacillus (AFB) stain* is found alphabetically under the A's as well as under the main entry *stain*. *Döderlein bacillus* is found in the D's as well as under the broad category *pathogen*, which includes a list of over a thousand organisms. Under *bacillus, bacteria, fungus, organism, parasite,* and *virus,* there is a *see pathogen* reference.

The extensive list of pathogens should be particularly helpful to students and inexperienced medical transcriptionists who find it difficult to determine the correct spelling of "bugs" dictated in medical reports. Physician dictators may not state what kind of organism a term is and thus the student does not know whether to look under *bacillus, bacteria, fungus, organism, parasite,* or *virus* (and usually ends up looking under every possibility before finding the correct term). The physician may dictate the formal name of an organism, such as *Escherichia coli* or *Clostridium difficile*, or part of a name (*Escherichia* or *Clostridium*), or an abbreviated form (such as *E. coli* or *"C. diff"*). All the terms are easily found in this book alphabetically as well as under the broad category *pathogen*.

The main entries *artery, bone, muscle, nerve,* and *vein* include phrases and descriptive terms related to those terms as they are dictated in patient reports, rather than the names of anatomical terms and eponyms which are instead listed in the Appendix in tabular form, with both the English and Latin forms given. The anatomical tables in the Appendix should be helpful to medical transcriptionists trying to find a correct spelling when it may not be clear if the term is in English or Latin, or whether the term is an artery or a muscle.

The fact that many physicians dictate strings of abbreviations and brief forms presents special difficulties for students and less experienced transcriptionists. Laboratory data is particularly difficult to transcribe, yet the accuracy of its transcription is essential to quality patient records. A table of laboratory tests that may be encountered in patient health records is provided in the Appendix, with examples of "normal" laboratory values. Of course, what is determined to be "normal" varies from laboratory to laboratory, and the values presented are intended for reference only.

A, a

A (alpha)
A albumin
AA (amyloid A) protein
AAT (alpha$_1$-antitrypsin)
Ab (antibody)
A band
abapical pole
abarticulation
Abbe-Zeiss counting cell
Abbott VP analyzer
ABC (aspiration biopsy cytology)
ABC peroxidase method of staining
ABC (avidin-biotin complex)
abdomen
  apertures of
  boatlike
  concave
  fascia of
  roof of
  scaphoid
abdominal aorta
abdominal aortic artery
abdominal aortic plexus
abdominal aponeurosis
abdominal apron
abdominal canal
abdominal cavity
abdominal contents
abdominal cramp
abdominal fissure
abdominal fistula
abdominal kidney
abdominal lymph node
abdominal muscle
abdominal ostium
abdominal pad
abdominal panniculus
abdominal pannus
abdominal pregnancy
abdominal pulse
abdominal raphe
abdominal reflex
abdominal region
abdominal ring
abdominal sac
abdominal stoma
abdominal viscera
abdominal wall venous pattern
abdominal zone
abdominis muscle
  rectus
  transversus
abdominocardiac reflex
abdominogenital

abdominopelvic cavity
abdominopelvic viscera
abdominoscrotal
abdominothoracic arch
abdominovaginal
abdominovesical
abducens nucleus
abducent nerve
abductor muscle
Abel bacillus
Abell-Kendall method
Abelson murine leukemia virus
Abercrombie degeneration
Abernethy fascia
Abernethy sarcoma
aberrant artery
aberrant bile duct
aberrant bundle
aberrant duct
aberrant ductule
aberrant ganglion
aberrant goiter
aberrant hemoglobin
aberrant tissue
aberration
abetalipoproteinemia, hereditary
ABGs (arterial blood gases)
A bile
abnormal capillary fragility
abnormal formation of connective
  tissue
abnormal hardening of tissue
abnormal increase in circulating
  leukocytes
abnormal mitochondrial protein
abnormal ossification
abnormal test result
abnormal whiteness of skin
abnormalities of development
abnormalities of urine
ABO and Rh blood typing
ABO blood group
ABO blood type
ABO factor
abomasal groove
abomasum
aborted fetus
abortion
  accidental
  ampullar
  artificial
  complete
  complications of
  habitual
  idiopathic
  imminent
  incomplete
  induced
  inevitable
  infected
  missed
  recurrent
  septic
  spontaneous
  therapeutic
  threatened
  tubal
abortion in progress
abortive pneumonia
abortus bacillus
ABP (androgen binding protein)
abraded wound
Abrams needle
abrasion
abruptio placentae
abscess
  acute
  alveolar
  ambolic
  amebic
  apical
  appendiceal
  arthrifluent
  bartholinian

abscess *(continued)*
- Bartholin (of vulvovaginal gland)
- bartholinitis
- Bezold
- bicameral
- bile duct
- biliary
- bone
- brain
- broad ligament
- Brodie
- bursal
- canalicular
- caseous
- cheesy
- cholangitic
- chronic
- circumtonsillar
- cold
- collar-button
- colonic
- crypt
- cutaneous
- dental
- dentoalveolar
- diffuse
- Douglas
- dry
- Dubois
- encapsulated
- epidural
- epiploic
- extradural
- fecal
- follicular
- frontal
- gas
- gingival
- gravitation
- helminthic
- hematogenous
- hepatic

abscess *(continued)*
- hot
- hypostatic
- iliopsoas muscle
- intradural
- intramastoid
- ischiorectal
- kidney
- lacrimal
- lacunar
- luetic
- lung
- lymphatic
- mammary
- mastoid
- metastatic
- metastatic tuberculous
- migrating
- miliary
- Munro
- orbital
- otic
- otogenous
- ovarian
- palatal
- pancreatic
- parametrial
- parametric
- paranephric
- parotid
- Pautrier
- pelvic
- pelvirectal
- perforating
- periapical
- periappendiceal
- periarticular
- pericoronal
- perinephric
- periodontal
- peripleuritic
- perirectal

abscess *(continued)*
- peritoneal
- peritonsillar
- periureteral
- phlegmonous
- phoenix
- Pott
- premammary
- prostatic
- psoas
- pulp
- pyemic
- radicular
- renal
- residual
- retrobulbar
- retrocecal
- retroperitoneal
- retropharyngeal
- retrotonsillar
- ring
- root
- satellite
- septicemic
- shirt-stud
- solitary cutaneous
- spermatic
- splenic
- stellate
- stercoral
- sterile
- stitch
- subaponeurotic
- subareolar
- subdiaphragmatic
- subdural
- subepidermal
- subfascial
- subgaleal
- subhepatic
- subpectoral
- subperiosteal

abscess *(continued)*
- subphrenic
- subscapular
- subungual
- sudoriparous
- superficial
- suprahepatic
- syphilitic
- thecal
- thymic
- Tornwaldt
- tropical
- tuberculous
- tubo-ovarian
- tympanitic
- tympanocervical
- tympanomastoid
- urethral
- urinary
- verminous
- vitreous
- wandering
- Welch
- worm

abscess culture
abscess formation
absence of myelin
absence of peripheral pulses
Absidia corymbifera
absolute count
absolute neutrophil count (ANC)
absolute scale
absolute temperature scale
absorption apparatus
absorption band
absorption cell
absorption fever
absorption line
absorption of tissue debris
absorptive cells of intestine
abutting
ACA (anticardiolipin antibody)

cantha
canthamoeba
canthion
canthocyte (spur cell)
canthokeratoderma
cantholysis
canthoma
canthosis, saw-toothed
cariasis
carine dermatosis
carodermatitis
carus
carus rhyzoglypticus hyacinthi
ccelerated hypertension
ccelerator factor
ccelerator fiber
ccelerator globulin (AcG)
ccelerator nerve
ccelerator urinae muscle
ccessioning
ccession number
ccessory adrenal
ccessory atrium
ccessory auricle
ccessory bone
ccessory breast
ccessory canal
ccessory cartilage
ccessory cell
ccessory cephalic vein
ccessory chromosome
ccessory cuneate nucleus
ccessory digit
ccessory flocculus
ccessory gland
ccessory hemiazygos vein
ccessory hepatic duct
ccessory lacrimal gland
ccessory ligament
ccessory meningeal artery
ccessory nasal cartilage
ccessory nerve
accessory nerve lymph node
accessory nipple
accessory obturator artery
accessory obturator nerve
accessory olivary nucleus
accessory organ
accessory pancreas
accessory pancreatic duct
accessory parotid gland
accessory phrenic nerve
accessory placenta
accessory plantar ligament
accessory process
accessory pudendal artery
accessory quadrate cartilage
accessory saphenous vein
accessory sinus
accessory spleen
accessory suprarenal gland
accessory thyroid gland
accessory tubercle
accessory vertebral vein
accessory visual apparatus
accessory volar ligament
accidental abortion
accidental proteinuria
accidental termination of pregnancy
accidental tissue
accommodate
accommodation reflex
accompanying vein
accretion line
Accu-Chek glucose monitor
accumulation analysis
accumulation of sphingomyelin in marrow histiocytes
accumulation of spinal fluid, abnormal
ACE (angiotensin converting enzyme)
A cell
acellular
acetabular artery
acetabular bone

acetabular fossa
acetabular labrum
acetabular notch
acetabulum
acetaldehyde test
Acetest
acetic acid
acetic acid stain
acetone body
acetone-insoluble antigen
acetone in urine test
acetonitrile
acetowhite epithelium
acetowhite reaction
acetowhite test
acetyl-activating enzyme
acetylcholine receptor antibody
acetylcholinesterase
acetylsalicylic acid
AcG, ac-g (accelerator globulin)
Ac-globulin (accelerator)
ACh (acetylcholine)
A chain
achalasia of esophagus
Achilles bursa
Achilles tendon
achlorhydria, gastric
acholic stool
acholuric jaundice
achondroplasia
achondroplastic dwarfism
AChRab (acetylcholine receptor)
  antibody
achrestic anemia
achromatic apparatus
achromatosis
achromia
achromic nevus
Achromobacter xylosoxidans
acid
  acetic
  acetylsalicylic

acid *(continued)*
  alpha amino
  amino
  aminolevulinic (ALA)
  aromatic amino
  ascorbic
  beta-hydroxybutyric
  bile
  branched chain amino
  carbonic
  choleic
  conjugated bile
  delta-aminolevulinic
  essential fatty
  ethylenediaminetetraacetic (EDTA)
  fatty
  fecal bile
  folic
  glacial acetic
  glucuronic
  homogentisic
  homovanillic (HVA)
  hydrochloric (HCl)
  lactic
  lipid-associated sialic
  medium chain fatty
  nitric
  organic
  osmic
  oxalic
  picric
  propionic
  pyruvic
  salicylic
  short chain fatty
  sialic
  sulfuric
  tartaric
  un-ionized
  uric
  valproic
  vanillylmandelic (VMA)

acid albumin
acid alcohol solution
acid aspiration pneumonitis
acid-base balance
acid-base reaction
acid cell
acid dye
acid elution test for fetal hemoglobin
acidemia
acid environment
acid-fast bacillus (AFB) (pl. bacilli)
acid-fast bacillus (AFB) stain
acid-fastness
acid-fast organism
acid-fast staining
acid fuchsin stain
acid gland
acid hematoxylin stain
acidic metabolite
acidified alcohol
acidified serum test for paroxysmal nocturnal hemoglobinuria
acid-lability test
acidophil (also acidophilic)
acidophil adenoma
acidophil body
acidophil cell
acidophil granule
acidophil leukocyte
acidosis
  diabetic
  lactic
  metabolic
  renal tubular
  respiratory
  starvation
  uremic
acid-peptic juice
acid perfusion test
acid phosphatase
  leukocyte
  prostatic

acid phosphatase *(continued)*
  semen
  tartrate resistant acid serum test
acid reflux test
acid serum test
acid-staining cell
acid-wash treatment
acinar architecture
acinar cell
acinar tissue
Acinetobacter calcoaceticus, var. *anitratus* (formerly *Herellea vaginicola*)
Acinetobacter calcoaceticus, var. *lwoffi* (formerly *Mima polymorpha*)
aciniform
acinitis
acinotubular gland
acinous cell
acinous cell carcinoma
acinous gland
acinus (pl. acini)
  cup-shaped
  flask-shaped
aclasis
acne
acnegenic
acneiform pustule
acne keloid
acne vulgaris
acortical artery
acoustic cell
acoustic crest
acoustic cyst
acoustic immittance test
acoustic meatus
acoustic nerve
acoustic neurilemoma
acoustic neuroma
acousticofacial crest
acousticofacial ganglion
acoustic papilla

acoustic stria
acoustic trauma
acoustic tubercle
acoustic vesicle
acquired aneurysm
acquired cuticle
acquired defect
acquired deficiency
acquired hemolyzing antibodies
acquired immune deficiency
  syndrome (AIDS)
acquired methemoglobulinemia
acquired nevus
acquired reflex
acquired tufted angioma
acral-lentiginous melanoma
Acremonium
Acremonium falciforme
Acremonium kiliense
Acremonium recifei
Acremonium restrictum
acrodermatitis
acrodermatitis continua
acrodermatitis enteropathica
acrodermatosis
acrokeratosis
acromegaly
acromial angle
acromial artery
acromial articular facies
acromial articular surface
acromial bone
acromial extremity
acromial process
acromial reflex
acromioclavicular disk
acromioclavicular joint
acromion
acromiothoracic artery
acrosclerosis
acrosomal cap
acrosomal granule
acrosomal vesicle
acrylamide/urea gel
ACTH (adrenocorticotropic hormone)
ACTH antibody
ACTH stimulation test
actin filament
actinic dermatitis
actinic keratitis
actinic keratosis
actinic prurigo
actinium emanation
Actinobacillus actinomycetemcomitans
Actinobacillus equuli
Actinobacillus hominis
Actinobacillus lignieresii
Actinobacillus suis
Actinomadura
Actinomyces
Actinomyces gonidiaformis
Actinomyces in suppurative and
  granulomatous infections
Actinomyces israelii
Actinomyces meyeri
Actinomyces naeslundii
Actinomyces odontolyticus
Actinomyces viscosus
actinomycosis
actinomycotic mycetoma
activated coagulation time (ACT)
activated fatty acid
activated partial thromboplastin
  substitution test
activated partial thromboplastin time
  (APTT)
activated protein C
activation analysis
activator, plasminogen
active congestion
active hyperemia
activity
  enzyme
  mitotic

acuminatum, condyloma
acute abscess
acute arteritis
acute benign pericarditis
acute bronchitis
acute compression triad
acute disseminated myositis
acute eosinophilic pneumonia
acute febrile neutrophilic dermatosis
acute fibrinous pericarditis
acute gastritis
acute glomerulonephritis
acute granulocytic leukemia
acute hemorrhagic cystitis
acute hemorrhagic pancreatitis
acute idiopathic polyneuritis
acute infectious gastroenteritis
acute intermittent porphyria (AIP)
acute interstitial myocarditis
acute interstitial pancreatitis
acute interstitial pneumonitis
acute isolated myocarditis
acute leukemia
acute lymphoblastic leukemia
  B-cell type
  Burkitt-like
  common type
  null cell type
  pre-B-cell type
  T-cell type
acute malaria
acute mastitis
acute mastoiditis
acute megakaryoblastic leukemia
acute monocytic leukemia
acute myelitis
acute myeloblastic leukemia
acute myelogenous leukemia (AML)
acute myelomonocytic leukemia
acute myoendocarditis
acute necrotizing encephalitis
acute nephritis
acute nephrosis
acute osteitis
acute pancreatitis
acute parenchymatous hepatitis
acute phase protein
acute phase reactant
acute pleurisy
acute pneumonia
acute porphyria
acute poststreptococcal glomerulo-nephritis
acute progressive myositis
acute promyelocytic leukemia
acute pyelonephritis
acute renal failure
acute rheumatic fever
acute rheumatic myocarditis
acute serum
acute suppurative parotitis
acute thyroiditis
acute tubular necrosis (ATN)
acute undifferentiated leukemia (AUL)
acute vascular purpura
acute yellow atrophy
acyl carrier protein
adamantinoma
Adamkiewicz, spinal artery of
Adam's apple
adaptive enzyme
adaptive hyperplasia
Addis count
Addison disease
addisonian crisis
Addison point
Addis test
adductor canal
adductor muscle
adductor reflex
adductor tubercle
adelomorphous cell
Aden fever
adeno-associated virus

adenocarcinoma
  acinous
  alveolar
  bronchogenic
  cervical
  clear cell
  colon
  cyst
  endometrial
  epithelium
  follicular
  liver
  lung
  moderately differentiated
  mucinous
  ovarian
  papillary
  polypoid
  poorly differentiated
  prostate
  serous
  undifferentiated
  urachal
  vaginal
  well-differentiated
adenocyst
adenocystoma
adenoidal
adenoiditis, follicular
adenoid pattern
adenoids
adenoid tissue
adenoma
  acidophil
  adrenal cortex
  basophil
  chromophobe
  colonic
  epithelial
  Hürthle cell (Huerthle)
  mammary
  parathyroid
adenomatous goiter
adenomatous hyperplasia
adenomatous polyp
adenomatous polyposis coli (APC)
adenomyosis
adenosine deaminase deficiency
adenosine monophosphate (AMP)
adenosine triphosphatase (ATPase)
adenosis
  mammary
  vaginal
adenovirus
adenovirus antibody titer
adenovirus antigen
adenovirus immunofluorescence
adenovirus type 8
adequal cleavage
adermia
adermogenesis
ADH (antidiuretic hormone)
adherent placenta
adhesed
adhesion
  bandlike
  banjo-string
  fibrous
  meningeal
  violin-string
adhesive inflammation
adhesive pericarditis
adhesive pleurisy
adhesive vaginitis
adipocere
adipocyte
adipokinetic hormone
adiponecrosis
adipose capsule of kidney
adipose cell
adipose degeneration
adipose fold
adipose fossa
adipose infiltration

adipose tissue
adiposis dolorosa
adiposity
adiposogenital degeneration
adiposus, panniculus
A disk
adjacent angle
adjuvant
admaxillary gland
admitting diagnosis
admixed
admixture
adnexal
adnexa mastoidea
adnexa oculi
adnexa uteri
adrenal androgen
adrenal antibody
adrenal atrophy
adrenal body
adrenal capsule
adrenal cortex
adrenal cortex adenoma
adrenal cortical deficiency
adrenal failure
adrenal gland
  accessory
  Marchand
adrenal hemorrhage
adrenal hypertension
Adrenalin
adrenaline
adrenaline acid tartrate
adrenal medulla
adrenal mineralocorticoids
adrenal tumor
adrenal weight factor
adrenocortical hyperplasia
adrenocortical steroid therapy
adrenocorticotropic hormone (ACTH)
adrenocorticotropic peptide
adrenocorticotropic releasing factor
adrenogenic tissue
adrenogenital syndrome
adrenotropic hormone
adsorption
adult-onset diabetes
adult-onset diabetes mellitus
adult-onset obesity
adult T-cell lymphoma (ATL)
adult T-cell lymphoma leukemia
adventitial cell
adventitial neuritis
adventitia, tunica
adventitious bursa
adventitious proteinuria
adynamic paralytic ileus
aerate
aeration
Aerobacter (old name for *Enterobacter*)
Aerobacter aerogenes
Aerobacter cloacae
Aerobacter liquefaciens
aerobe microorganism
aerobic bacteria
aerobic culture
Aerococcus
Aeromonas caviae
Aeromonas hydrophila
Aeromonas salmonicida
Aeromonas shigelloides
Aeromonas sobria
aestivoautumnal fever
AFB (acid-fast bacillus)
AFB culture
AFB stain
afferent arteriole
afferent fiber
afferent glomerular arteriole
afferent limb
afferent loop
afferent lymph vessel
afferent nerve

afferent vessel of kidney
affinity column
affinity for acidic stains
affinity for basic stains
affix
A fiber
Afipia felis
AFP (alpha-fetoprotein) test
African hemorrhagic fever
African lymphoma
African sleeping sickness
African tick-borne fever
afterbirth
Ag (antigen)
Ag (silver)
A/G (albumin-globulin) ratio
AGA (appropriate for gestational age)
agammaglobulinemia, congenital
aganglionic bowel
agar
  bile salt
  blood
  Bordet-Gengou
  chocolate
  cornmeal-Tween 80
  egg yolk
  laked blood
  MacConkey
  Nobel
  Sabouraud
agar culture medium
Agaricus
agarose gel
agarose gel electrophoresis
agar plate count
agar slant
age
  bone
  developmental
  gestational (GA)
aged normal serum
agenesis
agent
  antiadrenergic
  antifibrinolytic
  antifoaming
  diuretic
agger nasi cell
agglomeration of cells
agglutinating antibody
agglutination
  heterophile
  latex
  Widal
agglutination of cells
agglutination of latex beads
agglutination test for antibody
agglutination titer for brucellosis
agglutination titer for paratyphoid
agglutination titer for rickettsiae
agglutination titer for tularemia
agglutination titer for typhoid
agglutinin
  blood typing
  brucellosis
  chief
  cold
  cross-reacting
  erythrocyte
  febrile
  production of by immune system
  serum
  Weil-Felix
agglutinin to Rh positive cells in the Rh system
agglutinin to type A red blood cells in the ABO system
agglutinogen, erythrocyte
agglutinogens in red cells
aggregate dimension
aggregated lymphatic follicle
aggregated lymphatic nodule
aggregate gland
aggregate specimen

aggregations of lymphoid tissue
aging, consequences of
agitans, paralysis
agminated follicles
agminated gland
agnogenic myeloid metaplasia
agonal clot
agonal infection
agonist
agranular leukocyte
agranular mononuclear cell
agranular reticulum
agranulocytosis
Agrimonia eupatoria
agrypnodal coma
A hemoglobin
A_{1c} hemoglobin
A hemophilia
A hepatitis
AHG (antihemophilic globulin)
AIDS encephalopathy
AIHA (autoimmune hemolytic anemia)
AimV serum-free media
AIP (acute intermittent porphyria)
air-bone gap
airborne infection
air cell
  ethmoidal
  mastoid
air-dried smear
air embolism
airless mass
air sac
airspace-filling pattern
air vesicle
airway pattern
Ajellomyces capsulatus
Ajellomyces dermatitidis
akinesis, anterior wall
Al (aluminum)
AL patch test
AL protein (amyloid light chain)
ala, nasal
alanine aminotransferase (ALT)
  (formerly SGPT)
ala of ethmoid
ala of sacrum
ala of vomer
alar artery
alar bone
alar cartilage
alar fold
alar lamina
alar ligament
alar plate
alar process
alar spine
AlaSTAT latex allergy test
alba, linea
Albarran gland
Albarran test
Albers-Schoenberg disease
Albers-Schoenberg marble bone
albicans, corpus
albinism
albino
Albrecht bone
albuginea, tunica
albumin
  A
  acid
  alkali
  blood
  iodinated I 125 serum (also, ^{125}I)
  iodinated I 131 serum (also, ^{131}I)
  native
  serum
  urine
albumin/globulin (A/G) ratio
albuminocytologic dissociation
albuminoid
albuminous cell
albuminous degeneration
albuminous deposits

albuminous gland
albuminous granule
albumin test
albuminuria
Alcaligenes denitrificans
Alcaligenes faecalis
Alcaligenes odorans
Alcian blue
Alcock canal
alcohol
  acid
  acidified
  blood
  ethyl
  methyl
alcoholic cirrhosis
alcoholic coma
alcoholic formalin
alcoholic hepatitis
alcoholic hyalin
alcoholic pneumonia
alcoholic solution
alcohol intoxication
alcoholism
alcohol poisoning
alcohol-soluble protein
Alder-Reilly granules
aldolase test
aldosterone hormone
aldosterone test
aldosterone, urinary
aldosteronism
  primary
  secondary
aleukemic leukemia
Alexander leukodystrophy disease
algae, red
algid malaria
algid pernicious fever
algoid cell
algor mortis
alimentary apparatus
alimentary canal
alimentary glycosuria
alimentary mucosa
alimentary obesity
alimentary system
alimentary tract smear
aliphatic fatty acids
aliquot
alisphenoid bone
alisphenoids
alizarin stain
alkalemia
alkali albumin
alkali denaturation test
alkaline medium
alkaline phosphatase (ALP)
  leukocyte
  placental (PLAP)
  serum
alkaline phosphatase deficiency
alkaline phosphatase nitroblue
  tetrazolium (NBT)
alkaline phosphatase test
alkaloid test
alkalosis
  hypochloremic
  hypokalemic
  metabolic
  respiratory
alkaptonuria
ALL (acute lymphoblastic leukemia)
allantoic sac
allantoic stalk
allantoic vesicle
allantoid membrane
allantois
allelic gene
Allen-Doisy test
Allen test
allergen
allergic contact dermatitis
allergic dermatitis

allergic eczema
allergic granulomatosis
allergic inflammation
allergic pneumonia
allergic purpura
allergic reaction
allergic stomatitis
allergy
alloantibodies
alloantigen-presenting cell
allocortex
allogeneic disease
Almén test for blood
almond nucleus
alopecia
  androgenic
  cicatricial
  female pattern
  hereditary
  lipedematous
  male pattern
  moth-eaten
  patterned
  postoperative pressure
  postpartum
  pressure
  scarring
  traction
  traumatic
alopecia adnata
alopecia areata
alopecia capitis totalis
alopecia congenitalis
alopecia disseminata
alopecia follicularis
alopecia leprotica
alopecia liminaris frontalis
alopecia marginalis
alopecia medicamentosa
alopecia mucinosa
alopecia pityrodes
alopecia presenilis
alopecia senilis
alopecia symptomatica
alopecia syphilitica
alopecia totalis
alopecia toxica
alopecia triangularis
alopecia triangularis congenitalis
alopecia universalis
Al patch
alpha acid glycoprotein
alpha-adrenergic receptor
alpha amino acid
alpha amino nitrogen
alpha-amylase
alpha-amylose
$alpha_1$-antichymotrypsin (a1AC)
$alpha_1$-antitrypsin (AAT)
$alpha_1$-antitrypsin globulin
alpha-beta variation
alpha-blocker
alpha cell
alpha coma
alpha dinitrophenol
alpha-estradiol
alpha-fetoglobulin
alpha-fetoprotein (AFP)
  amniotic fluid
  fucosylated
  serum
alpha-fetoprotein test
alpha fiber
alpha globulin
alpha globulin antibodies
alpha-glucosidase deficiency
alpha granule
alpha heavy chain disease
alpha hemolysis
alpha-hemolytic streptococcus
alpha-hypophamine
alpha-ketoglutarate dehydrogenase
$alpha_1$-lipoprotein
alpha-naphthol esterase

alpha satellite biotinylated
  chromosome-specific probe
alpha-tocopherol (vitamin E)
alpha-trypsin inhibitor
Alphavirus, alphavirus
alphoid
ALS (amyotrophic lateral sclerosis)
ALT (alanine aminotransferase)
  (formerly SGPT)
Alternaria
Alternaria alternata
Alteromonas putrefaciens
Altmann-Gersh method
Altmann granule
Altmann solution
alum-carmine stain
alum-coated slide
aluminum (Al)
alveolar abscess
alveolar angle
alveolar arch
alveolar artery
alveolar body
alveolar bone
alveolar border of mandible
alveolar canal
alveolar cell
alveolar crest
alveolar dead space
alveolar duct
alveolar foramen
alveolar gland
alveolar hydatids
alveolar macrophage
alveolar mucosa
alveolar necrosis
alveolar nerve
alveolar osteitis
alveolar pattern
alveolar periosteum
alveolar point
alveolar process of maxilla
alveolar ridge
alveolar sac
alveolar septum
alveolar soft part sarcoma
alveolar space
alveolar supporting bone
alveolar wall
alveolar yoke
alveoli (pl. of alveolus)
alveolingual groove
alveolitis, extrinsic allergic
alveolobuccal groove
alveolobuccal sulcus
alveolodental canal
alveolodental ligament
alveolodental membrane
alveololabial groove
alveololabial sulcus
alveololingual groove
alveololingual sulcus
alveolonasal line
alveolus (pl. alveoli)
  dental
  glandular
  pulmonary
Alzheimer cell
Alzheimer disease
Alzheimer neurofibrillary degeneration
Alzheimer stain
AMA (antimitochondrial antibody)
amacrine cells of retina
Amanita
Amanita bisporigera
Amanita muscaria
Amanita ocreata
Amanita phalloides
Amanita verna
Amanita virosa
amastigote
amaurotic familial idiocy
amber streaks in lens
ambiguous external genitalia

ambolic abscess
ambulatory plague
ameba (amoeba)
amebiasis
amebic abscess
amebic dysentery
amebic pneumonia
ameboid astrocyte
ameboid cell
ameboid movement
amelanotic melanoma
amelanotic nevus
ameloblast
ameloblastic odontoma
ameloblastic sarcoma
ameloblastoma
American trypanosomiasis
Ames assay
Ameth index
AMEX method of processing and embedding
amino acid
  aromatic
  branched chain
  essential
amino acid cystine
amino acid nitrogen (AAN) test
amino acid screen
aminolevulinate dehydratase test
aminolevulinic acid (ALA) test
aminolevulinic-delta acid
aminopeptidase, serum leucine
aminotransferase, alanine (ALT)
AML (acute myelogenous leukemia)
Ammon horn
ammoniacal silver stain
ammonia dermatitis
ammonia nitrogen test
ammonia, synthesis of
ammonium biurate
ammonium chloride loading test
ammonium magnesium phosphate (triple phosphate)
ammonium silver carbonate
amniocentesis, genetic
amnioembryonic junction
amniogenic cell
amnion
amnionic
amnionitis
amnion ring
amniotic band
amniotic cavity
amniotic duct
amniotic fluid, meconium-stained
amniotic fluid embolism
amniotic fold
amniotic raphe
amniotic sac
Amoeba
amorphous debris
amorphous ground substance
amorphous material
amorphous phosphate
amorphous sediment
amorphous sediment in urine
amorphous urate
AMP (adenosine monophosphate)
ampere
amphiarthroses articulation (joint)
amphophil granule
amphophilic matrix
amplicon
ampulla (pl. ampullae)
  duodenal
  ductus deferens
  Henle
  rectal
  semicircular canal
  uterine tube
  Vater
ampullar (also, ampullary)

ampullar abortion
ampullar crest
ampullar limb
ampullar pregnancy
ampullar sulcus
amygdala
amygdaloid body
amygdaloid fossa
amygdaloid nucleus
amygdaloid tubercle
amylaceous corpuscle
amylase
  body fluid
  serum
  urinary
amylase/creatinine
amylase level, serum
amylase test
amyloid A protein
amyloid body
amyloid corpuscle
amyloid degeneration
amyloid kidney
amyloid light chain (AL) protein
amyloidosis
  primary
  renal
  secondary
amyloid precursor protein
amyloid protein
amyloid stain
amyotrophic lateral sclerosis (ALS)
amyotrophy, neuralgic
ANA (antinuclear antibody)
anabiotic cell
anabolic effect
anaerobe
anaerobic bacteria
anaerobic culture of pus or drainage from abscess
Anaerobiospirillum succiniciproducens
anal canal, involuntary sphincter of
anal cleft
anal column
anal crypt
anal disk
anal fascia
anal fissure
anal gland
anal intermuscular septum
anal intersphincteric groove
anal membrane
analogous tissue
anal orifice
anal pit
anal plate
anal pruritus
anal reflex
anal region
anal sac
anal sinus
anal sphincter
anal triangle
anal valve
anal vein
anal verge
analysis (pl. analyses)
  activation
  accumulation
  blood gas
  CDK4 amplification
  chemistry
  chromatin
  chromosomal
  DNA
  fetal chromosome
  gastric
  hormone receptor protein
  immunophenotypic
  qualitative
  quantitative
  Northern blot
  segregation
  semen

nalysis *(continued)*
- sequence
- sex chromatin
- Southern blot
- stratographic
- volumetric
- Western blot
- zoo blot

nalyte
nalyzer
- Abbott VP
- ASTRA
- Dade Paramax
- DuPont ACA
- Ektachem

naphylactic shock
naphylactoid purpura
naphylaxis
naplasia
naplastic cell
naplastic epithelial cell
naplastic tumor
nasarca
nastomoses (pl. of anastomosis)
nastomosing fiber
nastomosing veins
nastomosis (pl. anastomoses)
- arteriolovenular
- arteriovenous
- crucial
- longitudinal
- portacaval
- splenorenal
- supraoptic

nastomosis of arteries
nastomotic area, portal-systemic
nastomotic branch of inferior gluteal artery
nastomotic fiber
nastomotic ulcer
nastomotic vein
natomical dead space
anatomical neck
anatomical neck of humerus
anatomical root
anatomical snuff box
anatomical sphincter
anatomical tooth
anatomical tubercle
anatomic diagnosis
anatomic landmark
anatomic nervous system
anatomic pathology
ANC (absolute neutrophil count)
anchoring villus
"anchovy paste" material in hepatic abscess
"anchovy sauce" pus
ancillary
anconeal fossa
anconeus muscle
Ancylostoma americanum
Ancylostoma braziliense
Ancylostoma caninum
Ancylostoma dermatitis
Ancylostoma duodenale
ancylostomatic
ancylostomiasis
Anderson and Goldberger test
Anderson-Collip test
Anderson phenomenon
androgen, adrenal
androgen binding protein (ABP)
androgenic alopecia
androgenic hormone
androgenic zone
androgen level, urine
android pelvis
androstenediol
androstenedione test
anemia
- achrestic
- aplastic
- autoimmune hemolytic (AIHA)

anemia *(continued)*
  chronic disease
  congenital hemolytic
  Cooley
  hemolytic
  hereditary hemolytic
  hypochromic microcytic
  hypoplastic
  iron deficiency
  macrocytic
  Mediterranean
  megaloblastic
  normochromic
  normocytic
  pernicious
  secondary
  sickle cell
  sideroblastic
  spur-cell
anemia, hemolytic, after exposure to
  fava beans
  nitrofurans
  primaquine
  sulfonamides
anemia of chronic disease
anemic infarct
anemic nevus
anencephaly
anergic
anergy
anetoderma
aneuploid
aneuploidy chromosomal abnormality
aneurysm
  abdominal
  abdominal aortic (AAA)
  acquired
  aortic
  aortic sinus
  arterial
  arteriosclerotic
  arteriovenous

aneurysm *(continued)*
  atherosclerotic
  axial
  bacterial
  Bérard
  berry
  brain
  Charcot-Bouchard
  circumscript
  cirsoid
  compound
  congenital
  congenital aortic sinus
  congenital cerebral
  coronary artery
  coronary vessel
  cylindroid
  debulking of
  descending thoracic
  dissecting
  dissecting aortic
  distal aortic arch
  ductal
  ectatic
  embolic
  false
  fusiform
  hernial
  imperforate
  infected
  infraclinoid
  innominate
  intracavernous
  intracranial
  intramural coronary artery
  isthmus
  juxtarenal aortic
  late false
  lateral
  left ventricular
  luetic aortic
  mesh-wrapping of aortic

aneurysm *(continued)*
- miliary
- mixed
- mural
- mycotic
- mycotic suprarenal
- nodular
- orbital
- pararenal aortic
- Park
- pelvic
- peripheral
- phantom
- post infarction ventricular
- Potts
- pulmonary arteriovenous
- pulmonary artery compression ascending aorta
- pulmonary artery mycotic
- racemose
- Rasmussen
- renal
- renal artery
- Richet
- Rodriguez
- ruptured
- ruptured aortic
- ruptured cerebral
- ruptured atherosclerotic
- sacciform
- saccular
- sacculated
- serpentine
- Shekelton
- spindle-shaped
- splenic artery
- spontaneous infantile ductal
- spurious
- suprasellar
- syphilitic
- thoracic
- thoracic aorta

aneurysm *(continued)*
- thoracoabdominal
- traumatic
- true
- tubular
- Valsalva sinus
- varicose
- venous
- ventricular
- ventricular septal
- verminous
- windsock
- worm
- wrapping of abdominal aortic

aneurysmal bruit
aneurysmal dilatation
aneurysmal sac
ANF (atrial natriuretic factor)
angiitis
angina pectoris
angioblast
angioblastic cell
angiocentric immunoproliferative
angioedema
angiogenesis factor
angiokeratoma
angiokeratoma corporis diffusum
angiolipoma
angiolithic degeneration
angiolithic sarcoma
angioma (pl. angiomata)
- capillary
- cavernous
- cherry
- hemangioma
- lymphangioma
- petechial
- spider
- telangiectatic

angioma serpiginosum
angiomatosis, bacillary
angioma venosum racemosum

angiomyolipoma
angioneurotic edema
angiotensin converting enzyme (ACE)
angiotensin I test
angiotensin II hormone
angiotensin II test
angle
  acromial
  adjacent
  alveolar
  anopouch
  anorectal
  apical
  axial
  basilar
  beta
  biorbital
  buccal
  bucco-occlusal
  cardiohepatic
  carrying
  cavity line
  cavosurface
  cephalic
  cephalomedullary
  cerebellopontile
  cerebellopontine
  costal
  costophrenic
  costovertebral (CVA)
  craniofacial
  critical
  cusp
  disparity
  duodenojejunal
  epigastric
  ethmoid
  facial
  filtration
  Frankfort-mandibular incisor
  frontal
  gamma
angle *(continued)*
  hepatorenal
  infrasternal
  iridocorneal
  sacrovertebral
  splenorenal (splenic-renal)
  sternal
  subpubic
  subscapular
angle of clitoris
angle of convergence
angle of mandible
angle of refraction
angle of rib
angle of sternum
angle of trigone
angular aperture
angular artery
angular curvature
angular gyrus
angular ligament of wrist
angular movement
angular notch
angular vein
angulated
angulus of stomach
ANH (atrial natriuretic hormone)
anhepatic jaundice
anhidrosis
anhydride-induced immunologic respiratory disease
ani (see *levator ani muscle*)
Anichkov cell (also, Anitschkow)
aniline blue
animal bite infection
animal viruses
anion gap test
anisakiasis
Anisakis marina
anisocytosis
anisomorphic
anisonucleosis

anisotropic disk
anisotropic lipoid
Anitschkow cell (also, Anichkov)
ankle articulation
ankle bone
ankle joint
ankle region
ankylosing spondylitis
ankylosis
  bony
  fibrous
annular ligament of ankle
annular ligament of radius
annular ligament of stapes
annular ligament of trachea
annular ligament of wrist
annular pancreas
annulospiral organ
annulus (pl. annuli)
annulus fibrosus of intervertebral
  fibrocartilage
annulus inguinalis
annulus ovalis
annulus tendineus communis
anococcygeal body
anococcygeal ligament
anococcygeal nerve
anococcygeal raphe
anocutaneous line
anogenital band
anogenital raphe
anomalous
anomaly (pl. anomalies)
  Alder
  congenital
  developmental
  May-Hegglin
  Pelger-Huët nuclear
  Undritz
anonychia
anonymous artery
anonymous vein

anopouch angle
anorectal angle
anorectal junction
anorectal line
anorectal lymph node
anorectal ring
anorexia
anospinal center
anovular ovarian follicle
anoxemia test
anoxia
anoxic
ansa
  Haller
  Henle
  lenticular
  peduncular
  Reil
  Vieussens
ansa cervicalis
ansa lenticularis
anserine bursa
anserine bursitis
ansiform lobule
antagonist
antagonistic muscle
antebrachial cutaneous nerve
antebrachial fascia
antebrachial vein
antebrachiocarpal joint
antecubital fossa
antecubital region
antecubital space
anteflexed uterus
antegonial notch
antemortem clot
antemortem thrombus
antenatal diagnosis
anteprostatic gland
anterior abdominal wall
anterior annular ligament of wrist
anterior auricular artery

anterior auricular nerve
anterior band of colon
anterior basis bundle
anterior calcaneoastragaloid ligament
anterior cardiac vein
anterior cell
anterior cerebellar artery
anterior cerebral artery
anterior chamber
anterior choroidal artery
anterior ciliary artery
anterior circumflex artery
anterior clinoid process
anterior communicating artery
anterior condyloid canal of occipital bone
anterior condyloid foramen
anterior costotransverse ligament
anterior costovertebral ligament
anterior costoxiphoid ligament
anterior cruciate ligament
anterior crural nerve
anterior curvature
anterior cusp
anterior cutaneous branch
anterior cutaneous nerve
anterior descending artery
anterior ethmoidal nerve
anterior fontanelle
anterior fornix of vagina
anterior horn cells of spinal cord
anterior humeral circumflex artery
anterior inferior cerebellar artery
anterior inferior tibiofibular ligament
anterior intercostal artery
anterior interosseous artery
anterior interosseous nerve
anterior intraoccipital joint
anterior jugular vein
anterior labial commissure
anterior-lateral (anterolateral)
anterior layer of rectus sheath
anterior ligament of head of fibula
anterior ligament of Helmholtz
anterior ligament of knee
anterior ligament of malleus
anterior ligament of wrist
anterior longitudinal ligament
anterior mediastinum
anterior meningeal artery
anterior meningocele
anterior meniscofemoral ligament
anterior muscle, scalenus
anterior nares
anterior nasal aperture
anterior papillary muscle
anterior peroneal artery
anterior pillar of fauces
anterior pituitary-like hormone
anterior pituitary-like substance
anterior pulmonary nerve
anterior radioulnar ligament
anterior recess of ischiorectal fossa
anterior rectus fascia
anterior rectus sheath
anterior sacrococcygeal ligament
anterior sacroiliac ligaments
anterior sacrosciatic ligament
anterior semicircular canal
anterior spinal artery
anterior sternoclavicular ligament
anterior superior dental artery
anterior superior iliac spine
anterior surface of pancreas
anterior surface of prostate
anterior synechiae
anterior talotibial ligament
anterior temporal artery
anterior tibial artery
anterior tympanic artery
anterior uveitis of iris
anterior vagal trunk
anterior wall akinesis
anteroinferiorly

anterolateral (anterior-lateral)
anterolateral central artery
anterolateral column
anterolateral fontanelle
anterolateral groove
anterolateral striate artery
anterolateral sulcus
anterolateral surface
anteromedial central artery
anteromedial surface
anteromedial thalamostriate artery
anteromedian gap
anteromedian groove
anteroposterior (AP) diameter
anteverted uterus
anthracene laxative
anthracosis
anthracotic
anthrax bacillus
anthrax, inhalational
anthrax pneumonia
anthropoid pelvis
anti-A agglutinins in serum
anti-ACh receptor antibody
anti-AChR (antiacetylcholine receptor) antibody
antiacrodynia factor
antiadrenergic agent
antialopecia factor
antianemic factor
anti-antibody
anti-B agglutinins in serum
antiberiberi factor
antibiotic-containing disks
antibiotic sensitivity test(ing)
anti-black-tongue factor
antibody (Ab) (pl. antibodies)
  acetylcholine receptor (AChR)
  acquired hemolyzing
  ACTH (adrenocorticotropic hormone)
  adrenal

antibody *(continued)*
  AE1
  AE3
  agglutinating
  alpha-globulin
  anti-ACh receptor
  anti-AChR (antiacetylcholine receptor)
  anti-B
  anticardiolipin (aCA)
  anticentromere (ACA)
  anticolonic
  anticytoplasmic (ACPA)
  antidelta IgM
  antidermatitis factor
  anti-DNA
  anti-EA (early antigen) of Epstein Barr virus
  anti-ENA
  antifibrin
  anti-GBM
  antigliadin
  antiglioma monoclonal antibody kinase C
  anti-HA (hepatitis A)
  anti-HAV (hepatitis A virus)
  anti-HB (hepatitis B)
  anti-HB_c (hepatitis B core)
  anti-HB_e (hepatitis B "e")
  anti-HB_s (hepatitis B surface)
  anti-HEV (hepatitis E virus)
  antihuman globulin
  antihyaluronidase
  anti-idiotype
  anti-idiotypic
  anti-IL-2 receptor monoclonal
  anti-kidney
  anti-La
  antimitochondrial (AMA)
  anti-MPO
  anti-nRNP
  antinuclear (ANA)

antibody *(continued)*
  antiphospholipid
  anti-PR3
  anti-receptor
  anti-Rh
  anti-Ro
  anti-Scl-70
  anti-Sm
  anti-SS-A
  anti-SS-B
  anti-TBM
  antithyroglobulin
  anti-VCA (viral capsid antigen)
  A33 monoclonal
  biotinylated secondary
  CAM 5.2
  CC49 monoclonal
  CD5+ monoclonal
  cell-bound
  centromere
  CF (complement fixation)
  C-58 monoclonal
  complement fixation (CF)
  C100-3 hepatitis C virus (anti-HIV)
  cross-reacting
  cryptosporidiosis
  cytotrophic
  disease caused by
  Donath-Landsteiner
  Duffy blood antibody type
  eastern equine encephalitis
  E5 monoclonal
  EMA (epithelial membrane antigen)
  endomysial
  extractable nuclear (ENA)
  fluorescent
  fluorescently tagged
  fluorescent treponemal
  fungal
  GFAP (glial fibrillary acidic protein)
  glomerular basement membrane

antibody *(continued)*
  HA-1A monoclonal
  HAMA (human antimurine)
  HBe
  HIV
  HLA-DR monoclonal
  HLe-1 monoclonal
  idiotypic
  IgG
  IgM
  IgM anti-HAV
  IgM anti-HBc
  Ig2b kappa monoclonal
  inhibiting
  insulin
  intrinsic factor
  kinase C antiglioma monoclonal
  La (SS-B)
  Leu2a monoclonal
  Leu3a+3b monoclonal
  Leu4 monoclonal
  Leu5b monoclonal
  Leu17 monoclonal
  Leu23 monoclonal
  luteinizing hormone
  lym-1 monoclonal
  lymphocytotoxic
  milk protein
  mitochondrial
  monoclonal (MOAB, MoAb, MAB)
  MB1 monoclonal
  MSL-109 monoclonal
  MT2 monoclonal
  MT3 monoclonal
  Muromonab-CD3 monoclonal
  mycobacterial
  NCL-Arp monoclonal
  NCL-ER-LHZ monoclonal
  NCL-PGR monoclonal
  NSE (neuron-specific enolase)
  OKT3 monoclonal
  OKT4 monoclonal

antibody *(continued)*
  OKT8 monoclonal
  OPD4 monoclonal
  parietal cell
  PBC-associated
  pemphigus
  platelet
  PM-81 monoclonal
  production
  prolactin hormone
  Proteus OX-2
  Proteus OX-19
  Proteus OX-K
  Rh
  Ro (SS-A)
  scleroderma
  17-1A monoclonal SFHb
    (pyridoxilated stroma-free
    hemoglobin)
  6B6 monoclonal
  65-2A6 monoclonal
  Sjögren
  smooth muscle
  S-100 protein
  sperm
  staining
  teichoic acid
  testing
  3F8 monoclonal
  thyroglobulin
  thyroid microsomal
  thyrotropin hormone
  thyrotropin receptor
  TI-23 (CMV monoclonal a.)
  2A11 monoclonal
  UCHL1 monoclonal
  western equine encephalitis
antibody labeled with radioisotope
antibody technique, fluorescent
antibody titer
anticardiolipin antibody (aCA)
antichymotrypsin, $alpha_1$–
antichymotrypsin test
anticoagulant
  circulating
  coumarin
  Coumadin
  heparin
  lupus
anticoagulant heparin solution
anticoagulant-treated blood
anticolonic antibody
anticomplementary factor
anticytoplasmic antibody (ACPA) test
antidelta IgM antibody
anti-deoxyribonuclease-B titer
  (anti-DNAse titer)
anti-D immunoglobulin
antidiuretic hormone (ADH) test
antidiuretic hormone–water deprivation
  stimulation test
anti-DNA antibody
  Farr
  Ginsberg/Keiser
  indirect fluorescence
anti-DNA test
anti-double-stranded DNA test
anti-EA (Epstein-Barr) antibody
anti-ENA antibody
antifibrinolytic agent
antifoaming agent
anti-GBM antibody
antigen (Ag)
  acetone-insoluble
  adenovirus
  alpha-fetoprotein (AFP)
  antiproliferating cell nuclear
  Au (gold)
  Australian
  bile
  CA (cancer)
  C carbohydrate
  CA 15-3 antigenic tumor marker
  CA 19-9 carbohydrate

antigen *(continued)*
- CA 72-4 antigenic tumor marker
- CALLA (common acute lymphoblastic leukemia antigen)
- cancer (CA)
- capsular
- carcinoembryonic (CEA)
- CDE
- CD3
- CD45 leukocyte common
- Chr a
- common acute lymphoblastic leukemia (CALLA)
- conjugated
- delta (delta-Ag)
- Di
- ECA (enterobacterial common)
- EMA (epithelial membrane)
- ENA (extractable nuclear)
- enterobacterial common (ECA)
- epithelial membrane (EMA)
- erythrocyte
- extractable nuclear (ENA)
- febrile
- Forssman
- Goa (Gonzales blood)
- HBAg (hepatitis B antigen)
- hepatitis associated (HAA)
- hepatitis B
- hepatitis B core (HB_cAg)
- hepatitis B e (HB_eAg)
- hepatitis B surface (HB_sAg)
- hepatitis D virus
- HLA (human lymphocytic)
- HPA (*Histoplasma capsulatum*)
- inhalant
- latex particles coated with
- Ly
- Lyb
- membrane
- nonspecific
- p24

antigen *(continued)*
- pancreatic oncofetal (POA)
- PHA (phytohemagglutinin)
- polypeptide
- prostate specific (PSA)
- Rh (Rhesus factor)
- rheumatoid-associated nuclear (RANA)
- rotavirus
- serum hepatitis (SH)
- Sm
- streptococcal
- streptococcus M
- T-dependent
- T-independent
- Thy-1
- tissue
- tissue polypeptide (TPA)
- tumor
- VDRL
- von Willebrand factor (vWF)

antigen-antibody complex
antigen-antibody reaction
antigenically stable
antigenic change
antigenic complex
antigenic drift
antigenic profile
antigenic properties of blood
antigen labeled with radioisotope
antigen-presenting cell (APC)
antigen-reactive cell
antigen-responsive cell
antigen-sensitive cell
antigliadin antibody
antiglioma monoclonal antibody kinase C
antiglobulin
antiglobulin consumption test
antiglobulin test (AGT)
anti-glomerular basement membrane (anti-GBM) antibody disease

ntigonadotropic hormone
ntigravity muscle
nti-HA antibody
nti-HAV (hepatitis A virus) antibody
nti-HB antibody
nti-HB_c antibody (antibody to core antigen of hepatitis B virus)
nti-HB_e antibody (antibody to e antigen of hepatitis B virus)
nti-HB_s antibody (antibody to surface antigen of hepatitis B virus)
ntihelix (also, anhelix)
ntihemophilic factor
ntihemophilic globulin (AHG)
ntihemophilic plasma
ntihemorrhagic factor
nti-HEV (hepatitis E virus) antibody
ntihuman globulin antibody
ntihyaluronidase antibody
ntihyaluronidase titer (AH titer)
nti-idiotype antibody
nti-idiotype autoantibody
nti-IL-2 receptor monoclonal antibody
ntiketogenesis
nti-kidney antibody
nti-LA/SS-B test
ntimesenteric border of the distal ileum
ntimesenteric fat pad
ntimesenteric surface
ntimesocolic side of cecum
ntimicrobial removal device
ntimitochondrial antibody (AMA)
nti-Monson curve
nti-MPO antibody
ntineuritic factor
ntineuritic vitamin
nti-nRNP autoantibody
ntinuclear antibody (ANA)
ntinuclear factor
ntioncogene (see *tumor suppressor gene*)
antipellagra factor
antiphospholipid antibody
antiphospholipid syndrome
antiplasmin, alpha
antipodal cell
anti-Pr cold autoagglutinin
anti-PR3 antibody
antipyretic
antireceptor antibody
anti-Rh antibody
anti-Rh antiglobulins
anti-Ro/SS-A test
anti-Scl-70 autoantibody
antiseptic
antiserum (pl. antisera)
anti-Sm test
anti-SS-A antibody
anti-SS-B antibody
antisterility factor
antistreptolysin O titer (ASO titer)
anti-TBM antibody
antithrombin III (ATIII)
antithyroglobulin antibody
antitoxin
antitragicus muscle
antitragohelicine fissure
antitragus
antitrypsin
  $alpha_1$–
  PiZZ
antitrypsin globulin, alpha
antitrypsin test
anti-VCA (viral capsid antigen) antibody
antivenin of animal origin
antivenom (also, antivenin)
antivenomous serum
antiviral interferon
antiviral protein
Antoni type A neurilemoma
Antoni type B neurilemoma
antral gastric cell

antral gastritis
antral mucosa
antral pouch
antral sphincter
antrum
  aditus ad
  cardiac
  ethmoid
  gastric
  mastoid
  maxillary
  prepyloric
  pyloric
  stomach
  Willis
  Highmore
  pyloric
  tympanic
  Valsalva
antrum cardiacum
anuli fibrosi
anus
  imperforate
  preternatural
AoBP (aortic blood pressure)
aorta (pl. aortae)
  abdominal
  arch of
  ascending
  buckled
  calcified
  coarctation
  descending
  descending thoracic
  dynamic
  esophageal artery of
  kinked
  overriding
  shaggy
  supraceliac
  thoracic
  tortuous
aorta *(continued)*
  transverse
  primitive
  ventral
aortic aneurysm
aortic arch
aortic arch syndrome
aortic area
aortic artery
aortic blood pressure (AoBP)
aortic body
aortic bulb
aortic cusp
aortic foramen
aortic glands
aortic hiatus
aortic isthmus
aortic knob
aortic knuckle
aortic lymph node
aortic nerve
aortic notch
aortic opening
aorticorenal disease
aorticorenal ganglia
aortic orifice
aortic ostium
aortic plexus
aortic receptor
aortic sac
aortic semilunar valve
aortic septal defect
aortic septum
aortic sinus
aortic sinus aneurysm
aortic spindle
aortic sulcus
aortic valve
aortic valve stenosis
aortic valvular leaflet
aortic vestibule
aortitis, syphilitic

aortopulmonary septum
Apathy mounting medium
apatite
APC (adenomatous polyposis coli)
APC antioncogene
APC tumor suppressor gene
aperistalsis
aperture
  angular
  anterior nasal
  inferior pelvic
  inferior thoracic
  superior pelvic
  superior thoracic
apertures of abdomen
apex (pl. apices)
  bladder
  cordis
  duodenal bulb
  external ring
  fibrous
  fibula
  heart
  ischiorectal fossa
  lingual
  lung
  nose
  prostate
  pulmonis
apex of femur
apex pneumonia
aphakic eye
aphtha (pl. aphthae)
aphthoid
aphthosis
aphthous stomatitis
aphthous ulcer
apical abscess
apical angle
apical area
apical canaliculus
apical complex
apical dendrite
apical ectodermal ridge
apical foramen
apical gland
apical infection
apical ligament
apical lymph node
apical periodontal abscess
apical pneumonia
apical process
apical recess
apical segment
apical space
apical zone
apicoposterior segment
aplasia
aplastic anemia
aplastic anemia due to marrow
  suppression
aplastic anemia syndrome
aplastic lymph
apocrine adenosis
apocrine cell
apocrine gland
apocrine metaplasia of breast
apolar cell
aponeurosis (pl. aponeuroses)
  abdominal
  bicipital
  epicranial
  extensor
  external oblique muscle
  gluteal
  internal oblique muscle
  lingual
  lumbar
  lumbocostal
  palatine
  palmar
  palmaris
  pharyngeal
  plantar

aponeurosis *(continued)*
  plantaris
  suprahyoid
aponeurotic portion of diaphragm
apophyseal point
ApopTag molecular biological-histochemical system
apoptosis
apoptotic oligodendrocyte
aporic gland
apparatus
  absorption
  accessory visual
  achromatic
  alimentary
  Barcroft-Warburg
  Benedict-Roth
  central
  chromatic
  chromidial
  digestive
  Golgi
  Haldane
  juxtaglomerular
  lacrimal
  respiratory
  Tiselius
  urogenital
  vasomotor
  vestibular
appearance
  beefy
  cobblestone
  dewy
  granular
  ground-glass
  hobnailed (of liver)
  honeycomb(ed)
  meaty
  mottled
  nutmeg
  onionskin

appearance *(continued)*
  speckled
  steamy
  tigroid
appearance infarct
appendage
  auricular
  cecal
  epiploic
appendages of testis
appendectomy
appendiceal abscess
appendiceal lumen
appendiceal mass
appendiceal stump
appendicitis
appendicular artery
appendicular colic
appendicular lymph node
appendicular muscle
appendicular skeleton
appendicular vein
appendix (pl. appendices)
  auricular
  cecal
  ensiform
  epiploic
  inflammation
  mesentery of
  Morgagni
  orifice of
  paracecal
  preileal
  retrocecal
  retrocolic
  retroileal
  right auricular
  serpentine
  subcecal
  testis
  ventricle of larynx
  vermiform

ppendix *(continued)*
 vesicular
 xiphoid
ppendix of epididymis
ppendix of testis
pperceptive mass
ppetite juice
pple, Adam's
pple-green fluorescence
pple jelly nodules
pple-peel bowel
ppose
pposed
pposition
ppropriateness of treatment
pron
 abdominal
 vascular
pt test for differentiating fetal from adult hemoglobin
PTT (activated partial thromboplastin substitution test)
PUD cell (amine precursor uptake and decarboxylation)
pyrexia
quagenic pruritus
qua-Mount
queduct
 cerebral
 cochlear
 fallopian
 sylvian
 ventricular
queduct of cochlea
queduct of Sylvius
queduct of vestibule
queous humor
queous-influx phenomenon
queous solution
queous vein
rachidonic acid metabolites
rachnia
Arachnia propionica
arachnodactyly
arachnoidal foramen
arachnoidal membrane
arachnoid granulation
arachnoiditis, chronic adhesive
arachnoid matter
arachnoid membrane
arachnoid space
arachnoid villi
Aran-Duchenne muscular atrophy
Arantius body
Arantius canal
Arantius duct
Arantius ligament
Arantius nodule
Arantius ventricle
arbitrary unit
arborescence
arborescent
arborization of blood vessels (collateral circulation)
arbovirus
arc
 auricular
 binauricular
 bregmatolambdoid
 crater
 interauricular
 longitudinal
 nasobregmatic
 naso-occipital
 neural
 reflex
arcade
 gastroepiploic
 mitral
arcade of jejunum, arterial
arcade of Struthers
arch
 abdominothoracic
 alveolar

arch *(continued)*
- aortic
- arterial
- axillary
- branchial
- carotid
- carpal
- coracoacromial
- cortical
- costal
- crural
- dental
- diaphragmatic
- expansion
- fallopian
- femoral
- fibrous
- glossopalatine
- hyoid
- inguinal ligament
- jugular
- lateral lumbosacral
- lumbocostal
- mandibular
- medial lumbosacral
- nasal
- neural
- palatal
- palatoglossal
- palatopharyngeal
- palpebral
- pharyngeal
- pharyngopalatine
- plantar
- pubic
- Riolan
- superciliary
- tarsal
- tendinous
- Treitz
- venous dorsal
- visceral

arch *(continued)*
- Zimmermann
- zygomatic

arched crest
archenteric canal
arch formation, Gothic
architecture
- hepatic
- lobular

archival tissue
arch of aorta
arch of aortic artery
arch of atlas
arch of bone
arch of fauces
arch of foot
arch of pelvic fascia
arciform vein
arcuate artery
arcuate crest
arcuate eminence
arcuate fiber
arcuate ligament
arcuate line
arcuate nucleus
arcuate popliteal ligament
arcuate pubic ligament
arcuate vein
arcuate vessel
arcuate zone
arcus aortae (arch of aorta)
arcus senilis
ardent fever
area (see also *region*)
- aortic
- apical
- association
- auditory
- basal seat
- cochlear
- cribriform
- denture-bearing

area *(continued)*
  denture foundation
  denture-supporting
  dermatomic
  embryonic
  entorhinal
  excitable
  frontal
  fronto-orbital
  gastric
  gastrohepatic bare
  germinal
  pubo-obturator
  subhepatic
area of cardiac dullness
areatus
arenavirus
areola of bone
areolar connective tissue
areolar gland
areolar membrane
areolar sheet
areolar tissue
argentaffin cells of Kultschitzky
argentaffin granule
argentaffinoma
argentaffin stain
Argentinian hemorrhagic fever
Argentinian hemorrhagic fever virus
arginine 358 alpha$_1$-antitrypsin (Pittsburgh mutation)
arginine vasopressin (AVP)
arginosuccinicaciduria
ARGUS flow cytometer
argyrophil cell
argyrophil fiber
argyrophilic fibrillary tangle
argyrophil plaque
Arias-Stella cell
Arias-Stella reaction
A ring of esophagus
Arizona hinshawii
Armanni-Ebstein cell
Armanni-Ebstein disease
Armanni-Ebstein kidney
Armanni-Ebstein lesion
armed macrophage
Arneth classification of polymorphonuclear neutrophils
Arnold canal
Arnold-Chiari deformity
Arnold-Chiari malformation
Arnold ganglion
Arnold nerve
aromatic amino acid (AAA)
array, organoid
arrector pili muscle
arrest, cardiac
arrested growth lines
arrhenoblastoma
arsenic (As)
  blood
  hair analysis for
  nail analysis for
  urinary
arsenic poisoning
ART (automated reagin test)
arteria (see Table of Arteries)
arterial arcades of the jejunum
arterial arch
arterial blood
arterial blood gases (ABGs)
arterial bulb
arterial canal
arterial capillary
arterial carbon dioxide
arterial circle
arterial cone
arterial duct
arterial gases (blood)
arterial gland
arterial groove
arterial ligament
arterial line culture

arterial mesocardium
arterial nephrosclerosis
arterial obstruction
arterial oxygen
arterial oxygen saturation
arterial puncture
arterial stenosis
arterial stenosis from embolism
arterial stenosis without thrombosis
arterial transfusion
arterial vein
arteries (see Table of Arteries)
arteriococcygeal gland
arteriolar necrosis
arteriolar nephrosclerosis
arteriole
  afferent
  afferent glomerular
  capillary
  efferent
  efferent glomerular
arteriolitis in kidneys, necrotizing
arteriolovenular anastomosis
arteriolovenular bridge
arteriosclerosis
  cerebral
  coronary
  hyaline
  hypertensive
  infantile
  intimal
  medial
  Mönckeberg (Moenckeberg)
  peripheral
  presenile
  senile
arteriosclerosis obliterans
arteriosclerotic aneurysm
arteriosclerotic kidney
arteriosclerotic nephritis
arteriosclerotic plaque
arteriostenosis
arteriosus
  conus
  ductus
  embryonic truncus
  remnant of the ductus
arteriovenous anastomoses
arteriovenous fistula
arteriovenous shunt
arteritis
  acute
  giant cell
  infantile
  necrotizing
  syphilitic
  temporal
arterivirus
artery (pl. arteries)—descriptive terms (See Table of Arteries for anatomical terms.)
  aberrant
  Abbott
  accessory
  accompanying
  Adamkiewicz
  adipose
  afferent
  anastomosis of
  anastomotic
  angular
  anonymous
  anterior
  anterolateral
  arcuate
  articular
  ascending
  atrial
  auricular
  axillary
  azygos
  calcaneal
  carotid
  central

artery *(continued)*
- Charcot
- chief
- circumflex
- Cohnheim
- coiled
- collateral
- common
- communicating
- companion
- conducting
- copper-wire
- corduroy
- corkscrew
- deferential
- degeneration of
- descending
- dorsal
- Drummond
- efferent
- elastic
- end
- external
- great
- hardening of
- Heubner
- highest (superior)
- inferior
- inflammation of
- innominate
- intercostal
- interlobular
- intermediate
- internal
- interosseous
- intersegmental
- interventricular
- Kugel anastomotic
- labial
- labyrinthine
- lateral
- left

artery *(continued)*
- lesser
- long
- Louis
- lowest
- medial
- middle
- Müller (Mueller)
- Neubauer
- nutrient
- parietal
- perforating
- pipestem
- postcentral
- posterior
- posterolateral
- posteromedial
- precentral
- pre-Rolandic
- principal
- proper
- radial
- recurrent
- right coronary (RCA)
- Rolandic
- segmental
- short
- spinal
- screw
- sheath of
- sheathed
- straight
- superficial
- superior
- superior articular
- transverse
- vidian
- Wilkie
- Willis
- Zinn

arthralgia

arthrifluent abscess

Arthrinium
arthritic atrophy
arthritis
  gouty
  infectious
  juvenile rheumatoid
  rheumatoid
  septic
  tuberculous
arthritis panel including
  antinuclear antibody
  antistreptolysin O titer
  C-reactive protein
  erythrocyte sedimentation rate
  rheumatoid factor by latex agglutination
  serum uric acid
Arthroderma
arthrodial articulation
arthrodial cartilage
arthrodial joint
Arthropoda
arthropod-borne relapsing fever
arthropod-borne viruses
arthropod vectors
arthroscope
articular artery
articular capsule
articular cartilage, hyaline
articular chondritis
articular corpuscle
articular crescent
articular crest
articular disk
articular eminence
articular facet
articular fluid
articular fossa
articular labrum
articular lamella of bone
articular lip
articular margin
articular meniscus
articular muscle
articular nerve
articular network
articular pit
articular process of vertebrae
articular surface
articular system
articular tubercle of temporal bone
articular vascular circle
articulated skeleton
articulating surface
articulatio (pl. articulationes) (see *articulation*)
articulation (also, joint)
  acromioclavicular
  amphiarthroses
  ankle
  arthrodial
  atlantoaxial
  atlanto-occipital
  balanced
  ball-and-socket
  bicondylar
  brachiocarpal
  brachioradial
  brachioulnar
  calcaneocuboid
  capitular
  carpal
  carpometacarpal
  cartilaginous
  chondrosternal
  Chopart
  composite
  compound
  condylar
  condyloid
  confluent
  costocentral
  costochondral
  costosternal

articulation *(continued)*
costotransverse
costovertebral
coxal
coxofemoral
craniovertebral
cricoarytenoid
cricothyroid
crurotalar
cubital
cubitoradial
cuboideonavicular
cuneocuboid
cuneometatarsal
cuneonavicular
dental
dentoalveolar
diarthroses
digit
distal radioulnar
elbow
ellipsoidal
femoral
fibrous
glenohumeral
gliding
gomphosis
hip
humeral
humeroradial
humeroulnar
iliofemoral
iliosacral
immovable
incudomalleolar
incudostapedial
intercarpal
interchondral
intercostal
intercuneiform
intermetacarpal
intermetatarsal

articulation *(continued)*
interphalangeal
intertarsal
intervertebral
knee
laryngeal
lower extremity
lumbosacral
mandible
manubriosternal
maxillary
metacarpophalangeal
metatarsophalangeal
movable
multiaxial
occipitoatloid
ovoid
patellofemoral
peg-and-socket
petrobasilar
petro-occipital
phalangeal
pisiform bone
pisocuneiform
pivot
plane
proximal radioulnar
pubis
radiocarpal
radiohumeral
radioulnar
sacrococcygeal
sacroiliac
sacrum and coccyx
saddle
scapuloclavicular
schindylesis (wedge-and-groove joint)
shoulder
simple
spheroid (ball-and-socket joint)
sternal

articulation *(continued)*
sternoclavicular
sternocostal
sternum
subtalar
superior tibial
sutura
synarthrosis
synchondrosis
syndesmosis
synovial
talocalcaneal
talocalcaneonavicular
talocrural
talonavicular
tarsometatarsal
tarsus
temporomandibular
temporomaxillary
tibiofibular
tibiotarsal
transverse tarsal
trochoid (pivot joint)
xiphisternal
zygapophyseal
articulation by reciprocal reception
articulation of atlas with axis or epistropheus
articulation of atlas with occipital bone
articulation of auditory ossicles
articulation of Buisson
articulation of calcaneus and astragalus
articulation of digits of foot
articulation of digits of hand
articulation of hand
articulation of head of humerus
articulation of head of rib
articulation of hip
articulation of metacarpal bones
articulation of metatarsal bones
articulation of phalanges of foot
articulation of phalanges of hand
articulation of trunk
articulation of vertebral arches
articulator
artifact, suction
artifacts of resuscitation
artificial abortion
artificial eye
artificial heart
artificial kidney
aryepiglottic fold
aryepiglottic muscle
arylsulfatase test for differentiating species of rapid-growing mycobacteria
arytenoepiglottic
arytenoidal articular surface
arytenoid cartilage
arytenoid gland
arytenoid muscle
arytenoid swelling
As (arsenic)
asbestosis
ascariasis
Ascaris lumbricoides
ascending aorta
ascending aortic artery
ascending artery
ascending branch of uterine artery
ascending cervical artery
ascending colon
ascending degeneration
ascending frontal convolution
ascending lumbar vein
ascending lymphangitis
ascending myelitis
ascending nerve tracts
ascending neuritis
ascending oblique muscle
ascending palatine artery
ascending parietal convolution
ascending part

ascending pharyngeal artery
ascending process
ascending pyelonephritis
ascending ramus of ischium
ascending ramus of os pubis
Aschoff body
Aschoff cell
Aschoff-Rokitansky sinus
ascites
ascitic fluid
Ascoli precipitin test for anthrax
ascorbate-cyanide test
ascorbic acid
Aselli gland
Aselli pancreas
aseptate hyphae
aseptic fever
aseptic myocarditis of newborn
aseptic necrosis
aseptic wound
Ashby method
ashen tubercle
ashen wing
ashy dermatitis
ashy dermatosis
Asiatic cholera
Askanazy cell
Askin tumor
Ask-Upmark kidney
ASO (antistreptolysin O) titer
aspartate aminotransferase (AST)
  (formerly SGOT)
aspergillosis
Aspergillus
Aspergillus flavus
Aspergillus fumigatus
Aspergillus glaucus
Aspergillus niger
Aspergillus terreus
aspiration
  bronchial
  fine-needle (FNA)

aspiration *(continued)*
  lymph node
  marrow
  percutaneous epididymal sperm
  Vabra
aspirating needle
aspiration biopsy
aspiration biopsy cytology (ABC)
aspiration pneumonia
aspiration pneumonitis
aspiration trocar
aspirin tolerance test
asplenia
assay (see also *test*)
  biological activity
  CA-125
  Cardiac T Rapid
  competitive binding
  Clostridium difficile toxin
  1,25-dihydroxycholecalciferol
    (1,25-OH-D_3)
  enzyme
  enzyme-linked immunosorbent
    (ELISA)
  estrogen receptor
  fluorescent cytoprint
  Guthrie bacterial inhibitor (GBIA)
  hamster egg penetration
  histoculture drug response (HDRA)
  hormone
  25-hydroxyvitamin D (25-OH-D)
  immune complex
  Limulus amebocyte lysate
  lipoprotein
  microcytotoxicity
  PHA (phytohemagglutinin)
  plasma
  plasminogen activator inhibition
  progesterone receptor
  radioallergosorbent (RAST)
  radioceptor
  Raji cell

assay *(continued)*
  rapid flow cytometry
  Rio-rad protein
  sperm penetration
  stem cell
  T and B lymphocyte subset
  Vitamin D
assimilation pelvis
assimilation sacrum
association area
association cortex
association fiber
association tract
AST (aspartate aminotransferase) (formerly SGOT)
asteatosis
asterion
asteroid body
asthma
asthmaticus, status
Astler-Coller modification of Dukes classification of carcinoma
ASTRA analyzer
astragaloid bone
astragaloscaphoid bone
astragalus
astringent solution
astroblastoma
astrocyte
  ameboid
  proliferating
astrocytoma, gemistocytic
astroglia
astroglial cell
astroglial scarring
astrovirus
asymmetrical
asymmetry
asymptomatic gluten-sensitive enteropathy
asynchronism
asynchronous
asynchrony
asynergic
asynergy
atavistic epiphyses
ataxia, Friedreich
ataxic lymphopathy
atelectasis
atelectatic lung
atherogenic
atheroma
atheroma embolism
atheromatous degeneration
atheromatous plaque
atheromatous streaking
atherosclerosis
atherosclerotic
athlete's foot (tinea pedis)
athlete's heart
ATIII (antithrombin III)
atlantoaxial articulation
atlantoaxial joint
atlanto-occipital articulation
atlanto-occipital joint
atlanto-occipital membrane
atlas, arch of
atlas bone
atlas with axis, articulation of
atlas with epistropheus, articulation of
atlas with occipital bone, articulation of
atmospheric oxygen
ATN (acute tubular necrosis)
atopic dermatitis
atopic eczema
atopy
ATPase (adenosine triphosphatase)
atraumatic injury
atresia
  cardiac
  esophageal
atresia of ovarian follicle
atretic follicles
atretic ovarian follicle

atria (pl. of atrium)
atrial artery
atrial auricle
atrial auricula
atrial canal
atrial complex
atrial myxoma
atrial natriuretic factor (ANF)
atrial natriuretic hormone (ANH)
atrial septal defect
atrioventricular (AV or A/V)
atrioventricular band
atrioventricular block
atrioventricular bundle of His
atrioventricular canal
atrioventricular conduction
atrioventricular gradient
atrioventricular groove
atrioventricular nodal artery
atrioventricular nodal branch
atrioventricular node
atrioventricular node of His
atrioventricular opening of His
atrioventricular orifice
atrioventricular sulcus
atrioventricular trunk
atrioventricular valve
atrium (pl. atria)
  accessory
  left
  right
atrium dextrum of left heart
atrium dextrum of nasal fossa
atrium dextrum of primitive heart
atrium dextrum of right heart
atrophic change
atrophic gastritis
atrophic inflammation
atrophic kidney
atrophic pulp degeneration
atrophic vaginitis
atrophy
  acute yellow
  adrenal
  Aran-Duchenne muscular
  arthritic
  basal cell
  black
  blue
  bone
  breast
  brown
  cerebral
  cervical
  Charcot-Marie
  Charcot-Marie-Tooth
  circumscribed cerebral
  compensatory
  compression
  concentric
  correlated
  cortical
  Cruveilhier
  cutaneous
  degenerative
  Dejerine-Sottas
  Dejerine-Thomas
  denervated muscle
  disuse
  Duchenne-Aran muscular
  eccentric
  Eichhorst
  endocrine
  endometrial
  epidermal
  Erb
  exhaustion
  facial
  fatty
  Fazio-Londe
  gastric
  gastric mucosa

atrophy *(continued)*
- granular
- hepatic
- Hoffmann
- inflammatory
- interstitial
- ischemic muscular
- juvenile muscular
- lacrimal gland
- Landouzy-Dejerine
- laryngeal
- leaping
- Leber optic
- lingual
- lobar
- macular
- mammary
- multiple system
- muscular
- myelopathic muscular
- myopathic
- neural
- neuritic muscular
- neuromuscular
- neuropathic
- neurotrophic
- numeric
- optic
- otic
- pancreatic acini
- pathologic
- penile
- peroneal
- physiologic
- pigmentary
- post-traumatic
- postmenopausal
- pressure
- progressive choroidal
- progressive muscular
- progressive neuromuscular
- progressive spinal muscular

atrophy *(continued)*
- progressive subcortical
- progressive unilateral facial
- pseudohypertrophic muscular
- red
- renal
- rheumatic
- salivary gland
- senile
- serous
- simple
- spinal muscular
- splenic
- subacute
- subchronic
- Sudeck
- testicular
- thymic
- thyroid
- Tooth (Charcot-Marie-Tooth)
- toxic
- transneuronal
- unilateral facial
- vaginal
- vascular
- villous
- Vulpian
- Werdnig-Hoffmann spinal muscular
- white
- yellow
- Zimmerlin

atrophy of breast
atrophy of hair cells
atrophy of ovary
atrophy of pancreatic acini
atrophy of parenchyma of lacrimal and salivary glands
atrophy of skin, diffuse idiopathic
atrophy of tubular cells
atropine test
attenuation
attic recess

attolens aurem muscle
attrahens aurem muscle
atypia
  architectural
  cytologic
  koilocytotic
atypical bronchial pneumonia
atypical change
atypical interstitial pneumonia
atypical lymphocyte
atypical phenylketonuria
atypical pneumonia
atypical verrucous endocarditis
Au (gold) antigen
Auberger blood group
auditory area
auditory artery
auditory canal
auditory capsule
auditory cartilage
auditory cell
auditory cortex
auditory field
auditory ganglion
auditory meatus
auditory mucosa
auditory nerve
auditory nucleus
auditory ossicle
auditory pit
auditory plate
auditory process
auditory radiation
auditory receptor cell
auditory stria
auditory teeth of Huschke
auditory tooth
auditory tract
  cartilaginous portion of
  cushion of
  isthmus of
  pharyngeal orifice of

auditory tract *(continued)*
  pharyngeal ostium of
  tonsil of
  torus tubarius
auditory vein
auditory vesicle
Auerbach ganglia
Auerbach mesenteric plexus
Auerbach myenteric plexus
Auer body
Auer rod
augmented histamine test of gastric function
augmenting factor
augmentor fiber
augmentor nerve
AUL (acute undifferentiated leukemia)
auramine O dye
auramine–rhodamine fluorescent stain
auramine–rhodamine fluorochrome stain
auramine–rhodamine stain
aurantiasis
aurem muscle
  attolens
  attrahens
Aureobasidium pullulans
auricle
  accessory
  atrial
  cervical
auricle of left atrium
auricle of right atrium
auricula dextra
  cartilage of
  ligaments of
  muscles of
  nerves of
  vessels of
auricular appendage
auricular appendix
auricular arc

auricular artery
auricular canaliculus
auricular cartilage
auricular complex
auricular ganglion
auricular ligament
auricular lymph nodes
auricular nerve
auricular notch
auricular point
auricular reflex
auricular surface
auricular surface of ilium
auricular surface of sacrum
auricular triangle
auricular tubercle of Darwin
auricular vein
auriculo-infraorbital plane
auriculotemporal nerve
auriculoventricular groove
auscultation
auscultatory gap
Australian antigen
Australian Q fever
autemesia
autoagglutinin, anti-Pr cold
autoantibody, anti-idiotype
autoantigen
autochthonous malaria
autoclasis
autoclave
autoerythrocyte sensitivity test
autoerythrocyte sensitization syndrome
autograft
autohemolysis test
autoimmune disease
autoimmune hemolytic anemia (AIHA)
autoimmune hepatitis
autoimmune mechanism
autoimmune thyroiditis
autoimmunity
autoinfection
autoinoculation
autointerference
Autolet blood glucose test
autologous blood
autologous protein
autologous transfusion
autolysis, postmortem
autolytic enzyme
autolyze
automated reagin test (ART)
automatic cell
autonomic ganglion
autonomic motor neuron
autonomic nerve
autonomic nervous system
autonomic plexus
autoparenchymatous metaplasia
AutoPap 300 QC automatic PAP screener system
Autopath QC test
autophagic vacuole
autophagosome
autoprothrombin
autopsy (also called postmortem, postmortem examination, or “the post”)
  consent for
  coroner
  medicolegal
autopsy room
autopsy specimen
autopsy subject, names for
  the body
  the cadaver
  the deceased
  the decedent
  the patient
  the name of the late patient
  the remains
  the subject
autopsy surgeon
auxiliary ventricle of heart

avascular necrosis
avian excreta
avian leukosis viruses
avian malaria
avian tuberculosis
aviator's ear
avidin-biotin complex (ABC)
avidin-biotin peroxidase complex
avidin-biotinylated peroxidase complex
Avipoxvirus
A vitamin
AV (atrioventricular) node
AV (arteriovenous) shunt
avulsed wound
A wave
axial aneurysm
Ayala index
Ayre spatula
azoospermia
azotemia
Aztec ear
azurophilic granule

B, b

Babesia bigemina
Babesia microti
babesiosis
Bachman-Pettit test
Bachman test
bacillary angiomatosis
bacillary dysentery
bacillary embolism
bacillary hemoglobinuria
bacillary necrosis
bacille Calmette-Guérin
bacilli in urine
bacilluria
bacillus (pl. bacilli) (see *pathogen* for names of organisms)
bacitracin
backbone
back-flow of blood
back-to-back configuration
back tooth
backward curvature
BACTEC bottle
bacteremia
bacteria (pl. of bacterium) (see *pathogen* for names of organisms)
  acid-fast
  aerobic
bacteria *(continued)*
  anaerobic
  corkscrew-shaped
  defense against
  fibrillary
  funguslike
  gram-negative
  gram-positive
  helical
  intracellular
  pathogenic
  pus-forming
  pyogenic
  spiral-shaped
bacteria in stool
bacteria in urine
bacterial cellular protein
bacterial colonies
bacterial culture
bacterial culture media
bacterial dissociation
bacterial flora
bacterial gastroenteritis
bacterial infection
bacterial lipopolysaccharide
bacterial meningitis
bacterial myocarditis

bacterial nephritis
bacterial pericarditis
bacterial pneumonia
bacterial pneumonitis
bacterial protein
bacterial toxemia
bacterial toxins
bacterial vaginosis
bacterial virus
bactericidal concentration, minimum (MBC)
bacteriologic smear
bacteriological
bacteriology
bacteriolytic test
bacteriophage
bacteriophage plaque
bacterium (pl. bacteria) (see *bacteria*)
bacteriuria
Bacteroides (see *pathogen*)
Baehr-Lohlein lesion
Baerensprung erythrasma
Baermann concentration
bag, body
bagassosis
Bagros space
Baker cyst
baker's eczema
BAL (bronchoalveolar lavage)
balance
    acid-base
    electrolyte
balanced articulation
balanitis
balanitis xerotica obliterans
balanoposthitis
Balantidium coli
baldness (see *alopecia*)
    congenital
    female pattern
    male pattern
Balkan nephritis
ball-and-socket articulation
ball-and-socket joint
ballerina-foot pattern
balloon cell
balloon cell nevus
ballooning degeneration
ball valve
balsam mounting medium
Balser fatty necrosis
bamboo hair
band
    A
    absorption
    amniotic
    anogenital
    atrioventricular
    BB
    Bechterew
    Broca
    Bungner
    chromosome
    Clado
    contraction
    coronary
    Crooke-Russell
    delta
    diagonal
    Essick cell
    fibroelastic
    fibromuscular
    fibrous
    Gennari
    H
    Harris
    His
    Hunter-Schreger
    I
    iliotibial
    Ladd
    Lane
    longitudinal
    M

band *(continued)*
- Mach
- Maissiat
- matrix
- MB
- Meckel
- mesocolic
- MM
- moderator
- N-b
- oligoclonal
- omental
- pecten
- perioplic
- peritoneal
- pseudokeloidal
- Q
- R
- Reil
- septomarginal
- Silastic
- Simonart
- Soret
- Streeter
- tendinous
- transverse
- Z

band cell
bandlike adhesion
band neutrophil
band of Broca
band of colon
- anterior
- free

band of Giacomini
band of Gosset, spiral
band of Kaes-Bechterew
band-pass filter
band-shaped nucleus
band visualization
Bang bacillus
banjo-string adhesions
Bankart lesion
bank
- blood
- bone
- eye
- human milk
- skin
- tissue

Banti syndrome
Bárány caloric test
barber's pilonidal sinus
barbiturates, blood
Barcroft-Warburg apparatus
Bardinet ligament
Bard-Parker blade
bare area for colon
bare area of liver
barium meal
barium sulfate-absorbed plasma
Barkow ligaments
baroreceptor nerve
Barr body
Barr-Epstein virus
Barré-Guillain syndrome
barrel-shaped stone
Barrett epithelium
Bart abnormal hemoglobin
Bartholin abscess of vulvovaginal gland
Bartholin cyst
Bartholin duct
Bartholin gland
bartholinian abscess
Bartonella bacilliformis
basal body temperature (BBT)
basal bone
basal cell atrophy
basal cell carcinoma
basal cell epithelioma
basal cell layer
basal cell nevus
basal cell of skin

basal cell of vagina
basal cell papilloma
basal cell, swollen
basal corpuscle
basal epithelial hyperplasia
basal ganglia
basal granular cells
basal granule
basal lamina
basal layer
basal metabolism
basal nucleus
basal pigmentation
basal plate
basal plate cotyledon
basal ridge
basal rod
basal seat area
basal sphincter
basal squamous (basosquamous)
basal striation
basal surface
basal vein
basale, stratum
basalis decidua
basaloid cell
basaloma
base
  cement
  cranial
Basedow goiter
base excess test
base finger
baseline
baseline test
base material
basement lamina
basement membrane
basement tissue
base of bladder
base of ischiorectal fossa
base of lung
base plate or baseplate
basibregmatic axis
basic fuchsin
basic function
Basidiobolus ranarum
basihyal bone
basilar angle
basilar artery
basilar bone
basilar cartilage
basilar cell
basilar crest
basilar lamina
basilar membrane
basilar meningitis
basilar part
basilar plexus
basilar process
basilar sinus
basilar sulcus
basilar vertebra
basilic vein
basinasal line
basioccipital bone
basiotic bone
basipharyngeal canal
basis bundle, anterior
basisphenoid bone
basisphenoid vein
basket cell
basketweave pattern
baso (slang for basophil)
basopenia
basophil adenoma
basophil, beta
basophil cell
basophil degranulation test
basophil granule
basophil substance
basophilia
basophilic cell
basophilic cytoplasmic granules

basophilic leukemia
basophilic leukocyte
basophilic nuclear remnants in erythrocytes
basophilic stippling of erythrocytes
basosquamous (basal squamous)
basosquamous cell carcinoma
bath, flotation
bathing trunk nevus
bath itch
bath pruritus
battery of tests
Battey bacillus
battledore placenta
Bauhin gland
Bauhin valve
Baumé scale
BB bands
B bile
BB isoenzyme
BBT (basal body temperature)
BCAA (branched chain amino acid)
B (beta)
B cell
B-cell differentiating factor
B-cell lymphoma
B-cell monocytoid lymphoma
B-cell stimulatory factor
B chain
BCIP (5-bromo-4-chloro-3-indolyl phosphate)
bcl-2 gene (oncogene)
beach ear
beaded hepatic duct
beaked pelvis
beaker cell
beaklike projections of cartilage
Beale cell
Beale ganglion cells
Beau line
Bechterew band
Becker nevus
bed
  bladder
  capillary
  gallbladder
  hepatic
  liver
  nail
  portal vascular
  stomach
beef heart cardiolipin
beef heart infusion
beefy appearance
beefy red appearance of tongue
beefy texture
Behçet syndrome
BEI (butanol-extractable iodine)
bejel
bell clapper deformity
Bellini ligament
belly button
belly of muscle
B-emission counter
Bence Jones body
Bence Jones protein in urine
Bence Jones proteinemia
Bence Jones proteinuria
Bence Jones reaction
bench test
Benedict-Roth apparatus
Benedict test for glucose
benign epidermal tumor
benign false positive
benign familial chronic pemphigus
benign fibrous histiocytoma
benign hypertension
benign juvenile melanoma
benign lymphocytic meningitis
benign lymphoepithelial lesion
benign lymphoreticulosis
benign mucosal pemphigoid
benign neoplasm
benign nephrosclerosis

benign pigmented nevus
benign polyp
benign prostatic hyperplasia
benign recurrent hematuria
benign squamous papilloma
benign tertian malaria
bentiromide test
bentonite flocculation test
benzene nucleus
benzene poisoning
benzene ring
benzidine test for occult blood in urine or feces
Bérard aneurysm
Berger cells
Berger space
Bergmann cells
beriberi
berlock dermatitis
Bernard canal
Bernstein esophageal acid infusion test
berry aneurysm
berry cell
Berry ligaments
Berson test
Bertin bone
Bertin, columns of
Bertin ligament
berylliosis
beryllium dust
beryllium granuloma
Besnier-Boeck disease
Besnier-Boeck-Schaumann disease
Besnier prurigo
Bessey-Lowry unit
Best carmine stain
beta-adrenergic receptor
beta angle
beta basophil
beta blocker
beta-carotene cleavage enzyme
beta-cell
beta-endorphin
beta factor
beta fiber
beta fraction
beta globulin
beta granule
beta-HCG (human chorionic gonadotropin)
beta hemolysin
beta-hemolytic streptococcus
beta-hydroxybutyric acid
beta-lactamase
beta leukocyte
$beta_1$-lipoprotein
beta lipoprotein fraction
$beta_2$-microglobulin
beta particle
beta phage
Betascope 630 Biot Analyzer
beta substance
beta-thromboglobulin
Bethesda PAP smear classification
Bethesda system
Betke-Kleihauer stain
Bettendorff test for arsenic
Betz cell
Bevan-Lewis cell
bevel, cavosurface
Bezold abscess
B_T factor
B fiber
B5 fixative
BFP (biological false positive)
BGM cell
B hemophilia
B hepatitis
BHI (brain-heart infusion)
BHS-RFC A3 fluorescence microscope
Bial test
Bi antigen
biauricular axis
biaxial joint

bicameral abscess
bicameral uterus
bicanalicular sphincter
bicarbonate ion
bicarbonate, plasma
bicarbonate test
biceps brachii muscle
biceps tendon
Bichat canal
Bichat ligament
bicipital aponeurosis
bicipital bursitis
bicipital fascia
bicipital groove
bicipital rib
bicipital ridge
bicipital tuberosity
bicipitoradial bursa
bicondylar articulation
bicondylar joint
bicornuate uterus
bicuspid tissue
bicuspid tooth
bicuspid valve
Biebrich scarlet stain
Bielschowsky method
Bielschowsky stain
bifid rib
bifida, spina
Bifidobacterium
bifurcated ligament
bifurcation of lymph node
bifurcation of pulmonary trunk
Bigelow ligament
bigeminal body
bigeminal pregnancy
bilateral cortical necrosis
bilaterally
bilayer, outer lipoprotein
bile
  A
  B

bile *(continued)*
  C
  canaliculus
  extrahepatic
  gallbladder
  liver
  viscid
  viscous
  white
bile acid
  conjugated
  fecal
  total
bile acid pool
bile acid tolerance test
bile antigen
bile capillary
bile concretion
bile duct
  common (CBD)
  infundibulum
  interlobular
  preampullary portion of
  sphincter of
bile duct abscess
bile duct carcinoma
bile duct lumen
bile duct stone
bile esculin test
bile lake
bile papilla
bile pigment in basal ganglia
bile salts
bile sludge
bile solubility test for differentiation of pneumococci from other streptococci
bilharziasis
"bili" (slang for bilirubin)
biliary abscess
biliary apparatus
biliary calculus

biliary cirrhosis
biliary duct
biliary ductule
biliary fistula
biliary gland
biliary obstruction
biliary passage
biliary plexus
biliary radicle
biliary sludge
biliary structure
biliary tract
biliary tract stone
biliary tree
bilious diarrhea
bilious pneumonia
bilious remittent malaria
bilious vomiting
bilirubin
  conjugated
  deposition of unconjugated
  direct-reacting
  indirect-reacting
  serum
  total
  unconjugated
  urine
bilirubinate
bilirubin glucuronyltransferase
bilirubin infarct
bilirubin in urine
bilirubinuria (choluria)
Billheimer assay method
bilobate
bilobate placenta
bilobed (bi-lobed)
bilobed gallbladder
bilobular
bilobulate
bilocular joint
bilocular stomach
binary fission
binauricular arc
binding protein
Binz test for quinine in urine
biochemical profile
biochemical reaction
biochemistry
biological activity assay
biological false positive (BFP)
biological vector
biopsy (bx)
  aspiration
  bone marrow
  brain
  brush
  chorionic villus
  cold cup
  cone
  cytological
  dermis
  excisional
  exploratory
  fine-needle aspiration
  incisional
  Keyes punch
  mirror image breast
  needle
  needle core
  open
  punch
  shave
  skin
  stereotactic
  surface
  thin-needle
  Vabra aspirate
biopsy of myocardium via transvenous catheter
biopsy specimen
bioptome, Caves-Schutz-Stanford
Biopty cut needle
Biorad MRC 600 scanning system
Bio-rad protein assay

biorbital angle
biotin-dependent carboxylase deficiency
biotinylated secondary antibody
biparietal diameter (BPD)
bipartite patella
bipartite uterus
bipennate muscle
bipolar cell
bipolar retinal cell
Bipolaris australiensis
Bipolaris hawaiiensis
Bipolaris spicifera
Birbeck granule
bird's nest lesion
birefringence
birefringent crystal
birth canal
birth defect
birthmark, vascular
birth trauma
bisect
bisected
bisection
bismuth stomatitis
bite cell
bite plane
biuret test for serum proteins
biventral lobule
biventricular configuration
biventricular dilatation
biventricular hypertrophy
bizarre cell
bizarre mitotic figures
bizarre nuclei
Bizzozero red cell
BK DNA virus
black atrophy
black degeneration of brain
black eye
black fever
black induration
black light
black liver
black lung
black plague
black, Sudan
black tarry stool
black vomit
blackwater fever
bladder
  apex of
  base of
  exstrophy of
  hypertrophy
  hypotonic
  inflammation of
  neck of
  neurogenic
  papilloma of
  trigone of
  urinary
  uvula of
bladder bed
bladder capacity
bladder carcinoma
bladder cell
bladder diverticulum
bladder fundus
bladder tumor
bladder washing
blade bone
bland embolism
bland endometrium
Blandin and Nuhn gland
Blandin gland
blast cell
blast form
blastic lesion
blast injury
blastocyst
blastoderm
blastodermic disk
blastodermic layer

blastodermic vesicle
Blastomyces dermatitidis
blastomycetic dermatitis
blastomycosis
  European
  North American
  South American
blastoporic canal
Blastoschizomyces pseudotrichosporon
bleb
  cutaneous
  emphysematous
bleeding
  dysfunctional uterine (DUB)
  excessive
  postcoital
  postmenopausal
  purpuric
  recurrent
  widespread
bleeding from wounds, prolonged
bleeding gums
bleeding into a joint
bleeding polyp
bleeding time (BT)
  Duke
  Ivy
  Mielke
  Simplate
blennoid
blennorrhagia
blennorrhea, inclusion
blepharitis
blepharoplast
Blessig cyst
blighted ovum
blind foramen
blind gut
blindness
blind pouch
blind spot
blister cell
blistering
bloc (see *en bloc*)
Bloch scale
block
  atrioventricular
  cell
  occult
  paraffin
  tissue
  wax
blockade, ganglionic
blocked pleurisy
blocking and sectioning
blood
  anticoagulant-treated
  antigenic properties of
  arterial
  capillary
  circulating
  defibrinated
  degenerated
  donor
  extravasated
  hemolyzed
  iron-binding capacity of
  laky
  mass of congealed
  mixed venous
  nonoxygenated
  occult
  oxygen-carrying capacity of
  oxygenated
  peripheral
  platelet-poor (PPB)
  stagnation of
  sludged
  transfusion of incompatible
  typing and crossmatching of
  venous
  whole
blood agar, Bordet-Gengou
blood albumin

blood alcohol level
blood arsenic
blood barbiturate
blood-borne infection
blood-borne organism
blood-borne parasite
blood-brain barrier
blood cell
blood-clot lysis time (BLT)
blood clotting
blood coagulation
blood corpuscle
blood count
  complete
  differential
blood crystal
blood culture
blood ethanol
blood factor
blood fluke
blood-forming organ
blood-forming tissue
blood gas analysis
blood gases, arterial
blood gland
blood glucose
blood group (also, blood type)
  ABO
  Auberger
  autologous
  Cartwright
  Diego
  Dombrock
  Duffy
  high frequency
  I
  Kell
  Kidd
  Lewis
  low frequency
  Lutheran
  MNS
blood group *(continued)*
  P
  Rh
  Rh negative
  Rh positive
  Sutter
blood grouping
blood-influx phenomenon
blood lactic acid
blood lead level
bloodless field
blood loss
blood mole
blood pigment
blood plasma
blood plasma fraction
blood platelet
blood pool
blood pressure
blood serum
blood sludge
blood smear
blood specimen
bloodstained effusion
blood stream (also, bloodstream)
bloodsucking intestinal parasite
blood sugar test, fasting
blood tests (see Table, pp. 576-590)
blood-tinged fluid
blood-tinged sputum
blood transfusion, mismatched
blood type (see *blood group*)
blood typing
blood typing agglutinin
blood urea nitrogen (BUN)
blood vessel gland
blood volume
blood work
bloody diarrhea
bloody fluid
bloody spinal fluid
bloody stools

Bloom syndrome
blot, blotting
  Northern
  Southern
  Western
blotchy clumping of pigment
blotchy facial hyperpigmentation
blot-dot hybridization
Blount disease
blowing wound
blue aniline dye
blue aniline stain
blue atrophy
blue-black pigmentation (ochronosis) of cartilage, tendons, arterial intima
blue dome cyst
blue fever
blue-green pus
blue liver
blue nevus
blue ocular sclera
blue pus
blue pus bacillus
blue rubber bleb nevus
bluetongue virus
bluish macule
Blumenthal lesion
blunt trauma
B lymphocyte
Boas-Oppler bacillus
Boas point
boatlike abdomen
Bochdalek foramen
Bochdalek gap
Bockhart impetigo
Bodansky unit
Bodian method of staining
body (pl. bodies)
  acetone
  acidophilic
  adrenal
  alveolar

body *(continued)*
  Amato
  amyloid
  angularis
  anococcygeal
  aortic
  Arantius
  Arnold
  asbestos
  Aschoff
  asteroid
  Auer
  Barr
  Bence Jones
  bigeminal
  Bracht-Wachter
  Cabot ring
  Call-Exner
  carotid
  cavernous
  cell
  central
  chromaffin
  chromatin
  ciliary
  coccygeal
  colloid
  compressible cavernous
  conchoidal
  Councilman
  crystalloid
  cytoid
  Deetjen
  demilune
  dense
  Döhle (Doehl) inclusion
  Donovan
  Dutcher
  Ehrlich hemoglobinemic
  elementary
  epithelial
  esophageal

body *(continued)*
Exner-Call
fat
fibrin
foreign
fuchsin
fungal
geniculate
glomus
Guarnieri
Heinz
Heinz-Ehrlich
Herring
Hirano
Howell-Jolly
immune
inclusion
inner
Jolly
Jolly-Howell
ketone
Lafora
Leishman-Donovan
Lewy
Lewy inclusion
Lipschütz
lymphoglandular
lyssa inclusion
Mallory
Mallory malpighian
malpighian
Masson
Molluscum
Negri
Nissl
Pappenheimer
paravertebral
Pick
Pick inclusion
psammoma
Russell
Schaumann

body *(continued)*
Schmorl
Stieda
Toxoplasma
vermiform
vertebral
Weibel-Palade
Y
zebra
body bag
body cavity
body cell mass
body fluid
body fluid amylase
body fluid glucose
body louse
body of epididymis
body of femur
body of gallbladder
body of Retzius
body of sternum
body of vertebra
body stalk
body wall
Boeck disease
Boeck sarcoid
Boehmer hematoxylin
Boerhaave gland
Boettcher (see *Böttcher*)
boggy uterus
Bogros space
boil
Bolivian hemorrhagic fever
Bolivian hemorrhagic fever virus
Boll cell
Bollinger granule
bolster fingers
bone (see Table of Bones)
acetabular
acromial
alar
Albers-Schoenberg marble

bone *(continued)*
Albrecht
alveolar
alveolar supporting
ankle
arch of
areolae of
articular lamella of
articular tubercle of temporal
basal
basihyal
basilar
basioccipital
basisphenoid
Bertin
blade
breast
Breschet
brittle
bundle
calcaneal
calf
cancellous
cannon
capitate
carpal
cartilage
cavalry
central
chalky
cheek
coccygeal
coffin
collar
compact
convoluted
coronary
cortical
costal
coxal
cranial
cribriform

bone *(continued)*
cubital
cuboid
cuneiform
dead
dense
dermal
destruction of
devitalized portion of
dorsal talonavicular
ear
eburnated
elbow
endochondral
enetral
epactal
epihyal
epiphysis of
epipteric
episternal
erosion of epiphyseal
eburnated
ethmoid
exercise
exoccipital
facial
femoral
fibular
first cuneiform
flank
flat
Flower
fourth turbinated
fragile
freeze-dried
frontal
funny
Goethe
greater multangular
hamate
haunch
heel

bone *(continued)*
highest turbinated
hip
hollow
hooked
hyoid
hyperplastic
iliac
immature
incarial
incisive
inferior turbinated
inflammation of
innominate
intermaxillary
intermediate cuneiform
interparietal
intracartilaginous
intrachondral
intramembranous
irregular
ischial
ivory
ivorylike
jaw
jugal (zygomatic)
Krause
lacrimal
lamellar
lamellated
lateral cuneiform
lenticular
lentiform
lesser multangular
lingual
long
lunate
malar
marble
mastoid
maxillary
maxilloturbinal

bone *(continued)*
medial cuneiform
medullary
metacarpal
metastasis to
metatarsal
middle cuneiform
middle turbinated
multangular
nasal
navicular
necrotic
neoplasm of
new
newly woven
nonlamellar
nonlamellated
occipital
odontoid
orbicular
orbitosphenoidal
osteoporosis of
osteoporotic
palate
palatine
parietal
pedal
pelvic
penis
perichondral
periosteal
periotic
peroneal
petrosal
petrous
phalangeal
ping-pong
pipe
Pirie
pisiform
pneumatic
postsphenoid

bone *(continued)*
- preinterparietal
- premaxillary
- presphenoid
- pterygoid
- pubic
- pyramidal
- quadrilateral
- radial
- redness of
- replacement
- resurrection
- reticulated
- rider's
- Riolan
- rudimentary
- sacral
- sacred
- scaphoid
- scapular
- sclerotic
- scroll
- second cuneiform
- semilunar
- septal
- sesamoid
- shank
- shin
- short
- sieve
- skull
- sphenoid
- sphenoidal turbinated
- sphenoturbinal
- splint
- spoke
- spongy
- squamo-occipital
- squamous
- squamous-type
- stifle
- stirrup

bone *(continued)*
- substitution
- superior turbinated
- supernumerary
- suprainterparietal
- supraoccipital
- suprapharyngeal
- suprasternal
- supreme turbinated
- sutural
- tail
- tarsal
- temporal
- thigh
- thoracic
- three-cornered
- trabecular
- trapezium
- trapezoid
- triangular
- tuberculosis of
- turbinate
- turbinated
- tympanic
- tympanohyal
- ulnar
- unciform
- upper jaw
- vascular
- vesalian
- Vesalius
- vomer
- wedge
- weightbearing
- whettle
- woven
- xiphoid
- yoke
- zygomatic

bone abscess
bone age
bone architecture

bone atrophy
bone bank
bone calcification
bone canaliculus
bone cell
bone corpuscle
bone cortex
bone cyst
bone deformity
bone degeneration
bone dysplasia
bone erosion
bone fracture
bone fragment, jagged
bone infarct
bone lacuna
bonelet
bone marrow
bone marrow biopsy
bone marrow degeneration
bone marrow, differential count:
  lymphocytes
  metamyelocytes
  monocytes
  myeloblasts
  myelocytes: neutrophilic,
    eosinophilic, basophilic
  plasma cells
  polymorphonuclear basophils,
    eosinophils, neutrophils
  promyelocytes
  reticulum cells
bone marrow embolism
bone marrow failure
bone marrow study
bone marrow transplantation
bone matrix
bone medulla
bone mineral density
bone morphogenetic protein
bone pain
bone plate
bone resorption
bone salts
bone softening
bone splitting
bone spur
bone tissue, normal
bone tumor
bone wax
Bonnot gland
bony ankylosis
bony callus
bony eburnation
bony fossa
bony labyrinth
bony landmarks
bony palate
bony pelvis
bony proliferation
bony semicircular canal
bony thoracic cage
bony tissue
booster phenomenon on TB test
border
  alveolar
  brush
  crescentic
  interosseous
border cell
border disease virus
borderline diabetes
borderline hypertension
borderline leprosy
borderline malignancy
borderline normal
borderline test result
border of distal ileum, antimesenteric
border of heart
  inferior
  left
  right
  superior
border of mandible, alveolar

border zone
Bordet-Gengou agar
Bordet-Gengou bacillus
Bordet-Gengou blood agar
Bordet-Gengou phenomenon
Bordetella bronchiseptica
Bordetella parapertussis
Bordetella pertussis
Bornholm disease
Borrelia burgdorferi
Borrelia hermsii
Borrelia kochii
Borrelia mazzottii
Borrelia parkeri
Borrelia recurrentis
Borrelia turicatae
boss
bosselated
Boston exanthem
Botallo ligament
Botryodiplodia theobromae
botryoides sarcoma
botryomycosis
borderline normal
Böttcher (Boettcher)
Böttcher canal
Böttcher cell
Böttcher space
bottle, BACTEC
bottle-shaped hair cells
botulism
Bouin fixative
Bouin fluid
Bouin picroformol-acetic fixative
Bouin solution
boundary membrane
Bourgery ligament
bouquet fever
boutonneuse fever
boutonnière deformity
bowed tendon
bowel
  aganglionic
  apple-peel
  dead
  infarcted
  intussuscepted
  ischemic
  kink in
  large
  small
  strangulated
bowel axis
bowel contents
bowel disease with protein loss
bowel gases
bowel gas pattern
bowel loop
bowel lumen
bowel sounds
bowel stenosis
bowel stoma
bowel tones
bowel wall
Bowen disease
bowenoid cell
bowenoid papulosis
Bowen precancerous dermatosis
Bowie stain
bowing of long bones
bowleg, nonrachitic
Bowman capsule
Bowman disease
Bowman gland
Bowman membrane
Bowman space
boxer's encephalopathy
box, snuff
Boyden sphincter
Bozicevich test
BPD (biparietal diameter)
Br (bromine)

brachial artery
brachial fascia
brachial gland
brachial lymph node
brachial muscle
brachial neuritis
brachial plexus
brachial vein
brachii, biceps
brachii muscle
brachiocarpal articulation
brachiocephalic artery
brachiocephalic trunk
brachiocephalic vein
brachioradial articulation
brachioradial muscle
brachioradial tendon
brachioulnar articulation
Bracht-Wachter lesion
brachypellic pelvis
bradycardia
brain
  edematous
  inflammation of
  metastasis to
  respirator
  sand
  split
  wet
brain abscess
brain artery
brain biopsy
brain damage, irreversible
brain dead
brain death
brain degeneration
brain disease, demyelinating
brain fissure
brain-heart infusion (BHI)
brain heart infusion agar
brain laceration
brain mantle
brain stem
brain substance
brain sugar
brain swelling
brain tissue
brain tumor
brain wave
branch
  anterior cutaneous
  circumflex
  cutaneous lateral
  inferior cardiac
  perforating
  pudendal
branched chain alpha-ketoacids, block in decarboxylation of
branched chain amino acid (BCAA)
branched tubular glands of Littré
brancher (also, branching)
brancher enzyme
brancher enzyme deficiency
brancher factor
branches
  paired parietal
  paired visceral
  unpaired parietal
  unpaired visceral
branchial arch
branchial cartilage
branchial cell
branchial cleft
branchial cleft cyst
branchial cyst
branchial duct
branchial efferent column
branchial fistula
branchial groove
branchial pouch
branching enzyme
branching factor
branching filaments
branching pattern

branchiomeric muscle
branchiomotor nucleus
Branhamella catarrhalis (formerly *Neisseria catarrhalis*)
brass founder's fever
Braune canal
Brazilian spotted fever
bread-and-butter heart
bread-and-butter pericardium
breakbone fever
breakdown hemoglobin
breakdown of muscle tissue
breakdown of red blood cells
breast
  accessory
  biopsy of
  fibroadenoma of
  fibrocystic
  proemial
  shotty
breast atrophy
breast biopsy
breast bone (also, breastbone)
breast carcinoma
breast degeneration
breast inflammation
breast milk jaundice
breast neoplasm
breast tumor
breath analysis test
breath-holding test
bregmatic bone
bregmatic fontanel
bregmatolambdoid arc
Brenner tumor
Breschet bone
Breschet canal
Breslow classification of malignant melanoma
Breus mole
breviradiate cells
Brewer infarct
bridge
  arteriolovenular
  cell
  cytoplasmic
  intercellular
  mucosal
bridge corpuscle
bridge of nose
bridging epithelium
bridging necrosis
Brill-Zinsser disease
brim, pelvic
B ring of esophagus
Brinton disease
bristle cell
brittle bone
brittle diabetes
brittle mass
broadest muscle
broad fascia
broad flat nose
broad ligament abscess
broad ligament of uterus
broad ligament pregnancy
Broca area
Broca band
Broca center
Broca diagonal band
Broca pudendal pouch
Brockenbrough needle
Brodel white line
Broder criteria
Broders index of tumor malignancy
Brodie abscess
Brodie joint
Brodie knee
Brodie ligament
broken-down erythrocytes
Brolacin agar
bromine (Br)
bromosulfophthalein (also, sulfobromophthalein sodium) (BSP)

bromphenol test
bronchial artery
bronchial aspirate
bronchial asthma
bronchial brushing
bronchial fremitus
bronchial gland
bronchial mucosa
bronchial pneumonia
bronchial polyp
bronchial stenosis
bronchial tube
bronchial vein
bronchial washing
bronchic cell
bronchiectasis
bronchiolar edema
bronchiolar exocrine cell
bronchiolar spasm and edema
bronchiole
  conducting
  respiratory
  terminal
bronchiolitis obliterans organizing pneumonia
bronchiolitis, obliterative
bronchitis
  acute
  chronic
bronchoalveolar lavage (BAL)
bronchoalveolar lavage fluid
bronchobiliary fistula
bronchocavitary fistula
bronchoesophageal fistula
bronchoesophageal muscle
bronchogenic adenocarcinoma
bronchogenic carcinoma
bronchogenic cyst
bronchomediastinal lymph trunk
bronchomediastinal trunk
bronchopleural fistula
bronchopneumonia, hypostatic
bronchopulmonary dysplasia
bronchopulmonary lymph node
bronchopulmonary segment
bronchoscopic smear
bronchus (pl. bronchi)
  branch
  eparterial
  hyparterial
  inferior lobe
  inflammation of
  intermediate
  left main
  lobar
  main stem
  major
  middle lobe
  mucoid impaction of
  primary
  principal
  right lobe
  right main
  segmental
  superior
  superior lobe
bronchus intermedius
bronchus principalis sinister
bronchus principalis dexter
bronchus segmentalis
bronze diabetes
bronze edema
bronze pigmentation of skin
brood capsule
brood cell
Brooker periarticular heterotopic ossification (PHO)
broth, nutrient
brown adipose tissue
brown atrophy
Brown-Brenn Gram stain
brown fat
brown fat tissue
Brown-Hopp tissue Gram stain

brown induration
brown reaction product
brown stool
brown stria
brown-tail moth dermatitis
brown tissue
brown tumor
Brucella abortus
Brucella canis
Brucella melitensis
Brucella suis
brucellosis agglutinins
Bruch gland
Bruch membrane
Brücke line
Brunner gland
Brunn nest
Bruns glucose medium
brush biopsy
brush border
brushing, bronchial
Bruton disease
B_T factor
bubble gum dermatitis
bubonic plague
bucca (pl. buccae)
buccal angle
buccal artery
buccal cavity
buccal curve
buccal fat pad
buccal flange
buccal gingiva
buccal gland
buccal lymph node
buccal mucosa
buccal nerve
buccal occlusion
buccal region
buccal shelf
buccal smear
buccal surface
buccal ulcer
buccal vestibule
buccinator artery
buccinator crest
buccinator lymph node
buccinator nerve
buccocervical ridge
buccogingival ridge
bucconasal membrane
bucconeural duct
bucco-occlusal angle
buccopharyngeal fascia
buccopharyngeal membrane
buccopharyngeal part
buckled aorta
Bucky diaphragm
bud
  dorsal pancreatic
  end
  ventral pancreatic
budding platelet
Budin obstetrical joint
Buerger disease
buffalo hump
buffer capacity
buffered formalin
buffered neutral formalin
buffered solution
buffer, plasma
buffy coat
buffy coated cells
buffy coat smear
buffy coat smear test
Buhl desquamative pneumonia
Buisson, coxofemoral articulation of
bulb
  aortic
  arterial
  carotid
  dental
  duodenal
  end

bulb *(continued)*
  hair
  olfactory
bulbar conjunctiva
bulbar myelitis
bulbar ridge
bulbar septum
bulb artery, urethral
bulbi, phthisis
bulbi urethrae, arteria
bulbocavernosus muscle
bulbocavernous gland
bulb of penis
bulb of urethra
bulboid corpuscle
bulbosacral system
bulbospongiosus muscle of penis
bulbourethral artery
bulbourethral gland
bulb vestibule
bulging of bleb
bulging of mucosa between trabeculae
bulging of sac
bulging of sclera
bulky stool
bulla (pl. bullae)
Bullard hematoxylin
bullous emphysema
bullous fever
bullous impetigo of newborn
bullous pemphigoid
bull's-eye lesion
bumpy texture
BUN (blood urea nitrogen)
BUN/creatinine ratio
bundle
  aberrant
  atrioventricular (AV)
  collagen
  comma
  neurovascular
bundle bone
bundle of His, atrioventricular
Bungner band
Bunyamwera viruses
Bunyavirus encephalitis
Burdwan fever
buret (burette)
Burkitt lymphoma
Burkitt tumor
burned skin
burn infection
burn, powder
burns classification
Burns ligament
Burns space
Burow solution
burr cell
burrow
burrowing pus
bursa
  Achilles
  adventitious
  anserine
  bicipitoradial
  omental
bursal abscess
bursal equivalent tissue
bursitis
  anserine
  bicipital
  calcaneal
  chronic
  intertubercular
  olecranon
  prepatellar
  severe
  subacromial
  subdeltoid
  trochanteric
bursting of cells
bursting of red blood cells
Butchart staging classification
butter bacillus

butterfly rash
buttery texture
button, cell
buttonlike necrotic lesion at inoculation site
B virus hepatitis
B_1 vitamin
B_6 vitamin
B_{12} vitamin
Bwamba fever
B wave
bx (biopsy)
bypass graft
Byzantine arch palate

C, c

C (carbon)
C (Celsius)
C (cervical)
cablelike connection
Cabot ring body
cachectic fever
cachexia, malarial
cadaver
cadaveric
CAE (carcinoembryonic) antigen
caecum (cecum)
CA (cancer antigen)
CA 15-2 RIA test
CA 15-3 antigen
CA 15-3 antigenic tumor marker
CA 15-3 breast cancer tumor marker
CA 15-3 RIA test
CA 19-9 antigenic tumor marker
CA 19-9 carbohydrate antigen
CA 27.29 tumor marker
CA 50 tumor marker
CA 72-4 antigen
CA 72-4 antigenic tumor marker
CA 125 antigen
CA 125 assay
CA 125 cross-reactivity
CA 125 ovarian tumor marker
CA 125-11 tumor marker
CA 195 tumor marker
CA 549 breast cancer tumor marker
CA M26 tumor marker
CA M29 tumor marker
CA virus
caddy (dark, sandy mud) stool
café au lait spots on skin
cage
  bony thoracic
  osseocartilaginous thoracic
Cajal gold sublimate
Cajal, interstitial cells of
Cajal trichrome
cake kidney
Calabar swelling
calcaneal artery
calcaneal articular surface
calcaneal bone
calcaneal bursitis
calcaneal process
calcaneal region
calcaneal spur
calcaneal sulcus
calcaneal tendon
calcaneal tubercle
calcaneal tuberosity

calcaneoastragaloid ligament
calcaneocuboid articulation (or joint)
calcaneocuboid ligament
calcaneofibular ligament
calcaneonavicular ligament
calcaneotibial ligament
calcaneus and astragalus, articulation of
calcaneus bone
calcaneus, tendo
calcareous degeneration
calcareous infarct
calcareous infiltration
calcareous material
calcareous metastasis
calcareous pancreatitis
calcarine artery
calcarine fasciculus
calcarine fissure
calcarine sulcus
calciferous canal
calcification
  dystrophic
  metastatic
  Mönckeberg (Moenckeberg)
  normal
calcification line
calcification of bone
calcification of cysts
calcification of osseous matrix
calcific plaque
calcified aorta
calcified cartilage
calcified pericardium
calcified thrombus inside a vein
calcinosis
calcinosis cutis
calcinuric diabetes
calcitonin
calcitonin–calcium infusion stimulation test
calcitonin hormone
calcitonin test
calcium
  ionized
  total
calcium crystals
calcium deposition in osteoid tissue
calcium deposits
calcium infiltration
calcium oxalate
calcium oxalate calculus
calcium oxalate crystals in urine
calcium phosphate salt in bones and teeth
calcium pyrophosphate crystals in pseudogout
calcium resorption
calcium salts
  crystals of
  deposition of in kidney tissue
calculus (pl. calculi)
  alternating
  alvine
  articular
  biliary
  calcium oxalate
  cholesterol
  combination
  cystine
  decubitus
  encysted
  fibrin
  fusible
  gastric
  gallbladder
  gonecystic
  hemic
  hemp seed
  hepatic
  indigo
  intestinal
  joint
  lacrimal
  lacteal

calculus *(continued)*
- lung
- mammary
- matrix
- metabolic
- mulberry
- nasal
- nephritic
- oxalate
- pancreatic
- phosphate
- pocketed
- preputial
- prostatic
- renal
- salivary
- serumal
- shellac
- spermatic
- staghorn
- stomach
- stonelike
- struvite
- subgingival
- submorphous
- supragingival
- tonsillar
- urate
- urethral
- uric acid
- urinary
- urostealith
- uterine
- vesical
- vesicoprostatic
- xanthic

Caldani ligament
Caldwell-Moloy classification
calf bone
calf muscle
caliber of stool
calibration of testing instrument
calibration of testing method
calibration, standard
Calicivirus, calicivirus
California encephalitis virus
calix (pl. calices) (see *calyx*)
CALLA (common acute lymphoblastic leukemia antigen)
Call-Exner body
callosal convolution
callosal gyrus
callosal sulcus
callosity
callosomarginal artery
callosomarginal fissure
callous (adj.)
callus (noun)
- bony
- ensheathing

callus formation (*not* callous)
Calmette-Guérin bacillus
caloric deficiency in children
calorics
- cold water
- ice water

caloric test
Calot triangle
Calmette test
calvaria
calvaria dura mater
calvarium
Calvé-Perthes-Legg disease
calvities (baldness)
calyceal
calyces (pl. of calyx)
Calymmatobacterium granulomatis (formerly *Donovania granulomatis*)
calyx (pl. calyces) (also, calix)
- major
- minor
- renal

cameloid cell
CAM 5.2 antibody

Campbell ligament
Camper fascia
Camper ligament
camp fever
CAMP (Christie, Atkins, and Munch-Petersen) factor
CAMP test for Group B beta-hemolytic streptococci
Campylobacter cinaedi
Campylobacter coli
Campylobacter fennelliae
Campylobacter fetus (formerly *Vibrio fetus*)
Campylobacter gastroenteritis
Campylobacter jejuni
Campylobacter laridis
Campylobacter parahemolyticus
Campylobacter pylori
Campylobacter vulnificus
canal
  abdominal
  accessory
  adductor
  Alcock
  alimentary
  alveolar
  alveolodental
  ampulla of semicircular
  anal
  anterior condyloid
  anterior semicircular
  archenteric
  Arnold
  arterial
  artery of pterygoid
  atrial
  atrioventricular (AV)
  auditory
  basipharyngeal
  Bernard
  Bichat
  biliary (interlobular)

canal *(continued)*
  biliary (intralobular)
  birth
  blastoporic
  bony semicircular
  Böttcher
  Braune
  Breschet
  calciferous
  caroticotympanic
  carotid
  carpal
  caudal
  central
  cerebrospinal
  cervical (of uterus)
  cervical axillary
  cervicoaxillary
  ciliary
  Civinini
  Cloquet
  cochlear
  common atrioventricular
  condylar
  condyloid
  connecting
  Corti
  Cotunnius
  craniopharyngeal
  crural
  deferent
  dental
  dental root
  dentinal
  diploic
  Dorello
  Dupuytren
  ear
  endocervical
  endodermal
  ethmoid
  eustachian

canal *(continued)*
- external auditory
- facial
- fallopian
- femoral
- Ferrein
- flexor
- Fontana
- galactophorous
- ganglionic
- Gartner
- gastric
- genital
- greater palatine
- gubernacular
- Guyon
- gynecophoric
- hair
- Hannover
- haversian
- hemal
- Henle
- Hensen
- hernial
- Hirschfeld
- His
- Holmgren-Golgi
- Hoyer
- Huguier
- Hunter
- Huschke
- hyaloid
- hypoglossal
- iliac
- incisive
- incisor
- inferior dental
- infraorbital
- inguinal
- interdental
- interfacial
- intersacral

canal *(continued)*
- intestinal
- intracytoplasmic
- Jacobson
- Kovalevsky
- Kuersteiner
- lacrimal
- lateral
- lateral semicircular
- Lauth
- Leeuwenhoek
- Löwenberg (Loewenberg)
- mandibular
- marrow
- maxillary
- medullary
- mental
- Müller (Mueller)
- musculotubal
- nasal
- nasolacrimal
- nasopalatine
- neural
- neurenteric
- notochordal
- nutrient
- obstetric
- obturator
- olfactory
- optic
- orbital
- palatine
- palatomaxillary
- palatovaginal
- paraurethral
- parturient
- pelvic
- pericardioperitoneal
- perivascular
- persistent atrioventricular
- persistent common atrioventricular
- Petit

canal *(continued)*
- pharyngeal
- pleural
- pleuropericardial
- pleuroperitoneal
- portal
- posterior semicircular
- principal artery of pterygoid
- pterygoid
- pterygopalatine
- pudendal
- pulmoaortic
- pulp
- pyloric
- recurrent
- Reichert
- rigid
- Rivinus
- root (of tooth)
- Rosenthal
- sacculocochlear
- sacculoutricular
- sacral
- Santorini
- Schlemm
- scleral
- semicircular
- sheathing
- small (of chorda tympani)
- Sondermann
- sphenopalatine
- sphenopharyngeal
- spinal
- Stensen
- Stilling
- subsartorial
- Sucquet-Hoyer
- supraciliary
- supraoptic
- supraorbital
- tarsal
- temporal

canal *(continued)*
- Theile
- Tourtual
- tubal
- tubotympanic
- tympanic
- umbilical
- uniting
- urogenital
- uterine
- uterocervical
- uterovaginal
- utriculosaccular
- vaginal
- van Horne
- Velpeau
- ventricular
- Verneuil
- vertebral
- vesicourethral
- vestibular
- vidian
- Volkmann
- vomerine
- vomerobasilar
- vomerorostral
- vomerovaginal
- vulvar
- vulvouterine
- Walther
- Wirsung
- zygomaticofacial
- zygomaticotemporal

canal for tensor tympani muscle
canalicular abscess
canalicular duct
canalicular sphincter
canaliculus (pl. canaliculi)
- apical
- auricular
- bile
- bone

canaliculus *(continued)*
- cochlear
- haversian
- innominate
- intercellular

canalization
canal of Cuvier
canal of Guidi
canal of Guyon
canal of Hering
canal of Nuck
canal of Oken
canal of Recklinghausen
canal of Scarpa
canal of Schlemm
canal of Steno
canal of Stilling
canal of stomach
Canavan disease
Canavan–van Bogaert–Bertrand disease
cancellated bone
cancellous bone
cancellous tissue
cancer (see *carcinoma, sarcoma, tumor*)
- aniline
- betel
- chimney-sweep's
- clay pipe
- colloid
- contact
- cystic
- dendritic
- dye worker's
- hereditary
- latent
- melanotic
- mule-spinner's
- non-small cell lung
- occult
- paraffin
- pitch worker's
- scirrhous

cancer *(continued)*
- small-cell lung
- swamp
- tar
- tubular

cancer antigen (CA)
cancer cell
cancer embolism
cancer-inducing virus
cancerization
candela (cd)
Candida
Candida albicans
Candida guilliermondii
Candida krusei
Candida lusitaniae
Candida parapsilosis
Candida pseudotropicalis
Candida pulcherrima
Candida ravautii
Candida rugosa
Candida stellatoidea
Candida tropicalis
Candida viswanathii
candidal granuloma
candidal infection
candidiasis
candidosis
C&S (culture and sensitivity)
canicola fever
canine tissue
canine tooth
canis
canities
cannabinoids
cannon bone
CA 125 glycoprotein
caoutchouc pelvis
cap, cervical
capacity
- bladder
- buffer

capacity *(continued)*
- cranial
- forced vital (FVC)
- functional residual (FRC)
- heat
- hemoglobin-binding
- inspiratory
- iron-binding (IBC)
- lung
- maximum breathing
- oxygen
- residual
- respiratory
- thermal
- total iron-binding (TIBC)
- total lung (TLC)
- vital (VC)

capillary
- arterial
- bile
- continuous
- lymph
- sinusoidal
- venous

capillary angioma
capillary bed
capillary blood
capillary dilatation and proliferation
capillary embolism
capillary endothelial cell
capillary fenestrated
capillary fragility, abnormal
capillary fragility test
capillary gap method
capillary hemangioma
capillary hereditary fragility
capillary lake
capillary loops of glomerulus
capillary microaneurysms of retina
capillary nevus
capillary permeability factor
capillary pneumonia
capillary resistance test
capillary thrombosis
capillary tube
capillary valve
capillary vein
capillary vessel
capillary zone electrophoresis (CZE)
capitate bone
capitate facet
capitate hamate
capitate-hamate joint
capitate soft spot
capitate, volar
capitis, tinea
capitolunate joint
capitular articulation
capitular joint
capitulum bone
Capnocytophaga canimorsus
Capnocytophaga ochracea
Capripoxvirus
capsid
capsid formation
capsular antigen
capsular artery
capsular ligament
capsular nephritis
capsular polysaccharide
capsular space
capsular swelling
capsulatum
capsule
- adrenal
- articular
- auditory
- Bowman
- brood
- cartilage
- cricoarytenoid articular
- cricothyroid articular
- fatty renal
- fibrous

capsule *(continued)*
- fibrous renal
- Gerota
- Glisson
- hepatic
- joint
- organ
- splenic
- thyroid
- tough
- tough fibrous
- tumor

capsule cell
capsule of connective tissue
capsule of joint
capsule of liver
capture ELISA
caput medusae
caput succedaneum
carate
carbohydrate metabolism
carbohydrates, test on venous blood for
carbohydrate utilization test
carbolfuchsin stain
carbon (C)
carbon-containing fuels, combustion of
carbon dioxide (CO_2)
- arterial
- metabolism
- partial pressure of (PCO_2)
- pulmonary excretion of
- pulmonary retention of
- tests for
- total (TCO_2)

carbon dioxide gases
carbon dioxide tension
carbonic acid in blood
carbonization
carbon monoxide (CO)
carbon monoxide poisoning
carbon 13-labeled ketoisocaproate breath test
Carbowax embedding medium
carboxyhemoglobin in blood
carbuncle
carbunculosis
Carcassonne ligament
carcinoembryonic antigen (CEA) test
carcinoid syndrome
carcinoid tumor
carcinoma (see also *cancer, sarcoma, tumor*)
- acinous cell
- adenocystic
- adenoid cystic
- adenoid squamous cell
- adenosquamous
- adnexal
- adrenocortical
- aldosterone-producing
- aldosterone-secreting
- alveolar
- alveolar cell
- ameloblastic
- anaplastic c. of thyroid gland
- apocrine
- basal cell
  - alveolar
  - comedo
  - cystic
  - morphea-like
  - multicentric
  - nodulo-ulcerative
  - pigmented
  - sclerosing
  - superficial
- basaloid
- basosquamous cell
- bile duct
- bilharzial
- bladder
- breast
- bronchioalveolar
- bronchioloalveolar

carcinoma *(continued)*
- bronchogenic
- cerebriform
- cholangiocarcinoma
- cholangiocellular
- chorionic
- choroid plexus
- clear cell
- colloid
- comedo
- corpus
- cortisol-producing
- cribriform
- cylindrical
- ductal
- ductal carcinoma in situ (DCIS)
- ductal carcinoma of prostate
- duct cell
- eccrine
- embryonal
- embryonal cell
- endometrial
- epidermal, epidermoid
- exophytic
- extrahepatic bile duct
- fibrolamellar
- follicular
- gastric
- gelatinous
- genital
- giant cell
- giant cell c. of thyroid gland
- glandular
- glans, intraepidermal
- granulosa cell
- hepatic
- hepatocellular
- hereditary
- Hürthle cell
- hypernephroid
- infantile embryonal
- infiltrating ductal

carcinoma *(continued)*
- infiltrating lobular
- inflammatory c. of breast
- intraductal
- intraepidermal
- intraepithelial
- invasive
- invasive lobular
- juvenile embryonal
- Kulchitzky cell
- large cell
- lenticular
- leptomeningeal
- lobular
- lobular c. in situ (LCIS)
- Lucké
- medullary
- melanotic
- meningeal
- Merkel cell
- metastatic
- metatypical
- microinvasive
- micropapillary
- moderately well-differentiated
- mucinous
- mucoepidermoid
- mucous
- nasopharyngeal
- neuroendocrine c. of skin
- noninfiltrating lobular
- oat cell
- osteoid
- Paget
- pancreatic
- papillary
- papillary c. of thyroid gland
- poorly differentiated
- preinvasive
- prickle cell
- primary
- primary intraosseous

carcinoma *(continued)*
- rectosigmoid
- renal cell
- residual
- retinoblastoma hereditary human
- scar
- schistosomal bladder
- schneiderian
- scirrhous
- sebaceous
- signet ring
- small cell
- small cell lung c. (SCLC)
- small round cell
- spindle cell
- squamous
- squamous cell (SCC)
- staging of cervical
- string cell
- systemic effects
- terminal duct
- thyroid
- trabecular c. of skin
- transitional cell
- tubular
- undifferentiated
- undifferentiated c. of thyroid gland
- undifferentiated squamous cell
- uterine cervix
- uterine corpus
- verrucous
- villous
- well-differentiated

carcinoma in situ
- ductal (DCIS)
- lobular (LCIS)

carcinoma en cuirasse

carcinoma ex mixed tumor

carcinoma ex pleomorphic adenoma

carcinomatosis

carcinomatous pericarditis

carcinosarcoma

cardia
- crescent of
- gastric

cardia of stomach

cardiac aneurysm

cardiac anomaly

cardiac antrum

cardiac area of stomach

cardiac arrest

cardiac atresia

cardiac branch

cardiac cirrhosis

cardiac congestion

cardiac dilatation

cardiac dullness

cardiac edema

cardiac failure

cardiac ganglion

cardiac gland

cardiac histiocyte

cardiac hormone

cardiac hypertrophy

cardiac impression on liver

cardiac index

cardiac isoenzymes (see *isoenzymes*)

cardiac liver

cardiac lung

cardiac mucosa

cardiac muscle fiber

cardiac muscle, striated

cardiac muscle tissue

cardiac nerve, parasympathetic

cardiac notch

cardiac obstruction

cardiac opening

cardiac orifice

cardiac output

cardiac part

cardiac plexus

cardiac polyp

cardiac prominence

cardiac reflex

cardiac segment
cardiac shadow
cardiac skeleton
cardiac stomach
cardiac tamponade
Cardiac T Rapid Assay
cardiac troponin T marker in blood
cardiac valve, vegetations of
cardiac valvular abnormality
cardiac valvular defect
cardiac valvular lesion
cardiac valvular stenosis
cardiac vein
cardinal ligament of uterus
cardinal point
cardinal vein
Cardiobacterium hominis
cardioesophageal (CE) junction
cardiogenic embolism
cardiogenic plate
cardiogenic shock
cardiohepatic angle
cardiohepatic triangle
cardiomegaly
cardiomyopathy, hypertrophic
cardiorrhexis
cardiovascular silhouette
caries, dental
carinal lymph node
carina of the trachea
carinatum, pectus
cariniform cartilage
carmine
carnassial tooth
carneous degeneration
Carney complex
Carnoy fixative
Carnoy solution
carotene absorption test
carotene-containing vegetables and fruits
carotene test
carotenoderma
carotenoids
caroticoclinoid ligament
caroticotympanic artery
caroticotympanic canal
caroticotympanic nerve
carotid arch
carotid artery
carotid gland
carotid sheath
carotid sinus
carotid sinus nerve
carpal arch
carpal artery
carpal articular surface
carpal articulation
carpal bone
carpal canal
carpal groove
carpal joint
carpal tunnel
carpometacarpal articulation
carpometacarpal joint
carpometacarpal ligament
carpus bone
carrier cell
carrier electrophoresis
carrier protein
Carr-Price test
carrying angle
Carter fever
cartilage
  accessory
  accessory nasal
  alar
  arthrodial
  articular
  arytenoid
  auditory
  auricular
  basilar
  branchial

cartilage *(continued)*
- calcified
- cariniform
- cells of
- cellular
- ciliary
- circumferential
- conchal
- connecting
- corniculate
- costal
- cricoid
- cuneiform
- diarthrodial
- elastic
- ensiform
- epiglottic
- epiphyseal
- falciform
- fibroelastic
- fibrous
- floating
- hyaline
- hyaline articular
- loss of elasticity of
- pitted
- roughened
- scored
- thinned
- yellow

cartilage bone
cartilage capsule
cartilage cell
cartilage corpuscle
cartilage lacuna
cartilage matrix
cartilage model
cartilaginous articulation
cartilaginous joint
- primary
- secondary
- symphysis

cartilaginous part
cartilage plate, epiphyseal
cartilage space
cartilaginous portion of auditory tube
cartilaginous septum
cartilaginous tissue
cartilaginous viscerocranium
cartilago (pl. cartilagines)
cartwheel pattern
Cartwright blood group
caruncle, hymenal
cascade, diagnostic
cascara
caseating
caseation
caseous abscess
caseous necrosis
caseous nephritis
caseous pneumonia
Casoni intradermal test for hydatid disease
Casoni skin test
Caspersson type B cell
casserian ligament
Casser ligament
cast (pl. casts)
- abnormal c. in urine
- epithelial
- granular c. in urine
- homogeneous c. in urine
- hyaline
- RTE (renal tubular epithelial)
- waxy c. in urine

casting
Castle intrinsic factor
castrate cell
castration cell
catabolic
catabolism of fatty acids
catacrotic pulse
catadicrotic pulse
catagen phase of hair growth

catalase test
cataract
  congenital
  senile
cataract needle
catarrh
catarrhal fever
catarrhal inflammation
catarrhal pneumonia
catarrhal stomatitis
cat-bite fever
catecholamines
  fractionated
  free
  plasma
  total
  urinary
caterpillar cell
"cath" (slang for catheter, catheterized)
cathepsin D
catheter
  central venous pressure (CVP)
  Foley
  indwelling
  fluid-filled
  intracranial pressure (ICP)
  urinary bladder
catheter fever
catheter-induced embolism
catheterized specimen
cation
cationic protein
cat-scratch disease
cat-scratch fever
CA II flow cytometer
cauda equina
caudal
caudal canal
caudal flexure
caudal ligament
caudal neuropore
caudal neurosecretory system
caudal pancreatic artery
caudal pharyngeal complex
caudal retinaculum
caudal sheath
caudal vertebra
caudate lobe of liver
caudate nucleus
caudate process
cauliflower ear
cauliflower-like polyp
caval cuff, suprahepatic
caval fold
cavalry bone
cavalryman osteoma
caval valve
caveolated cell
cavernosa penis, corpora
cavernosum, corpus
cavernous angioma
cavernous artery
cavernous body
cavernous groove
cavernous hemangioma
cavernous nerve
cavernous part
cavernous plexus
cavernous sinus
cavernous tissue
cavernous vein
Caves-Schutz-Stanford bioptome
caviar lesion
cavitary dilatation of central canal of spinal cord
cavitary fluid
cavitary myelitis
cavitation
cavity
  abdominal
  abdominopelvic
  amniotic
  axillary
  body

cavity *(continued)*
  buccal
  chcst
  cleavage
  cotyloid
  cranial
  crown
  endometrial
  epamniotic
  epidural
  funnel-shaped
  glenoid
  joint
  medullary
  oral
  pericardial
  peritoneal
  pleural
  retroperitoneal
  thoracic
  tubular
  uterine
cavity line angle
cavity margin
cavity of tunica vaginalis
cavity wall
cavosurface angle
cavosurface bevel
cavum (pl. cava)
CBC (complete blood count)
  hematocrit
  hemoglobin
  MCH (mean corpuscular hemoglobin)
  MCHC (mean corpuscular hemoglobin concentration)
  MCV (mean corpuscular volume)
  RBC (red blood cell) count
  WBC (white blood cell) count
CBD (common bile duct)
C bile
C_4 binding protein
cc (cubic centimeter)
C carbohydrate antigen
CCAT (conglutinating complement absorption test)
C cell
CCK (cholecystokinin)
CCK-PZ (cholecystokinin-pancreozymin)
C_3 complement
C_4 complement
CD (cluster of differentiation)
CDC (Centers for Disease Control)
CDC classification of HIV infection
CD4 count
CD4 lymphocyte count (T4)
CD4+ lymphocyte
CD14 membrane protein
CD45 leukocyte common antigen
CDE antigen
"C. diff" (slang for *Clostridium difficile*) toxin assay
CDK4 amplification analysis
CDLHb (diaspirin-cross-linked hemoglobin)
CE (cardioesophageal) junction
CEA (carcinoembryonic antigen)
cecal appendage
cecal appendix
cecal artery, ileocolic
cecal fold
cecal foramen
cecal recess
cecal volvulus
cecum (also, caecum)
  antimesocolic side of
  subhepatic
Cedecea
Cedecea davisae
Cedecea lapagei
Cedecea neteri
Celani method

celiac artery
celiac axis
celiac disease
celiac ganglion
celiac gland
celiac lymph node
celiac plexus
celiac sprue
celiac trunk
celite-absorbed plasma
cell
- A (alpha)
- absorption
- absorptive
- accessory
- acid
- acidophil
- acidophilic
- acid-staining
- acinar
- acinous
- acoustic
- adenomorphous
- adipose
- adventitial
- agger nasi
- agglomeration of
- agglutination of
- air
- albuminous
- algoid
- alloantigen-presenting
- alpha
- alveolar
- Alzheimer
- amacrine
- ameboid
- amniogenic
- anabiotic
- anaplastic
- anaplastic epithelial
- aneuploid

cell *(continued)*
- angioblastic
- anterior
- anterior ethmoidal air
- anterior horn
- antigen-presenting (APC)
- antigen-reactive
- antigen-responsive
- antigen-sensitive
- antral gastric
- apocrine
- apolar
- APUD (amine precursor uptake and decarboxylation)
- argentaffin
- argyrophil
- argyrophilic
- Arias-Stella
- Armanni-Ebstein
- Aschoff
- Askanazy
- astroglia
- atrophy of hair
- atypical
- auditory
- auditory receptor
- automatic
- B (beta)
- balloon
- band
- basal granular
- basaloid
- basilar
- basket
- basophil
- basophilic
- beaker
- Beale
- Beale ganglion
- Berger
- Bergmann
- berry

cell *(continued)*
beta
Betz
Bevan-Lewis
BGM
bipolar
bipolar retinal
bite
bizarre
Bizzozero red
bladder
blast
blister
blood
Boll
bone
border
Böttcher (Boettcher)
bottle-shaped hair
bowenoid
branchial
breakdown of red blood
breviradiate
bristle
bronchial mucosal
bronchic
bronchiolar exocrine
brood
burr
bursting of
C
Cajal
Cajal interstitial
cameloid
cancer
capillary endothelial
capsule
carrier
cartilage
Caspersson type B
castration
caterpillar

cell *(continued)*
caveolated
CD45RO+
cement
central
centroacinar
chalice
chief
chromaffin
chromophobe
chromophobic
chromosomal structure of
ciliated
Clara
Clarke
Claudius
clear
cleavage
cleaved
clonogenic
clue
clump
clumping of
cochlear hair
collenchyma
column
columnar
columnar epithelial
columnar sustentacular
commissural
compound granule
cone
connective-tissue
contractile fiber
contrasuppressor
cordlike arrangement of
corneal
Corti
corticotroph-lipotroph
cover
crescent
cribrate

cell *(continued)*
- Crooke
- cuboid
- cuboidal
- cuboidal epithelial
- cuboidal glandular
- cultured
- Custer
- cylindrical
- cytomegalic
- cytotoxic
- cytotoxic T
- cytotrophoblastic
- D (delta)
- damaged nerve
- dark
- Daudi
- daughter
- Davidoff
- dead nerve
- decidual
- decoy
- deep
- deficient production of red blood
- definition
- degenerating nerve
- Deiters
- delomorphous
- delta
- demilune
- dendritic
- dendritic reticular
- denture
- devitalized nerve
- Dogiel
- dome
- donor
- Dorothy Reed
- Downey
- duct
- ductal
- dust

cell *(continued)*
- dyskeratotic
- ECL (enterochromaffin-like)
- effector
- egg
- electrolytic
- elementary
- embryonic
- embryonic mesenchymal
- enamel
- enamel-forming
- encasing (also incasing)
- endocervical
- endodermal
- endometrial
- endothelial
- enterochromaffin
- enteroendocrine
- entodermal
- ependymal
- epidermic
- epithelial
- epithelial reticular
- epithelioid
- erythrocyte progenitor
- erythroid
- ethmoid air
- ethmoidal
- excitable
- external pillar
- exudation
- Fananás
- fasciculata
- fat
- fat-storing
- fatty granule
- Ferrata
- fiber
- Finkeldey-Warthin
- flagellate
- flat
- floor

cell *(continued)*
- foam
- follicular
- follicular epithelial
- follicular ovarian
- foreign
- foreign body giant
- formative
- foveolar
- fuchsinophil
- fusiform
- G
- galvanic
- gametoid
- gamma
- ganglion
- gastrin-secreting
- Gaucher
- Gegenbaur
- gemistocytic
- germ
- germinal
- ghost
- giant
- giant Betz
- Gierke
- gitter
- Gley
- glia
- glial
- glitter
- globoid
- glomerular
- glomus
- goblet
- Golgi epithelial
- Goormaghtigh
- granular
- granule
- granulocytic white
- granulosa
- granulosa lutein

cell *(continued)*
- grape
- great alveolar
- ground-glass
- guanine
- gustatory
- gyrochrome
- hair
- hairy
- Haller
- heart-disease
- heart-failure
- heart-lesion
- heckle
- Heidenhain
- HeLa
- helmet
- helper (inducer)
- helper/inducer T cell
- helper T
- hemolymphatic
- hemolyzed red blood
- HEMPAS
- Hensen
- hepatic parenchymal
- heteromeric
- hexagonal
- hilar
- hilus
- hobnail
- Hodgkin
- Hofbauer
- homozygous typing (HTC)
- horizontal
- horn
- horny
- Hortega
- host
- Hürthle
- hyperchromatic
- I (inclusion)
- immature

cell *(continued)*
immature red blood
immature white blood
immunologically activated
immunologically competent
incasing (also encasing)
inclusion
indifferent
inflammatory
inflammatory response
initial
injured nerve
innocent bystander
intercalary
intercapillary
interdigitating
interfollicular
intermediate
internal pillar
interstitial
irritability of nerve
irritation
islet
Ito
juvenile
juxtaglomerular
K (killer)
karyochrome
keratinized
keratinized epithelial
killer T
koilocytotic
Kulchitsky
Kupffer
L
lacis (meshwork)
lacrimoethmoid
lacunar
LAK
Langerhans
Langhans
Langhans giant

cell *(continued)*
large
large cleaved
large granule
large noncleaved
lattice
LE (lupus erythematosus)
Leishman chrome
lepra
Leydig
light (of thyroid)
lining
Lipschütz
littoral
liver
Loevit
lupus erythematosus (LE)
luteal
lutein
luteinizing theca
lymph
lymphadenoma
lymphoid
lymphokine-activated killer (LAK)
lymphoreticular
lysis of
macroglia
male sex
malignant
malpighian
Marchand wandering
marrow
Martinotti
mast
mastoid
mastoid air
matrix
Mauthner
McCoy
megakaryocyte progenitor
megaspore mother
melanin-containing

cell *(continued)*
memory
meningothelial
Merkel
Merkel-Ranvier
Merkel tactile
mesangial
mesenchymal
mesoglial
mesothelial
metaplastic squamous
Mexican hat
Meynert
microglia
microglial
middle
middle ethmoidal air
midget bipolar
migratory
Mikulicz
mirror-image
mitral
monocytoid
monomorphous oval
mononuclear
Mooser
mossy
mother
motor
Mott
mucin-secreting columnar
mucoalbuminous
mucoserous
mucous
mucous neck
mucus-secreting
mulberry
Müller radial (Mueller)
multinucleated giant
multinucleate globoid
multipolar
mural

cell *(continued)*
muscle
mycosis
myeloid
myeloma
myoepithelial
myoepithelioid
myoid
myointimal
Nageotte
natural killer (NK)
neoplastic
nerve
nerve sheath
Neumann
neurilemma
neuroendocrine
neuroendocrine transducer
neuroepithelial
neuroglia
neuroglial
neuromuscular
neurosecretory
nevus
nevus-type giant
Niemann-Pick
NK (natural killer)
non-alpha, non-beta pancreatic islet
non-beta
nonclonogenic
nonglandular
nonmalignant
non-nerve
nonspecialized
nucleated
nucleated red blood
null
nurse
oat
OKT
olfactory
olfactory receptor

cell *(continued)*
- oligodendroglia
- Onodi
- Opalski
- osseous
- osteochondrogenic
- osteogenic
- osteoprogenitor
- oval
- oxygen-carrying material of red blood
- oxyntic
- oxyphil
- P
- pacemaker
- packed human blood
- packed red blood
- pagetoid
- Paget
- palisade
- pancreatic islet
- panel
- Paneth granular
- papillary
- parafollicular
- paraganglionic
- paraluteal
- paralutein
- parenchymal
- parent
- parietal
- Pelger-Huët
- peptic
- pericapillary
- peripolar
- perithelial
- peritubular contractile
- permissive
- pessary
- phagocytic stellate
- phalangeal
- pheochrome

cell *(continued)*
- photo
- photoreceptor
- physaliphorous
- Pick
- pigment
- pillar
- pineal
- plasma
- platelike
- pleomorphic
- pluripotent
- pluripotential
- pneumatic
- PNH (paroxysmal nocturnal hemoglobinuria)
- polar
- polychromatic
- polychromatophil
- polygonal
- polyhedral
- polymorphic pigment-producing
- polyplastic
- posterior
- posterior ethmoidal air
- PP (pancreatic polypeptide)
- pre-B
- precursor
- prefollicle
- pregnancy
- pregranulosa
- pre-T
- prickle
- primary embryonic
- primitive
- primitive granulosa
- primitive reticular
- primitive wandering
- primordial
- primordial germ
- principal
- prokaryotic

cell *(continued)*
- prolactin
- proliferating
- pseudo-Gaucher
- pseudounipolar
- pseudoxanthoma
- ptyocrinous
- pulmonary endothelial
- pulmonary epithelial
- pulpar
- Purkinje
- pus
- pyramidal
- pyrrol
- quiescent
- RA (ragocyte)
- radial
- Raji
- reactive
- reactive mesothelial
- recipient
- red blood
- Reed
- Reed-Sternberg
- Renshaw
- reserve
- residential
- resting
- retina (amacrine)
- resting wandering
- restructured
- reticular
- reticularis
- reticuloendothelial
- reticulum
- rhagiocrine
- Rieder
- Rindfleisch
- rod
- rod nuclear
- Rohon-Beard
- Rolando

cell *(continued)*
- root
- rosette-forming
- Rouget
- round
- S
- Sala
- sarcogenic
- satellite
- scalelike
- scavenger
- Schilling band
- Schultze
- Schwann
- sclerenchyma
- secretory
- segmented
- seminal
- sensitized
- sensory
- sentinel
- septal
- seromucous
- serous
- Sertoli
- sex
- Sézary
- shadow
- sheep red blood (sRBC)
- shrinking of
- sickle
- signet ring
- silver
- skein
- skeletogenous
- slender elongated
- small
- small cleaved
- small granule
- smooth-muscle
- smudge
- solitary

cell *(continued)*
- somatic
- somatostatin
- specialized
- sperm
- spermatogenic
- sphenoid
- spider
- spindle
- spindle-shaped
- splenic
- spur
- squamous
- squamous alveolar
- squamous epithelial
- stab
- staff
- standard
- star
- star-shaped
- stellate
- stem
- Sternberg
- Sternberg-Reed
- strap
- structure of
- superficial
- supporting
- suppressor
- suppressor T
- surface mucous
- sustentacular
- swelling of
- swollen basal
- sympathetic formative
- sympathicotropic
- sympathochromaffin
- syncytial
- synovial
- T (thymus, thymus-dependent, or thymus-derived lymphocytes)
- T cytotoxic

cell *(continued)*
- T effector
- T helper
- T lymphocyte
- T4 helper
- T8 suppressor
- tactile
- tanned red (TRC)
- target
- tart
- taste
- TDTH
- teardrop
- tendon
- Tg
- theca
- theca lutein
- thymus-dependent (T cells)
- thymus-independent (B cells)
- tightly packed round
- Tiselius electrophoresis
- Tm
- totipotent
- touch
- Touton giant
- transducer
- transepithelial migration of chronic inflammatory
- transitional
- transitional epithelial
- TRC (tanned red cell)
- tufted
- tunnel
- Türk
- tympanic
- tympanic air
- type I alveolar
- type II alveolar
- Tzanck
- umbrella
- undegenerated nerve
- undifferentiated

cell *(continued)*
undifferentiated columnar epithelial
undifferentiated mesenchymal
unipolar
urothelial
vacuolated
vacuolation of
vasoformative
veil
veiled
Vero
vestibular hair
veto
Virchow
virus-transformed
visual receptor
vitreous
volume of packed
von Kupffer
wandering
Warthin
Warthin-Finkeldey giant
wasserhelle
water-clear
white blood (WBC)
WI-38 (Wistar Institute)
wing
xanthoma
yolk
zymogen
zymogenic
cell aggregations, normal
cell assay test, Raji
cell block of paraffin
cell block, opening
cell bodies, chromatolysis
cell body of motor neuron
cell-bound antibody
cell bridge
cell button
cell center
cell cluster
cell count
cell count of cerebrospinal fluid
cell count of urine
cell culture
cell death
cell layer
cell line
cell-mediated immunity
cell membrane
cell nest
celloidin
Cellosolve dehydrating agent
cell plate
cell polarity
cell prep, LE (lupus erythematosus)
cell sac
cell-serum mixture in saline
cell sheet
cell strand
cell tubule
cellular blue nevus
cellular bone marrow
cellular debris
cellular embolism
cellular immunity
cellular infiltrate
cellularity, scant
cellular organelle
cellular polyp
cellular repair
cellular tissue
cellulitis of scalp, dissecting
cellulitis, periurethral
cellulocutaneous
cellulose
cellulosity
cell wall
celom, extraembryonic
celomic bay
celomic pouch
Celsius scale (C)
cement base

cement cell
cement corpuscle
cement line
cement substance
cementodentinal junction
cementum
center
  anospinal
  Broca
  ciliospinal
  diaphyseal
  epiotic
  germinal
  ossification
  swallowing
center cell
centigrade scale
centigram (cg)
centigray (cGy)
centiliter (cL)
centimeter (cm)
centimole (cmol)
central apparatus
central artery of retina
central bone of ankle
central canal of spinal cord
central canal of vitreous
central canal of cochlea
central cell
Central European tick-borne fever
central gray substance
central groove
central incisor
central lesion
central lobule
central lymph node
central myelitis
central necrosis
central nervous system
central perineal tendon
central pit
central pneumonia
central sulcus
central tegmental fasciculus
central tegmental tract
central tendon of diaphragm
central tendon of perineum
central vein of liver lobule
central venous pressure (CVP) catheter
central zone of amyloid
centralis retinae, arteria
centrifugation
centrifuge
centrilobar pancreatitis
centrilobular congestion
centrilobular emphysema
centrilobular necrosis of liver
centrilobular region of liver
centripetal nerve
Centri-Sep spin column
centroacinar cell
centrocyte
centrodistal joint
centromedian nucleus
centromere antibody
centromere, chromosomal
centromeric index
centrosome
centrum
CEP (congenital erythropoietic porphyria)
cephalic angle
cephalic flexure
cephalic pole
cephalic triangle
cephalic vein
cephalic ventricle
cephalocaudal axis
cephalomedullary angle
ceramide trihexosidase
ceramide trihexosidase deficiency
ceratocricoid ligament
ceratopharyngeal part
c-erb protein

cercariae of avian schistosomes in skin
cercarial dermatitis
cerebellar artery
cerebellar cortex
cerebellar fissure
cerebellar fossa
cerebellar notch
cerebellar pyramid
cerebellar sulcus
cerebellomedullary cistern
cerebellopontine angle
cerebellopontine angle meningioma
cerebellopontine recess
cerebellorubral tract
cerebellothalamic tract
cerebellum
cerebral aqueduct
cerebral arteriosclerosis
cerebral artery
cerebral atrophy
cerebral concussion
cerebral congestion
cerebral contusion
cerebral cortex
cerebral cranium
cerebral cyst
cerebral death
cerebral edema
cerebral embolism
cerebral fissure
cerebral flexure
cerebral hemisphere
cerebral infarction
cerebral malaria
cerebral meningitis
cerebral parenchyma
cerebral part
cerebral petechiae
cerebral pneumonia
cerebral sulcus
cerebral surface
cerebral vein
cerebral ventricle
cerebral vesicle
cerebromacular degeneration (CMD)
cerebroretinal degeneration
cerebrospinal axis
cerebrospinal canal
cerebrospinal fluid (CSF)
cerebrospinal fluid glucose
cerebrospinal fluid glutamine
cerebrospinal fluid lactic acid
cerebrospinal fluid otorrhea
cerebrospinal fluid pressure
cerebrospinal fluid protein
cerebrospinal fluid volume
cerebrospinal meningitis
cerebrospinal system
cerebrovascular accident (CVA)
cerebrum
  first ventricle of
  lateral ventricle of
  second ventricle of
  third ventricle of
ceroid-laden macrophage
ceruloplasmin
ceruminous gland
cervical adenocarcinoma
cervical aortic knuckle
cervical artery
cervical atrophy
cervical auricle
cervical axillary canal
cervical canal
cervical cap
cervical chain
cervical condyloma
cervical cone biopsy
cervical cytology
cervical disk
cervical dysplasia
cervical erosion
cervical eversion
cervical fascia

cervical flexure
cervical ganglion, uterine
cervical gland
cervical incompetence
cervical interspinal muscle
cervical intraepithelial neoplasia (CIN)
cervical ligament
cervical line
cervical loop
cervical margin
cervical motion tenderness (CMT)
cervical mucus
cervical nerve
cervical os
cervical paratracheal lymph node
cervical part
cervical pleura
cervical plexus
cervical polyp
cervical pregnancy
cervical rib
cervical rotator muscle
cervical sinus
cervical smear
cervical spine
cervical stenosis
cervical stump
cervical transformation zone
cervical triangle
cervical ulcer
cervical vein
cervical vertebra
cervical vesicle
cervical zone
cervicalis, ansa
cervicitis
cervicoaxillary canal
cervicothoracic ganglion
cervicovaginal artery
cervix (pl. cervixes, cervices)
  biopsy of
  cone biopsy of
cervix *(continued)*
  conization of
  fish-mouth
  incompetent
  uterine
C_1 esterase
C_1 esterase inhibitor
C factor
CF (complement fixation)
CF antibody
C fiber
C-14 cholate breath
cg (centigram)
cGMP (cyclic guanosine-3-5'-monophosphate)
cGy (centigray)
Chaetoconidium
Chagas disease
chain (pl. chains)
  A
  B
  branched
  heavy
  kappa
  light
  long
  monoclonal light
  polypeptide
  short
chain amino acid, branched
chain disease, heavy alpha
chain fatty acid (see also *fatty acid*)
  medium
  short
chain reaction, polymerase
chalazion
chalice cell
chalky bone
chamber
  anterior
  pulp
Champy fixative

chancre, syphilitic
chancriform pyoderma
chancroid
change
  antigenic
  atrophic
  koilocytotic cellular
  malignant
  post-radiation
  pregangrenous
  radiation cell
  reparative
  solar degenerative
channel
  gastric
  pancreaticobiliary common
  pyloric
Charcot-Bouchard aneurysm
Charcot cirrhosis
Charcot intermittent fever
Charcot joint
Charcot-Leyden crystals
Charcot-Marie atrophy
Charcot-Marie-Tooth atrophy
Charcot triad
charring
Chassaignac space
Chauffard point
Chaussier line
check ligaments
Chédiak-Higashi granules
Chédiak-Steinbrinck-Higashi syndrome
cheek
  gluteal
  infraorbital
cheek bone
cheek gland
cheek muscle
cheek tooth
cheesy abscess
cheesy discharge
cheesy necrosis
cheesy nephritis
cheesy pneumonia
cheesy pus
cheilitis
cheiloschisis
cheilosis
"chem 6" (SMA-6)
"chem 12" (SMA-12)
"chem 20" (SMA-20)
chemical cleavage
chemical debris
chemical dermatitis
chemical diabetes
chemical irritant
chemical pneumonitis
chemical poisoning
chemical poison
chemical test
chemistry, blood
chemistry panel
chemistry profile
C hemoglobin
chemotactic response
chemotactic sexual hormone
chemotaxis
chemotherapy code
Chemstrip bG dipstick
Chemstrip urine dipstick
chenodeoxycholic acid, total
chenodeoxycholylglycine, conjugated
C hepatitis
cherry angioma
chest tube
chest wall
chevron bone
Chiari-Arnold malformation
Chiari reticulum
chiasm, optic
chiasmatic cistern
chiasmatic sulcus
Chiba aspiration biopsy needle
chicken fat clot

chickenpox (varicella)
chickenpox immunoglobulin
Chick-Martin test
chiclero ulcer
chief agglutinin
chief artery
chief cell
chief complaint
chikungunya virus
chilblain
Child classification of hepatic risk criteria
Child-Pugh A, B, C, classification
Child-Turcotte classification
chills
chip, prostate (prostatic)
chisel
  Councilman
  Virchow bone-splitting
chlamydia
Chlamydia pneumoniae
Chlamydia psittaci
Chlamydia trachomatis
Chlamydiazyme test
chloasma
chloracne
chloride
  mercuric
  serum
  sweat
  urine
chloride test
chloroazotemic nephritis
chloroform poisoning
chlorpalladium
choana (pl. choanae)
choanal polyp
cholangiole
chocolate agar
chocolate cyst
Chodosh macroscopic appearance
choked disk disease
cholangiocarcinoma
cholangiogram
cholangitic abscess
cholangitis
cholecystectomy
cholecystitis
cholecystoduodenal fistula
cholecystoduodenal ligament
cholecystoduodenocolic fold
cholecystokinin (CCK)
cholecystokinin-pancreozymin (CCK-PZ)
choledochous duct
choledochal sphincter
choledochoduodenal junction
choledocholithiasis
choledochopancreatic ductal junction
choleic acid
cholelithiasis
cholemic nephrosis
cholera
cholestasis
cholestatic jaundice
cholesteatoma
Cholestec L-D-X system to measure total cholesterol and glucose
cholesterol
  serum
  total
cholesterol cleft
cholesterol crystals
cholesterol deposition
cholesterol embolism
cholesterol gallstone
cholesterol granuloma
cholesterol pleurisy
cholesterol pneumonitis
cholesterolosis
cholic acid, total
cholinergic fiber
cholinergic receptor
cholinesterase II test

choluria (bilirubinuria)
choluric jaundice
chondritis, articular
chondrocyte
chondroid tissue
chondroma
chondropharyngeal part
chondrosarcoma
chondrosternal articulation
chondroxiphoid ligament
Chopart articulation
Chopart joint
chorda (pl. chordae)
chorda saliva
chorda tendinea (pl. chordae tendineae)
chorda tympani nerve
chordal tissue
chordoma
chorea, Huntington
chorioallantoic graft
chorioallantoic membrane
chorioallantoic placenta
chorioamnionitis
choriocapillary layer
choriocarcinoma
chorioepithelioma
choriomeningitis, lymphocytic
chorionic disk
chorionic gonadotropic hormone
chorionic gonadotropin in urine
chorionic growth hormone
chorionic plate
chorionic sac
chorionic tissue
chorionic villi biopsy
chorionic villus (pl. villi)
chorioretinitis
choristoma
choroidal nevus
choroidal ring
choroid artery
choroid coat
choroiditis
choroid layer
choroid plexus
choroid plexus papilloma
choroid vein
Chr a antigen
Christchurch (Ch^1) chromosome
Christian-Hand-Schüller disease
Christmas disease
Christmas factor
chromaffin body
chromaffin cell
chromaffinoma
chromaffin reaction
chromaffin tissue
chromate
chromatic apparatus
chromatic fiber
chromatic granule
chromatin analysis, sex
chromatin body
chromatin, clumped
chromatin nucleolus
chromatin particle
chromatin pattern
chromatin reservoir
chromatin test for genetic sex
  determination
chromatography
  gas
  high-performance liquid
  high-pressure liquid
  ion-exchange
  liquid
  paper
  thin-layer
chromaffinoma
chromatolysis of cell bodies
chromatophore
chromatophorotropic hormone
chromatosis
chromic acid

chromidial apparatus
chromium, radioactive
chromium red blood cell survival test
Chromobacterium violaceum
chromoblastomycosis
chromocenter
chromogenic enzyme substrate test
chromogranin A
chromomycosis
chromophil (also chromophilic)
chromophil granule
chromophil substance
chromophobic adenoma
chromophobic cell
chromophobic granule
chromophytosis
chromoprobe
chromosomal abnormality
  aneuploidy
  deletion
  inversion
  reduplication
  translocation
chromosomal analysis
chromosomal centromere
chromosomal disorder
chromosomal gap
chromosomal structure of cell
chromosome
  accessory
  Christchurch (Ch 1)
  fragile X
  giant
  Philadelphia
  ring
chromosome analysis
chromosome band(ing)
chromosome in situ hybridization
chromosome satellite
chronic abscess
chronic acholuric jaundice
chronic active hepatitis
chronic adhesive arachnoiditis
chronic bacillary diarrhea
chronic bone marrow failure
chronic bowel disease with protein loss
chronic bronchitis
chronic bullous dermatosis of childhood
chronic constrictive pericarditis
chronic diffuse sclerosing osteomyelitis
chronic eczema
chronic eosinophilic pneumonia
chronic Epstein-Barr virus infection
chronic exposure to loud noise
chronic familial jaundice
chronic fibrous thyroiditis
chronic fissure
chronic focal sclerosing osteomyelitis
chronic gastritis
chronic glomerulonephritis
chronic granulocytic leukemia
chronic hypertrophic myocarditis
chronic idiopathic
chronic inflammation
chronic interstitial myocarditis
chronic interstitial salpingitis
chronic leukemia
chronic lymphocytic leukemia (CLL)
chronic meningitis
chronic myelitis
chronic myelomonocytic leukemia
chronic myocarditis
chronic nephritis
chronic nutritional deficiency
chronic obstructive pulmonary disease (COPD)
chronic osteitis
chronic pancreatitis
chronic passive congestion
chronic pernicious myocarditis
chronic persistent hepatitis
chronic pleurisy
chronic pneumonia

chronic pneumonitis
chronic pyelonephritis
chronic ulcer
chronicity
chronicum migrans, erythema
Chrysosporium
Chrysosporium parvum
Churg-Strauss syndrome
chyle
chyle cistern
chyle corpuscle
chyle lymph
chyle vessel
chyliferous vessel
chyliform pleurisy
chylomicron
chylous pleurisy
chyme, fat-containing
Ciaccio gland
cicatricial alopecia
cicatricial horn
cicatricial kidney
cicatricial pemphigoid
cicatricial tissue
cicatrix
cicatrization
CIE (counterimmunoelectrophoresis)
cilia
ciliary artery
ciliary body
ciliary canal
ciliary cartilage
ciliary crown
ciliary disk
ciliary fold
ciliary ganglion
ciliary ganglionic plexus
ciliary gland
ciliary ligament
ciliary margin
ciliary muscle
ciliary process
ciliary ring
ciliary vein
ciliary zone
ciliary zonule
ciliated cell
ciliated columnar epithelium
ciliated epithelium
ciliospinal center
cimicosis
CIN (cervical intraepithelial neoplasia)
  classification
Cinna-Biotecx protocol
circinata, psoriasis
circinate
circle
  arterial
  articular vascular
circle of Willis artery
circular electrode mark
circular fiber
circular fold
circular layer
circular muscle coat
circular sinus
circular sulcus
circular swirl
circular syncytium
circular vortex
circulating anticoagulant
circulating blood
circulating leukocyte
circulating lymphocyte
circulation
  capillary
  collateral
  cross
  extracorporeal
  increased local
circulatory collapse
circulatory compromise
circulatory disorder
circulatory impairment

circulatory stasis
circulatory system
circumanal gland
circumcised
circumcision
circumference
circumferential cartilage
circumferential fibrocartilage
circumferential lamella
circumflex artery
circumflex branch
circumflex fibular artery
circumflex nerve
circumflex scapular artery
circumflex vein
circum-marginate
circumoral pallor
circumpennate muscle
circumrenal
circumscribe
circumscribed cerebral atrophy
circumscribed pleurisy
circumscribed pyocephalus
circumtonsillar abscess
circumvallate papilla
circumventricular organ
circus senilis
cirrhosis
- acholangic biliary
- acute juvenile
- alcoholic
- atrophic
- bacterial
- biliary
- calculus
- cardiac
- Charcot
- congestive
- Cruveilhier-Baumgarten
- decompensated
- diffuse septal
- fatty

cirrhosis *(continued)*
- hepatic
- Indian childhood
- Laënnec
- macrolobular
- microlobular
- malarial
- metabolic
- micronodular
- multilobular
- nutritional
- periportal
- pigment
- pipe stem
- portal
- posthepatitic
- postnecrotic
- primary biliary
- pulmonary
- secondary biliary
- septal
- stasis
- syphilitic
- Todd
- toxic
- unilobular
- vascular

cirrhosis of liver
cirrhosis of lung
cirrhotic gastritis
cirrhotic inflammation
cirsoid aneurysm
cirsoid placenta
cirsoid varix
cistern
- basal
- cerebellomedullary
- chyle

cisterna of endoplasmic reticulum
cisternal puncture
citrate
citrate test

citrated plasma
Citrobacter
Citrobacter amalonaticus
Citrobacter diversus
Citrobacter freundii
citrovorum factor
citrulline test
Civinini canal
Civinini ligament
CK-BB (CK_1) isoenzyme
CK enzyme (also, CPK)
CK isoenzyme
CK-MB isoenzyme (CK_2)
CK-MM (CK_3) isoenzyme
cL (centiliter)
Cladosporium
Cladosporium bantianum
Cladosporium carrionii
Cladosporium cladosporioides
Cladosporium trichoides
Cladosporium werneckii
Clado ligament
clam digger's itch
Clapton line
Clara cell
Clarite mounting medium
Clark classification of malignant melanoma
Clarke cell
classical hemophilia
classical osteosarcoma
classic dengue
classic interstitial pneumonia
classic phenylketonuria
classification (see also *grade*, *stage*)
- Arneth c. of polymorphonuclear neutrophils
- Astler-Coller modification of Dukes c. of carcinoma
- Bethesda PAP smear c.
- Breslow c. of malignant melanoma
- Broders tumor index

classification *(continued)*
- Brooker periarticular heterotopic ossification (PHO)
- burns
- Butchart staging c.
- Caldwell-Moloy c.
- CDC c. for HIV infection
- chemotherapy code
- Child c. of hepatic risk criteria
- Child-Pugh A, B, C
- Child-Turcotte
- CIN (cervical iantraepithelial neoplasia)
- Clark c. of malignant melanoma
- DeBakey aortic c.
- Delbet fracture c.
- Denver chromosome c.
- diabetes mellitus c.
- Dubin and Amelar varicocele c.
- Dukes c. of carcinoma
- Erlanger and Gasser peripheral nerve c.
- FAB c. of acute nonlymphoid leukemia
- FIGO staging of adenocarcinoma of endometrium
- Floyd peripheral nerve c.
- Frykman c. of hand fractures
- Gell and Coombs hypersensitivity reactions
- HIV c. of children
- Hoehn and Yahr staging of Parkinson disease
- House-Brackmann facial weakness
- Hunt and Hess neurological c.
- Hyams grading of esthesioneuroblastoma
- International C. of Diseases for Oncology (ICD-O)
- Jackson and Parker c. of Hodgkin disease
- Jansky human blood groups

classification *(continued)*
- Jewett c. of bladder carcinoma
- Judet epiphyseal fracture c.
- Karnofsky status c.
- Keith-Wagener c. of retinopathy
- Kiel c. of non-Hodgkin lymphoma
- Klatskin tumor c.
- Lancefield c. of hemolytic streptococci into groups
- leukemia c.
- Lukes-Butler c. of non-Hodgkin lymphoma
- Lukes-Collins c. of non-Hodgkin lymphoma
- microinvasive carcinoma c.
- Modic disk abnormality c.
- morphologic c.
- MSTS (Musculoskeletal Tumor Society) staging system
- multiaxial
- murmur grades
- Neer shoulder fractures I, II, III
- NYHA (New York Heart Association) c. of congestive heart failure
- Olerud and Molander fracture c.
- osteoarthritis grading
- Pauwels femoral neck fracture
- Rappaport lymphoma
- Reese-Ellsworth c. of retinoblastoma
- Rye c. of Hodgkin disease
- Singh-Vaughn-Williams arrhythmia
- TNM (tumor size, nodal involvement, metastatic progress) c.
- van Heuven anatomic c. of diabetic retinopathy
- Wiberg c. of patellar types
- Wolfe breast carcinoma c.

Claudius cell
clavate papilla
clavicle bone
clavicle, midpoint of
clavicular artery
clavicular facet
clavicular notch
clavicular part
clavipectoral fascia
clavipectoral triangle
clay-colored stool
clean-catch urine
clean-catch urine specimen
clean-voided urine specimen
clearance
- creatinine
- insulin
- urea

clear cell
clear cell adenocarcinoma of cervix or vagina
clear cell carcinoma of vagina
clear cell carcinoma of vagina and cervix among DES daughters
clearing factor
clearing of tissue specimen
clear margin
clear medium
clear tissue
clear urine
cleavage
- adequal
- determinate
- discoidal
- enamel
- equatorial

cleavage cavity
cleavage cell
cleavage line
cleavage spindle
cleaved cell
CLED (cystine, lactose, electrolyte deficient)
cleft
- anal
- branchial

cleft *(continued)*
  cholesterol
  facial
  first visceral
  gill
  pudendal
cleftlike space
cleft lip
cleft palate
cleistothecia
climbing fiber
clinical diagnosis
Clinistix
Clinitest
clinoid plate
clinoid process
clitoral artery
clitoral hypertrophy
clitoris
  angle of
  crus of
  deep artery of
  frenulum of
  glans of
  prepuce of
clival meningioma
CLL (chronic lymphocytic leukemia)
cloacal membrane
cloacal plate
clomiphene test
clone
cloning
clonogenic cell
clonorchiasis
Clonorchis sinensis
C-loop, duodenal
Cloquet canal
Cloquet fascia
Cloquet ganglion
Cloquet gland
Cloquet ligament
Cloquet space
closed comedo
closed gland
closed loop
closed-loop obstruction
closing membrane
Clostridium
Clostridium bifermentans
Clostridium botulinum
Clostridium butyricum
Clostridium cadaveris
Clostridium difficile (slang "C. diff")
Clostridium difficile toxin assay
Clostridium histolyticum
Clostridium innocuum
Clostridium novyi
Clostridium paraputrificum
Clostridium perfringens
Clostridium putrificum
Clostridium ramosum
Clostridium septicum
Clostridium sordellii
Clostridium sphenoides
Clostridium sporogenes
Clostridium subterminale
Clostridium tertium
Clostridium tetani
Clostridium welchii
closure of skull, failure of
clot
  agonal
  antemortem
  blood
  chicken
  chicken fat
  currant jelly
  distal
  external
  friable
  heart
  internal
  laminated
  marantic

clot *(continued)*
- organized
- passive
- plastic
- postmortem
- proximal
- retraction of
- spider-web
- stratified
- washed

clot lysis test
clot retraction test
clotting factor
clotting time (also, coagulation)
- activated
- Lee-White
- plasma

clot tube
cloudy gray streaks in lens
cloudy "snowflake" opacities
cloudy swelling
cloudy urine
clubbed finger
clubbed penis
clubbing of digits
clublike dermal papillae
club-shaped bacillus
clue cell
clump cell
clumped chromatin
clumping of cells
clumping of white blood cells
clumps and nests
cluster of cells with large nuclei
cluster of differentiation (CD)
Clutton joint
cm (centimeter)
cmol (centimole)
CMT (cervical motion tenderness)
c-myc protein
CNS (central nervous system) tumor
CO (carbon monoxide)
"coag" (slang for coagulation)
coagulase-negative staphylococcus
coagulase test
coagulate
coagulated protein
coagulation
- acquired disorder of
- blood
- diffuse intravascular (DIC)
- congenital disorder of
- disseminated intravascular (DIC)
- electric
- massive

coagulation defect
coagulation factor
- failure to form
- factor I (fibrinogen)
- factor II (prothrombin)
- factor III (tissue thromboplastin)
- factor IV (calcium)
- factor V (proaccelerin)
- factor VI (stable)
- factor VII (proconvertin)
- factor VIII (antihemophilic)
- factor IX (plasma thromboplastin component)
- factor X (Stuart-Prower)
- factor XI (plasma thromboplastin antecedent)
- factor XII (Hageman)
- factor XIII (fibrin stabilizing)

coagulation factor assay
coagulation necrosis
coagulation of tissue by excessive heat
coagulation panel
- bleeding time
- clot retraction
- clotting time
- partial thromboplastin time
- plasma assay
- platelet count
- prothrombin time

coagulation time (also, clotting)
  activated
  Lee-White
  plasma
coagulation time test
coagulopathy
coarctate retina
coarctation of aorta
coarse azurophilic granules
coarse basophilic stippling in
  cytoplasm of neutrophils
coarse features
coarsely granular
coarsening of hair
coarsening of skin
coat
  buffy
  choroid
  circular muscle
  longitudinal muscle
cobalamin
cobalt, radioactive
cobblestone appearance
cobblestone granulations of conjunctiva
Cobelli gland
Coca-Cola urine
coccal infection
cocci (pl. of coccus)
coccidioidal meningitis
coccidioidin test
Coccidioides immitis
coccidioidin skin test
coccidioidomycosis
coccidiosis
coccobacillus
coccus (pl. cocci), gram-negative
coccygeal body
coccygeal bone
coccygeal ganglion
coccygeal gland
coccygeal joint
coccygeal muscle
coccygeal nerve
coccygeal part
coccygeal plexus
coccygeal sinus
coccygeal vertebra
coccygeal whorl
coccygeus muscle
coccyx, tip of
cochlea, aqueduct of
cochlear aqueduct
cochlear area
cochlear artery
cochlear canal
cochlear canaliculus
cochlear duct
cochlear hair cell
cochleariform process
cochlear joint
cochlear labyrinth
cochlear nerve
cochlear nucleus
cochlear part
cochlear recess
cochlear root
cockscomb (also, coxcomb)
cockscomb of cervix
cockscomb papilloma
Code 500
Code Blue
codfish vertebra
codocyte
codominant gene
coeliac (also celiac)
coenzyme factor
cofactor
coffee-grounds material
coffin bone
coffin formation
coffin joint
cohesion
cohesive
coiled artery

coil gland
coin lesion
coin lesion of lungs
coil of intestine
coil of jejunum
coinfection with hepatitis B
cold abscess
cold agglutinin pneumonia
cold agglutinins
cold cone biopsy
cold cup biopsy
cold erythema
cold hemolysin
cold, injury due to
cold nodule
cold pressure test
cold-rigor point
coldsore (herpes simplex)
cold-target DNA
cold water calorics
coli
  E. (*Escherichia*)
  melanosis
  taeniae
colibacillemia
colibacillosis, enteric
coli granuloma
colic, appendicular
colic artery
colic flexure
colic impression
colic omentum
colic plexus
colic sphincter
colic surface
colic vein
coliform bacilli
coliform bacteria
colistin
colitis
  collagenous
  granulomatous

colitis *(continued)*
  hemorrhagic
  ischemic
  microscopic
  radiation
  regional
  transmural
  ulcerative
collagen bundle
collagen disease
collagen fiber
collagen fibril
collagenic fibers, matrix of
collagenous connective tissue
collagenous fiber
collagen pus
collar bone
collar-button abscess
collar chain
collateral artery
collateral branch
collateral branches of intercostal nerve
collateral circulation
collateral digital artery
collateral eminence
collateral fissure
collateral ligament
collateral radial artery
collateral route
collateral sulcus
collateral trigone
collateral ulnar artery
collateral vessel
collecting system
collecting tubule
collecting vessel
collenchyma cells
Colles fascia
Colles ligament
Colles space
colliculi of midbrain
colliculitis

colliculus
  facial
  seminal
colliquation
  ballooning
  reticular
colliquative diarrhea
colliquative necrosis
colliquative proteinuria
colloidal gel
colloidal gold test
colloid body
colloid corpuscle
colloid degeneration
colloid goiter
colloid material
colloid system
coloboma iridis
colon
  anterior band of
  ascending
  descending
  distal
  free band of
  giant
  iliac
  inflammation
  irritable
  lateral reflection of
  lead-pipe
  left
  mesosigmoid
  midsigmoid
  pelvic
  perisigmoid
  right
  sigmoid
  transverse
colon adenocarcinoma
colon polyp
colon bacillus
colonic abscess
colonic adenoma
colonic diverticulitis
colonic diverticulum
colonic fistula
colonic loop
colonic myenteric plexus
colonic pit
colonic polyp
colonies, bacterial
colonization infection
colonization of urinary tract
colony count, urine
colony-stimulating factor (CSF)
color and caliber of stool
color and consistency of skin
color and distribution of head and body hair
Colorado tick fever
Colorado tick fever virus
coloration
colorectal mucosa
colorimetry
colorless gas
colorless reaction
Coloscreen test for occult blood in stool
colostomy
colostrum corpuscle
colovaginal fistula
colovesical fistula
colposcope
colposcopic diagnosis
Columbia blood agar
column
  affinity
  anal
  anterolateral
  Bertin
  branchial efferent
  renal
  variceal
columnar cell

columnar epithelial cells
columnar epithelium
columnar layer
columnar metaplasia
columnar metaplasia of epithelium
columnar sustentacular cells
column cell
column of Bertin
column typing
coma
  agrypnodal
  alcoholic
  alpha
  diabetic
  hepatic
  hyperosmolar nonketotic
  irreversible
  Kussmaul
  metabolic
  uremic
coma scale
coma vigil
Comamonas terrigena
combined pregnancy
combined sclerosis
combined system disease
Combistix
combustion of carbon-containing fuels
comedo (pl. comedones)
  closed
  open
comedo-type DCIS (ductal carcinoma in situ)
comedocarcinoma
comedomastitis
comedo nevus
comma bundle
comma degeneration
comma tract (interfascicular fasciculus)
comminuted fracture
commissural cell
commissural fiber
commissural neuron
commissure, anterior labial
committed cell
common acute lymphoblastic leukemia antigen (CALLA)
common atrioventricular canal
common basal vein
common bile duct (CBD)
common bile duct stone
common cardinal vein
common carotid artery
common carotid plexus
common cold virus
common duct
common duct stone
common facial vein
common fibular nerve
common gall duct
common hepatic duct
common iliac artery
common iliac lymph node
common iliac node
common interosseous artery
common palmar digital nerve
common peroneal nerve
common plantar digital artery
common plantar digital nerve
common ring tendon
common synovial flexor sheath
common tendinous ring
communicans
  gray ramus
  white ramus
communicating artery
community-acquired infection
community-acquired pneumonia
compact bone
compact osteoma
compact tissue
companion artery of sciatic nerve
companion lymph node
companion vein

compartment
 infracolic
 supracolic
compatibility testing (cross-match)
compensatory atrophy
compensatory hyperplasia
compensatory hypertrophy
competent cell, immunologically
competitive binding assay
complement, C_3
complementary hypertrophy
complementary strand
complement chemotactic factor
complement fixation (CF) test
complement-fixing antibody
complement-mediated depletion
complete abortion
complete blood count (see *CBC*)
complete protein
complex
 aberrant
 AIDS dementia
 AIDS-related (ARC)
 amyotrophic lateral sclerosis–parkinsonism–dementia
 antigen-antibody
 antigenic
 apical
 atrial
 auricular
 avidin-biotin (ABC)
 avidin-biotin peroxidase
 avidin-biotinylated peroxidase
 Carney
 caudal pharyngeal
 C_1 q immune
 Eisenmenger
 gastroduodenal artery
 HLA (human lymphocyte antigen)
 immune
 junctional
 Meyenburg

complex *(continued)*
 MHC (major histocompatibility)
 nipple-areola
 streptavidin-biotin peroxidase
 Tacaribe
 thrombin-antithrombin III (TAT)
 triangular fibrocartilage
 von Meyenburg
complications of abortion
component
composite articulation
composite joint
composite odontoma
composition, homogeneous
compound aneurysm
compound articulation
compound gland
compound granule cell
compound joint
compound lipid
compound nevus
compound pregnancy
compound protein
compound tubuloalveolar gland
compressible cavernous body
compression atrophy
compression myelitis
compressor muscle
concanavalin A
concave abdomen
concealed penis
concentrated human red blood corpuscle
concentration
 mean corpuscular hemoglobin
 minimum inhibitory (MIC)
 minimum lethal (MLC)
concentration test, Fishberg
concentration test for renal function
concentric atrophy
concentric lamella
concentric rings

concentrically laminated concretions
concentrically laminated mass
conception, products of
concha (pl. conchae)
  inferior nasal
  middle nasal
  superior nasal
conchal cartilage
conchal crest
conchiolin osteomyelitis
conchoidal body
concretion
  bile
  fecal
  prostatic
concretion of abnormal substances
concussion, cerebral
concussion myelitis
condensing osteitis
conducting bronchiole
conducting system
conduction, atrioventricular
condylar articulation
condylar axis
condylar canal
condylar emissary vein
condylar fossa
condylar joint
condylar process
condyle cord
condyle path
condyloid articulation
condyloid canal
condyloid foramen, anterior
condyloid joint
condyloid process
condyloma (pl. condylomata)
  cervical
  flat
  pointed
condyloma acuminatum (pl. acuminata)
condyloma latum (pl. condylomata lata)
condylomatous
cone
  arterial
  retinal
cone-and-plate viscometer
cone biopsy of cervix
cone cell
cone disk
cone fiber
configuration
  back-to-back
  biventricular
  stellate
cone granule
confluent articulation
confluent reticulated papillomatosis
confocal epifluorescence microscope
confocal laser scanning microscopy
confocal microscopy
congenital adrenal hyperplasia
congenital agammaglobulinemia
congenital aneurysm
congenital anomaly
congenital baldness
congenital cataract
congenital defect
congenital deficiency of galactosyl-ceramidase
congenital erythropoietic porphyria (CEP)
congenital goiter
congenital hemolytic anemia
congenital hemolytic jaundice
congenital malaria
congenital malformation of the eye
congenital megacolon
congenital methemoglobinemia
congenital nephritis
congenital nevus
congenital porphyria
congenital pulmonary arteriovenous fistula

congenital rubella pneumonitis
congenital syphilis
congenital toxoplasmosis
congential hemolytic anemia
congested kidney
congestion
 active
 cardiac
 centrilobular
 cerebral
 chronic passive
 functional
 hepatic
 hypostatic
 intravascular
 neurotonic
 passive
 pulmonary
 splenic
 vascular
 venous
congestion of tissues with blood
congestive cirrhosis
congestive heart failure
conglobate gland
conglutinating complement absorption test (CCAT)
Congolian red fever
Congo red stain test for amyloidosis
congruent point
conical bulging of cornea
conical masses
conical papilla
conidia, diamond-shaped
Conidiobolus coronatus
Conidiobolus incongruus
conization of cervix
conjoined tendon
conjoint tendon
conjugate axis
conjugate foramen
conjugate ligament
conjugated antigen
conjugated bile acid
conjugated bilirubin
conjugated protein
conjugative plasmid
conjunctiva
 cobblestone granulations of
 edema of
 lymphocytic aggregations of
 mucopurulent exudate of
 papillary hypertrophy of
conjunctival artery
conjunctival cul-de-sac
conjunctival gland
conjunctival layer
conjunctival ring
conjunctival sac
conjunctival scrapings
conjunctival test
conjunctival varix
conjunctival vein
conjunctivitis
 granulomatous
 inclusion (of newborn)
 noninfectious
 ulcerative
 vernal
connecting canal
connecting cartilage
connecting tubule
connective tissue
 areolar
 dense
 fibril
 loose
 peribronchial
 regular
 reticular
 subcutaneous
connective-tissue cell
connective-tissue covering of cartilage
connective-tissue disorder

connective-tissue fiber
connective-tissue matrix
connective-tissue nevus
connective-tissue stroma
Conn syndrome
conoid ligament
conoid process
conoid tubercle
consecutive aneurysm
consent, autopsy
consistency of stool
consolidation, pulmonary
consolidative pneumonia
constituents of umbilical cord
constitutive protein
constricting
constrictive pericarditis
contact area zone
contact dermatitis
contact patch test
contact-type dermatitis
contagiosum
  impetigo
  molluscum
contagious ecthyma (orf)
contagious pustular dermatitis
contamination
contents
  abdominal
  bowel
  digestive tract
  gastric
  intestinal
continuous capillary
contour line
contracted kidney
contracted pelvis
contracted tendon
contractile fiber cells
contractile vacuole
contraction band
contraction band necrosis
contraction, peristaltic
contraction stress test (CST)
contracture deformity
contracture, Volkmann
contrast medium (pl. media)
contrasuppressor cell
control
  negative
  positive
control gene
contused wound
contusion, cerebral
contusion of brain
contusion of muscle
contusion pneumonia
conus
convalescent serum
convergence, angle of
convex border of stomach
convexity, cortical
convexity meningioma
convoluted bone
convoluted gland
convoluted part
convoluted seminiferous tubule
convoluted tubule
convolution
  ascending frontal
  ascending parietal
  callosal
convulsant threshold
Cook aspiration biopsy needle
cooled-knife method
Cooley anemia
Coomassie blue
Coombs test
  direct
  indirect
Cooper ligament
COPD (chronic obstructive pulmonary disease)
Cope needle

copious discharge
copious rice-water diarrhea
copious watery diarrhea
Coplin jar
copper (Cu)
  excessive absorption of
  impaired excretion of
copper-containing plasma globulin
copper grid
copper line
copper poisoning
copper sulfate method
copper-wire artery
coprine toxin
Coprinus cinereus
coproporphyrin test
coproporphyrin, urinary excretion of
coracoacromial ligament
coracobrachial muscle
coracoclavicular ligament
coracohumeral ligament
coracoid process
coracoid tuberosity
cor bovinum
cord
  condyle
  dental
  false vocal
  gangliated
  genital
  germinal
  hepatic
  medullary
  spermatic
  spinal
  three-vessel umbilical
  two-vessel umbilical
  umbilical
  vocal
cordate pelvis
cord bladder
cordiform pelvis
cordis, apex
cordlike arrangements of cells
cordlike trunk
cords in parallel bundles
cord structure
corduroy artery
core, necrobiotic
corium
corkboard
corkscrew artery
corkscrew-shaped bacterium
cornea
  conical bulging of
  fibrosis in
  inflammation of the
  opaque
  vascularization in
corneal cell
corneal corpuscle
corneal layer
corneal lens
corneal margin
corneal opacity
corneal scarring
corneal section
corneal space
corneal tube
corneal ulcer
corneal ulceration
Corner-Allen test
corneum, stratum
corniculate cartilage
corniculate tubercle
corniculopharyngeal ligament
cornification
cornified layer
cornmeal-Tween 80 agar
cornu (pl. cornua), sacral
cornual myelitis
cornual pregnancy
cornua of spinal cord
cornua of uterus

coronal plane
coronal pulp
coronal section
coronal suture
coronal zone
corona of glans
coronary arteriosclerosis
coronary artery embolism
coronary artery of heart
coronary artery of stomach
coronary band
coronary bone
coronary groove
coronary ligament of knee
coronary ligament of liver
coronary node
coronary plexus
coronary sinus
coronary sulcus
coronary tendon
coronary valve
coronary vein
coronavirus
coroner's autopsy
coroner's case
corporis, tinea
corpse
corpse fat
cor pulmonale
corpus albicans
corpus cavernosum
corpuscle
  amylaceous
  amyloid
  articular
  axile
  axis
  basal
  blood
  bone
  bridge
  bulboid

corpuscle *(continued)*
  cartilage
  cement
  chyle
  colloid
  colostrum
  concentrated human red blood
  corneal
  Dogiel
  dust
  exudation
  fat
  genital
  ghost
  Hassall
  malpighian
  Meissner
  pus
  Zimmermann
corpuscular lymph
corpus luteum
corpus luteum cyst
corpus spongiosum
corpus spongiosum penis
correlated atrophy
Corrigan line
Corrigan pneumonia
corrugated
corrugator muscle
cortex (pl. cortices)
  adrenal
  auditory
  bone
  cerebellar
  cerebral
  dysgranular
  frontal
  lymphatic
  ovarian
  pale
  renal
Corti arch

cortical arch
cortical artery
cortical atrophy
cortical bone
cortical convexity
cortical cyst
cortical defect
cortical hormone
cortical nodule
cortical osteitis
cortical part
cortical plate
cortical substance
cortical surface
cortical tissue
Corti canal
Corti cell
corticobinding globulin (CBG)
corticosterone test
corticobulbar tract
corticomedullary demarcation
corticomedullary junction
corticonuclear fiber
corticopontine tract
corticoreticular fiber
corticospinal fiber
corticospinal tract
corticosteroid-binding globulin
corticosterone test
corticostriatal-spinal degeneration cell
corticotropic hormone
corticotropin-releasing factor
corticotropin-releasing hormone
Corti fiber
Corti ganglion
Corti pillar
Corti rod
cortisol, free
cortisol hormone
Corti tunnel
Corynebacterium acnes
Corynebacterium bovis
Corynebacterium diphtheriae
Corynebacterium equi
Corynebacterium haemolyticum
Corynebacterium minutissimum
Corynebacterium pseudodiphtheriticum
Corynebacterium pseudotuberculosis
Corynebacterium ulcerans
Corynebacterium xerosis
coryza
cosmetic dermatitis
costal angle
costal arch
costal arch reflex
costal artery
costal bone
costal cartilage
costal facet
costal groove
costal margin
costal notch
costal part
costal pit
costal pleura
costal pleural reflection
costal pleurisy
costal process
costal surface
costal surface of lung
costal tuberosity
costeocartilaginous
costoaxillary vein
costocentral articulation
costocentral joint
costocervical artery
costocervical trunk
costocervical trunk artery
costochondral articulation
costochondral joint
costochondral junction
costoclavicular ligament
costoclavicular line

costocolic ligament
costodiaphragmatic recess of pleura
costomediastinal recess
costomediastinal sinus
costophrenic angle
costophrenic septal line
costosternal articulation
costosternal joint
costotransverse articulation
costotransverse foramen
costotransverse joint
costotransverse ligament
costovertebral angle (CVA)
costovertebral articulation
costovertebral joint
costovertebral junction
costovertebral ligament
costoxiphoid ligament
cothromboplastin
cotton-fiber embolism
cotton-mill fever
cotton-wool patch, spot
Cotunnius canal
Cotunnius space
cotyledon, basal plate
cotyloid cavity
cotyloid joint
cotyloid ligament
cotyloid notch
couch grass
cough
  paroxysmal
  whooping
coughing up blood from respiratory tract
cough plate
Coumadin anticoagulant
coumarin anticoagulant
Councilman body
Councilman chisel
Councilman lesion
counseling, genetic
count
  absolute
  absolute neutrophil (ANC)
  Addis
  CD4 (T4) lymphocyte
  cell (of cerebrospinal fluid)
  cell (of urine)
  colony (of urine)
  complete blood (CBC)
  differential
  differential white blood
  differential white blood cell
  indirect platelet
  lamellar body density (LBD)
  platelet
  red blood cell (RBC)
  reticulocyte
  urine colony
  white blood cell (WBC)
counter, B-emission
counterimmunoelectrophoresis (CIE)
counterstain
counting cells
Courvoisier gallbladder
cover cell
covering, fascial
covering of spermatic cord
covering of umbilical cord
coverslip
CO_2–withdrawal seizure test
cow kidney
cowl muscle
Cowper gland
Cowper ligament
coxa
coxal articulation
coxal bone
coxal joint
coxcomb (see *cockscomb*)
Coxiella burnetii
coxofemoral articulation of Buisson
Coxsackie virus (also, coxsackievirus)

coxsackievirus A
coxsackievirus B
coxsackievirus myocarditis
C-peptide (connecting peptide)
CPK (creatine phosphokinase) (also, CK, creatine kinase)
CPK-MB (CK_2) isoenzyme
C_3 proactivator
CPT (Current Procedural Terminology) codes
C_1q immune complex
crackling
cramp, muscle
cranial base
cranial bone
cranial capacity
cranial cavity
cranial flexure
cranial fontanelle
cranial fossa
cranial meninges
cranial meningocele
cranial nerves (I through XII)
cranial part of accessory nerve
cranial root
cranial sinus
cranial suture (joint)
cranial synchondrosis
cranial synostosis
cranial vault
cranial vertebra
craniofacial angle
craniofacial axis
craniofacial notch
craniometric point
craniopharyngeal canal
craniopharyngeal duct
craniopharyngioma
craniosacral system
craniovertebral articulation
crater arc
C-reactive protein (CRP)
crease
  ear lobe
  inguinal
  midline abdominal
  palmar
  skin
  torso
crease wound
creatine kinase (CK)
creatine phosphokinase (CPK)
creatinine clearance
creatinine test
creatinine, urinary
creeping eruption
cremasteric artery
cremasteric fascia
cremaster muscle
crenated
crepitant
crepitation
crepitus
crescent, articular
crescent cell
crescentic border
crescentic lobule
crescent of cardia
crescent of foramina
crescent-shaped structure
crest
  acoustic
  acousticofacial
  alveolar
  ampullary
  arched
  arcuate
  articular
  basilar
  buccinator
  conchal
  deltoid
  dental
  ethmoidal

crest *(continued)*
  falciform
  frontal
  ganglionic
  gingival
  iliac
  pubic
  sacral
  urethral
CREST syndrome
  calcinosis
  Raynaud phenomenon
  esophageal dysfunction
  sclerodactyly
  telangiectasia
cresyl blue
cresyl blue brilliant
cresyl fast violet
cretinism
Creutzfeldt-Jakob disease
creviced appearance
crevicular epithelium fluid
cribrate cell
cribriform
cribriform area
cribriform bone
cribriform fascia
cribriform pattern
cribriform plate
cribriform tissue
cricoarytenoid articular capsule
cricoarytenoid articulation
cricoarytenoid joint
cricoesophageal tendon
cricopharyngeal diverticulum
cricopharyngeal ligament
cricopharyngeal part
cricopharyngeal sphincter
cricosantorinian ligament
cricothyroid artery
cricothyroid articular capsule
cricothyroid articulation
cricothyroid joint
cricothyroid ligament
cricothyroid membrane
cricothyroid muscle
cricotracheal ligament
cricotracheal membrane
cricovocal membrane
Crigler-Najjar syndrome
Crimean-Congo hemorrhagic fever
  virus
Crimean fever
crisscrossing cords
crista galli
crista terminalis
"crit" (slang for hematocrit)
criteria, Broder
Crithidia luciliae
critical angle
critical organ
CRM (cross-reacting material)
cRNA (complementary RNA)
Crohn disease
cromolyn sodium
Crooke cell
Crooke hyaline degeneration
Crooke-Russell band
cross-bridges
cross-circulation
crossed embolism
crossed eye
crossed pyramidal tract
crossed reflex
cross-infection
crossing over (also, crossover)
cross-linking
crossmatch
  HLA (human lymphocyte antigen)
  major
  minor
  pretransplant
  type and
crossmatching

crossover (also, crossing over)
cross-reacting agglutinin
cross-reacting antibody
cross-reacting material (CRM)
cross-reactivation
cross-reactivity
cross-reference
cross-resistance
cross-section (noun, verb)
cross-sectional (adj.)
cross-sensitization
croup-associated virus (CA v.)
croupous inflammation
croupous lymph
croupous membrane
croupous nephritis
croupy
crown cavity
crown, ciliary
crown-heel length
crown-rump length
crown tubercle
CRP (C-reactive protein)
^{51}Cr red cell survival
CRST syndrome (see *CREST*)
crucial anastomosis
cruciate eminence
cruciate ligament
cruciate ligament of atlas
cruciate ligament of knee
cruciate ligament of leg
cruciate muscle
cruciform eminence
cruciform ligament
cruciform part
crumbly
crura (plural of crus)
crura of diaphragm
crura of penis
crural arch
crural canal
crural fossa
crural nerve
crural ring
crural septum
crural sheath
crural triangle
cruris, tinea
crurotalar articulation
crus (pl. crura)
  lateral
  left
  medial
  right
crush kidney
crush syndrome
crus penis, crus of penis
crust (scab)
crusting center
crust of exudate
Cruveilhier atrophy
Cruveilhier-Baumgarten cirrhosis
Cruveilhier fascia
Cruveilhier joint
Cruveilhier ligament
cryofibrinogen
cryoglobulin
cryostat
crypt
  anal
  enamel
  epithelium
  ileal
  Lieberkühn
  Morgagni
  tonsillar
crypt abscess
cryptitis, anal
cryptococcal meningitis
cryptococcosis
Cryptococcus
Cryptococcus albidus
Cryptococcus laurentii
Cryptococcus luteolus

Cryptococcus neoformans
Cryptococcus neoformans pneumonia
cryptogenic pyemia
cryptorchidism
cryptosporidiosis
Cryptosporidium
crystal (pl. crystals)
  asthma
  blood
  Böttcher
  calcium
  calcium pyrophosphate dihydrate (CPPD)
  Charcot-Leyden
  cholesterol
  coffin lid
  dumbbell
  hydroxyapatite
  liquid
  Lubarsch
  thorn-apple
  urate
  Virchow
  whetstone
crystal violet
crystal violet stain
crystallization
crystalloid
crystals in urine
crystals of calcium salts
Crystodigin
CSF (cerebrospinal fluid)
CSF glucose
CSF protein
CST (contraction stress test)
cu mm (cubic millimeter)
Cu (copper)
cubic centimeter (cc)
cubic millimeter (cu mm or mm^3)
cubital articulation
cubital bone
cubital fossa
cubital joint
cubital lymph node
cubital nerve
cubital tunnel
cubitoradial articulation
cubitus valgus
cuboidal articular surface
cuboidal epithelial cell
cuboidal epithelium
cuboidal glandular cell
cuboid bone
cuboid cell
cuboideonavicular articulation
cuboideonavicular joint
cuboideonavicular ligament
cuff
  musculotendinous
  rectal muscle
  rotator
  suprahepatic caval
cuffing, perivascular
cuirass, tabetic
cul-de-sac, conjunctival
cul-de-sac of Douglas
cul-de-sac smear
Culex mosquito
Cult-Dip Plus bacteriological culture test
culture
  abscess
  aerobic
  anaerobic
  arterial line
  bacterial
  blood
  cell
  cervical
  cerebrospinal fluid
  diphtheria
  disk
  fungal
  mixed leukocyte

culture *(continued)*
  mixed lymphocyte (MLC)
  nasopharyngeal
  radioisotopic
  Sabouraud
  spinal fluid
  sputum
  stool
  throat
  tissue (TC)
  Tween-albumin broth
  urine
  Vero cell
  viral
culture and sensitivity (C&S)
cultured cells of human lymphoblastoid line
culture medium (pl. media)
  agar
  bacterial
  laked sheep blood, kanamycin, vancomycin
  sheep red blood cells (sRBC)
  sRBC and phenylethyl alcohol
  tryptic soy agar with sRBC, colistin, and nalidixic acid
cuneate fasciculus
cuneate nucleus
cuneiform bone, first
cuneiform cartilage
cuneiform lobe
cuneiform tubercle
cuneocerebellar tract
cuneocuboid joint
cuneocuboid ligament
cuneometatarsal articulation
cuneometatarsal joint
cuneonavicular articulation
cuneonavicular joint
cuneonavicular ligament
cup ear
cupola, pleural
cupular blind sac
cupulate part
curdlike discharge
curdlike excrescence
curdy pus
curet (also, curette)
curet lesion
curettage
  endocervical
  endometrial
curetting
curled edge
Curling ulcer
currant jelly clot
currant jelly stool
current, electrotonic
Curschmann spiral
cursory examination
Curtis–Fitz-Hugh syndrome
curvature
  angular
  anterior
  backward
  gingival
curvature of stomach
  greater
  lesser
curve
  anti-Monso
  buccal
  glucose tolerance
  sigmoid
curve of duodenum
curving of diaphyses
Curvularia geniculata
Curvularia lunata
Curvularia pallescens
Curvularia senegalensis
Curvularia verruculosa
Cushing disease
Cushing phenomenon
Cushing syndrome

Cushing ulcer
cushion of auditory tube
cushion, polar
cusp
  anterior
  aortic
  noncoronary
  posterior
  septal
  valve
cusp angle
cuspidate tooth
cuspid tooth
cusp of valve
Custer cells
custocolic fold
cutaneomucous muscle
cutaneous abscess
cutaneous angiomata
cutaneous atrophy
cutaneous bleb
cutaneous branch
cutaneous cervical nerve
cutaneous cyst
cutaneous defect
cutaneous ellipse
cutaneous emphysema
cutaneous erosion
cutaneous fissure
cutaneous gland
cutaneous horn
cutaneous larva migrans
cutaneous leishmaniasis
cutaneous lymphangioma
cutaneous muscle
cutaneous nerve
cutaneous nodule
cutaneous papilloma
cutaneous pigmentation
cutaneous pit
cutaneous plaque
cutaneous ridge
cutaneous schistosomiasis
cutaneous test
cutaneous tissue
cutaneous tuberculin test
cutaneous tumor
cutaneous twig
cutaneous ulcer
cutaneous vein
cutaneous wound
cutaneous zone
cuticle
  acquired
  dental
  enamel
cutis anserina (goose flesh)
cutis hyperelastica
cutis marmorata (marble skin)
cutis laxa
  acquired
  congenital
cutis rhomboidalis nuchae
cutis verticis gyrata (gyrate scalp)
cut surface
cutter tissue
Cuvier, canal of
CVA (cerebrovascular accident)
CVA (costovertebral angle)
C vitamin
CVP (central venous pressure) catheter
C wave
cyanide–nitroprusside test
cyanide poisoning
cyanide test
cyanmethemoglobin
cyanocobalamin
cyanosis
cyanotic induration
cyanotic kidney
cyclical changes
cyclic AMP (adenosine monophosphate)
cyclodextrin agar

cylindrical cells
cylindrical punch
cylindric epithelium
cylindroid aneurysm
cyst
  acoustic
  Baker
  Bartholin
  benign
  bland
  Blessig
  blue dome
  bone
  branchial
  branchial cleft
  bronchogenic
  calcification of
  cerebral
  chocolate
  corpus luteum
  cortical
  cutaneous
  dentigerous
  dermoid
  endometrial
  epidermal
  epidermal inclusion
  epithelial
  fluid-filled
  follicular
  functional ovarian
  ganglion
  germinal inclusion
  hemorrhagic
  hydatid
  inclusion
  joint
  lutein
  mammary
  meibomian
  mesothelial
  milk-filled

cyst *(continued)*
  morgagnian
  mucous
  müllerian
  multilocular
  multiloculated
  myxoid
  nabothian
  neoplastic
  non-neoplastic
  ovarian
  ovarian follicular
  pancreatic
  parasite
  paratubal
  parovarian
  pearl
  pericardial
  pilar
  pilonidal
  pineal
  pituitary
  primordial
  prostatic
  renal
  retention
  sebaceous
  serosal
  solitary bone
  tarsal
  testicular
  theca-lutein
  thin-walled
  thyroglossal duct
  unilocular
  wolffian
cyst adenocarcinoma
  mucinous
  serous
cystadenoma
Cysteine Albimi media
cysteine proteinase

cysteine test (see *cystine*)
cystic adenomatoid malformation
cystic artery
cystic degeneration
cystic duct
cystic duct lumen
cysticercosis
cystic eye
cystic fibrosis
cystic fistula
cystic fluid
cystic gall duct
cystic goiter
cystic kidney
cystic lymph node
cystic mastitis
cystic medial necrosis
cystic meningioma
cystic mole
cystic ovary
cystic plexus
cystic polyp
cystic swelling in a meibomian gland
cystic teratoma
cystic vein
cystine (also, cysteine)
cystine, amino acid
cystine calculi in urinary tract
cystine, lactose, electrolyte deficient (CLED)
cystine metabolism abnormalities
cystine stones
cystinuria
cystitis
  acute hemorrhagic
  hemorrhagic
  honeymoon
  interstitial
  radiation
cystocholedochal junction
cystochrome system
cystoduodenal ligament
cystohepatic triangle
cystoid degeneration
cystosarcoma phyllodes
cyst wall
Cytobrush
cytochromes
cytocrine secretion
cytogenetics
cytoid body
cytokeratin immunoreactivity
cytokine
cytokinesis
cytological biopsy
cytologically bland leiomyoma
cytologic atypia
cytologic diagnosis
cytologic report
cytologic smear
cytology
  cervical
  exfoliative
cytolysis
cytolysosome
cytomegalic cell
cytomegalic inclusion disease virus
cytomegalovirus
cytomegalovirus disease
cytomegalovirus encephalitis
cytomegalovirus pneumonitis
cytometer
  ARGUS flow
  CA II flow
  Cytoron Absolute flow
  ELITE Analyzer flow
  Epics Profile II flow
  FACScan flow
  PAS III flow
cytometry
cytopathic
cytoplasm
  eosinophilic
  eosinophilic homogeneous

cytoplasm *(continued)*
  foamy
  granular
  pale
  scanty
cytoplasmic bridge
cytoplasmic granule
cytoplasmic inclusion
cytoplasmic inclusion body
cytoplasmic matrix
cytoplasmic/nuclear ratio
cytoplasmic ratio
cytoplasmic staining
cytoplasmic stippling
cytoplasmic vacuole
Cytoron Absolute flow cytometer
cytoskeletal pathology
cytosol
cytosolic concentration
cytosolic fraction
cytospin preparation
Cytospray
cytotoxic cell
cytotoxic T cell
cytotoxic T lymphocyte
cytotoxicity
  antibody-dependent cell-mediated (ADCC)
  complement-mediated
  lymphocyte-mediated
cytotropic antibody test
cytotrophoblast
cytotrophoblastic cell
CZE (capillary zone electrophoresis)

D, d

D (delta)
D (dorsal)
dacryocyte (teardrop cell)
Dactylaria
Dade Paramax analyzer
dag (decagram)
DAKO AEC substrate/chromogen
DAKO glycergel
DAKO liquid DAB substrate/
  chromogen
DAKO target retrieval solution
daL (decaliter)
Dalen-Fuchs nodule
dam (decameter)
damage
  irreparable
  predator
damaged nerve tissue
damaged tissue
damol (decamole)
dancer's foot malformation
Dane and Herman keratin stain
Dane particle
Danlos-Ehlers syndrome
Danysz phenomenon
DA pregnancy test
Darier disease
dark cells
darkfield examination
darkfield microscope
dark green stool
dark stool
dark urine
Darrow red stain
dartoid tissue
dartos muscle
Darwin auricular tubercle
darwinian ear
darwinian tubercle
datum plane
Daudi cell
daughter cell
Davenport stain
Davidoff cell
Davidsohn differential absorption test
dawn phenomenon
Dawson encephalitis
Day test
DBP (vitamin D-binding protein)
DCC (deleted in colon carcinoma)
  tumor suppressor gene
D cell of pancreas
DCIS (ductal carcinoma in situ)
d-dimer (or D-dimer) test

dead
  brain
  pronounced
dead bowel
dead fetus in utero (DFU)
dead nerve
dead pulp
dead space
dead tooth
dead tract
deafness due to otosclerosis
deamidizing enzyme
death
  apparent
  black
  brain
  cell
  cerebral
  cot
  crib
  fetal (early, intermediate, late)
  functional
  genetic
  liver
  local
  molecular
  natural
  programmed cell
  SIDS (sudden infant d. syndrome)
  somatic
  sudden cardiac
  sudden infant d. symdrone (SIDS)
  unattended
  unsuspected cause of
  voodoo
death syndrome, sudden infant (SIDS)
DeBakey aortic classification
debilitated patient
debrancher (debranching) enzyme
debrancher (debranching) factor
Debré phenomenon
debrided
debridement tissue
debris
  amorphous
  cellular
  chemical
  fibrin
  fibrinous
  foreign
  keratin
  laminated keratotic
  necrotic
  pasty
  semisolid sebaceous
decagram (dag)
decalcification
decaliter (daL)
decamer
decameter (dam)
decamole (damol)
decapitation factor
Decaprime II
decay
decedent
decidua
  basal
  parietal
decidual cell
decidual fissure
deciduate placenta
deciduous membrane
deciduous skin
decigram (dg)
deciliter (dL)
decimeter (dm)
decimole (dmol)
decolorizer (see *stain*)
decompensated cirrhosis
decomposition
decoy cells
decubitus ulcer
deep artery of clitoris
deep auricular artery

deep brachial artery
deep cell
deep cervical artery
deep dorsal sacrococcygeal ligament
deep epigastric artery
deep external pudendal artery
deep fascia
deep fascia of penis
deep femoral artery
deep iliac circumflex artery
deep lingual artery
deep lingual vein
deep lymph vessel
deeply pigmented lesions in retina
deep palmar arch artery
deep penis artery
deep perineal pouch
deep plantar artery
deep plexus
deep posterior sacrococcygeal ligament
deep temporal artery
deep transverse metacarpal ligament
deep transverse metatarsal ligament
deep volar branch of ulnar artery
defect
    acquired
    aortic septal
    atrial septal
    birth
    coagulation
    congenital
    cortical
    fibrous cortical
    filling
    luteal phase
    neural tube
    pear-shaped
    pressure cone
    retention
    salt-losing
    septal
    ventricular septal
defective synthesis of hemoglobin
defective virus
deferens, ductus
deferent canal
deferent duct
deferential artery
deferential plexus
defibrinated blood
deficiency
    acquired immune
    adenosine deaminase
    adrenal cortical
    biotin-dependent carboxylase
    cobalamin
    congenital
    galactokinase
    immune
    iron
    oxygen
    plasma clotting factor
    platelet
    protein C
    thiamine
    transcobalamin 2
    vitamin
deficient production of red blood cells
definitive diagnosis
deformans
    osteitis
    osteochondrodystrophia
deformity
    Akerlund
    Arnold-Chiari
    bell clapper
    bone
    boutonnière
    contracture
    gibbous
    Erlenmeyer flask
    funnel-like
    gunstock
    Haglund

deformity *(continued)*
- J-sella
- keyhole
- lobster-claw
- Madelung
- mermaid
- parachute
- phrygian cap
- reduction
- seal-fin
- silver-fork
- Sprengel
- swan-neck
- torsional
- whistling
- Whitehead

deformity of bony digits
degenerate blood clot
degenerated blood
degenerating fibrils within neurons
degenerating neurons
degeneration
- Abercrombie
- adipose
- adiposogenital
- albuminous
- Alzheimer neurofibrillary
- amyloid
- angiolithic
- ascending
- atheromatous
- atrophic pulp
- axonal
- ballooning
- black
- bone
- bone marrow
- brain
- breast
- calcareous
- carneous
- cerebromacular (CMD)

degeneration *(continued)*
- cerebroretinal
- colloid
- comma
- corticostriatal-spinal
- Crooke hyaline
- cystic
- cystoid
- descending
- Doyne familial colloid
- Doyne honeycomb
- dystrophic
- earthy
- elastoid
- esophageal
- fascicular
- fatty
- fibrillary
- fibrinoid
- fibrinous
- fibroid
- gelatiniform
- glassy
- glistening
- glycogenic
- Gombault
- granulovacuolar
- gray matter
- heart
- hematohyaloid
- hepatic
- hepatolenticular
- hyaline
- hydropic
- lipoidal
- liquefaction
- liver
- macular
- malignant
- Mönckeberg
- mucinoid
- mucinous

degeneration *(continued)*
mucoid
mucous
muscular
myelinic
myxomatous
nerve
nerve cell
nerve tissue
neuronal
Nissl
optic
otic
pancreas
parenchymatous
periodontal
pigmental
pigmentary
primary progressive cerebellar
progressive
red
renal tubular
retinal
retrograde
rim
Rosenthal
sclerotic
secondary
senile
solar
spinal
spongiform
spongy
Stargardt macular
striatonigral
subacute combined
testicular
thyroid
trabecular
transneuronal
traumatic
Türck

degeneration *(continued)*
vacuolar
wallerian
Zenker waxy
degeneration of retinal ganglion cells
degeneration of sarcoplasm, vacuolar
degeneration of white substance of spinal cord
degenerative arthritic change
degenerative atrophy
degenerative changes
degenerative disk disease
degenerative joint disease (DJD)
degenerative liver
degenerative nephritis
degenerative osteoarthritis
degenerative spine disease
degenerative spondylosis
degenerative spur
deglutition mechanism
deglutition pneumonia
Degos disease
Dehio test
dehydration
dehydration fever
dehydrocholate test for speed of blood circulation
dehydroepiandrosterone (DHEA) test
dehydroepiandrosterone sulfate ($DHEA-SO_4$) test
dehydrogenase, alpha-ketoglutarate
deiterospinal tract
Deiters cell
Dejerine-Landouzy dystrophy
Dejerine-Landouzy muscular dystrophy
Dejerine-Sottas atrophy
Dejerine-Thomas atrophy
Delafield fluid
Delafield hematoxylin
Delafield hematoxylin stain
Delafield solution

delayed resolution of pneumonia
Delbet fracture classification
deletion
  chromosomal abnormality of
  interstitial
  terminal
delicate
delimited
delineate
delineation
delirium
delivery, postmortem
delomorphous cell
Del Rio Hortega method
delta-aminolevulinic acid
delta antigen (delta-Ag)
delta band
delta cell
delta granule
delta hepatitis (hepatitis D)
delta wave
deltoid artery
deltoid crest
deltoid eminence
deltoideopectoral trigone
deltoid impression
deltoid ligament
deltoid muscle
deltoid reflex
deltoid region
deltoid tuberosity
demarcation, corticomedullary
demifacet
demilune body
demilune cell
demineralized material
demyelinating disease of brain
demyelination and gliosis in central nervous system
demyelination of cerebral white matter
demyelination, segmental
demyelinization
denatured protein
dendrite, apical
dendritic cell
dendritic keratitis
dendritic process
dendritic reticular cell
denervated muscle atrophy
dengue
  classic
  hemorrhagic
  Philippine
dengue hemorrhage fever
dengue-like disease
dengue shock syndrome
dengue virus
Denis Browne superficial inguinal pouch
Denonvilliers fascia
Denonvilliers ligament
dens
dense connective tissue
density, bone mineral
dental abscess
dental alveolus
dental arch
dental artery
dental articulation
dental bulb
dental canal
dental caries
dental cord
dental crest
dental cuticle
dental fiber
dental follicle
dental groove
dental lamina
dental lymph
dental material
dental mottling
dental neck
dental nerve

dental plaque
dental polyp
dental process
dental pulp
dental ridge
dental root
dental root canal
dental sac
dental shelf
dental tubercle
dental tubule
dental tumor
dentate fascia
dentate fissure
dentate gyrus
dentate ligament of spinal cord
dentate line
dentate margin
dentate nucleus
dentate suture
dentatothalamic tract
denticulate hymen
denticulate ligament
dentigerous cyst
dentin
dentin globule
dentinal fiber
dentinal fluid
dentinal papilla
dentinal pulp
dentinal sheath
dentinal tubule
dentinocemental junction
dentinoenamel junction
dentoalveolar abscess
dentoalveolar articulation
dentoalveolar gomphosis
dentoalveolar joint
dentofacial zone
dentogingival lamina
denture basal surface
denture-bearing area
denture cell
denture foundation area
denture foundation surface
denture impression surface
denture occlusal surface
denture polished surface
denture-supporting area
denture-supporting structure
Denucé ligament
denudation
denude
denuded
Denver chromosome classification
Denys-Leclef phenomenon
D enzyme
11-deoxycortisol hormone
(Compound S)
11-deoxycorticosterone (DOC)
deoxyribonuclease (DNase) test
deoxyuridine suppression test
deparaffinization
dependent edema
dependent lividity
Depex mounting solution
depigmentation
depigmented lesion
depletion of colloid
depletion of fat stores
deposit, albuminous
deposition
collagen
fibrin
hemosiderin
melanin
pigment
deposition of calcium salts in kidney
tissue
deposition of mineral salts
deposition of mucoid material in
muscle
deposition of mucoid material in
subcutaneous tissue

deposition of unconjugated bilirubin
deposition of yellow or brown pigment
  granules in cytoplasm
depressed ejection fracture
depressed marrow
depressor fiber
depressor muscle
depressor nerve
depressor reflex
depth
de Quervain disease
de Quervain thyroiditis
derived protein
dermabrasion
dermal bone
dermal chromatophores
dermal lymphatic involvement
dermal melanocytoma
dermal microabscess
dermal nevus
dermal papilla (pl. papillae)
dermal sinus
dermal stria
dermal system
dermal tissue
dermal wart
dermatitis
  actinic
  allergic
  allergic contact
  ammonia
  Ancylostoma
  ashy
  atopic
  berlock
  blastomycetic
  brown-tail moth
  bubble gum
  cercarial
  chemical
  contact
  contact-type

dermatitis *(continued)*
  contagious pustular
  cosmetic
  dhobie mark
  diaper
  eczematous
  exfoliativa neonatorum
  exfoliative
  exudative
  exudative and lichenoid
  exudative discoid
  factitial
  grass
  industrial
  infectious eczematous
  insect
  irritant
  Jacquet
  Leiner
  lichenoid
  livedoid
  mango
  marine
  meadow
  meadow grass
  nickel
  nummular eczematous
  occupational
  onion mite
  papular (of pregnancy)
  papulovesicular
  perfume
  periocular
  perioral
  photoallergic contact
  phototoxic
  pigmented purpuric lichenoid
  plant
  poison ivy
  poison oak
  poison sumac
  precancerous

dermatitis *(continued)*
  primary irritant
  proliferative
  radiation
  rat-mite
  rhus
  sabra
  sandal strap
  scaly erythematous
  Schamberg
  schistosome
  seborrheic
  solar
  stasis
  swimmer's
  trefoil
  uncinarial
  verminous
  vesicular
  washerman's mark
  x-ray
dermatitis aestivalis
dermatitis atrophicans
dermatitis bullosa
dermatitis bullosa striata pratensis (grass)
dermatitis calorica
dermatitis combustionis (burn)
dermatitis congelationis (frostbite)
dermatitis gangrenosa infantum
dermatitis herpetiformis
dermatitis hiemalis
dermatitis medicamentosa (drug eruption)
dermatitis nodosa
dermatitis nodularis necrotica
dermatitis papillaris capillitii
dermatitis pediculoides ventricosus
dermatitis repens
dermatitis simplex
dermatitis vegetans
dermatitis venenata
dermatitis verrucosa
dermatofibroma
dermatofibrosarcoma
dermatofibrosarcoma protuberans
dermatofibrosis
dermatofibrosis lenticularis disseminata
dermatome
dermatomic area
dermatomycosis
dermatomyositis
dermatopathology
Dermatophilus
Dermatophilus congolensis
dermatophytic fungi
dermatophytid
dermatophytosis
dermatosis (pl. dermatoses)
  acarine
  acute febrile neutrophilic
  ashy
  Bowen precancerous
  chronic bullous
  dermolytic bullous
  digitate
  dyschromic
  industrial
  scaly
  transient acantholytic
  ulcerative
dermis
  papillary
  papillary layer of
  reticular
dermoepidermal interface
dermoepidermal junction
dermoid cyst
dermoid system
dermolytic bullous dermatosis
dermotropic virus
DES (diethylstilbestrol)
descemetocele
Descemet membrane

descending aorta
descending aorta artery
descending artery
descending branch of occipital artery
descending branch of uterine artery
descending colon
descending degeneration
descending duodenum
descending lymphangitis
descending neuritis
descending nucleus
descending palatine artery
descending part
descending pyelonephritis
descending scapular artery
descending thoracic aorta
descending tract
Deschamps needle
desiccate
desiccation
Desjardins point
desmoplakin protein
desmoplasia
desmoplastic malignant melanoma
desmoplastic response
desmoplastic stroma
desmosomal junction
desquamated cells
desquamation
desquamative interstitial pneumonia
desquamative pneumonia
destruction of tissue
detached retina
detachment, retinal
determinate cleavage
detrusor muscle
development, abnormalities of
developmental age
developmental anomaly
developmental groove
developmental line
Deventer pelvis
deviating eye
Devic disease
devitalized pulp
devitalized tissue
devoid
dewaxed
dewy appearance
dexamethasone single dose overnight suppression test
dexamethasone suppression test
dextran sulfate
dextrocardia
dextrose test
Dextrostix
DFA-TP test (direct fluorescent antibody-*Treponema pallidum* test)
DF-2 bacillus
DFU (dead fetus in utero)
dg (decigram)
D hemoglobin
D hepatitis
dhobie mark dermatitis
DI (diabetes insipidus)
diabetes
- adult onset
- borderline
- brittle
- bronze
- calcinuric
- chemical
- drug-induced
- gestational
- growth-onset
- insulinopenic
- juvenile onset
- ketosis-prone
- ketosis-resistant
- latent
- lipoatrophic
- lipogenous
- maturity-onset
- maturity-onset d. of youth (MODY)

diabetes *(continued)*
  maternal
  metahypophysial
  Mosler
  neurogenic
  obesity-associated
  overt
  pancreatic
  phosphate
  preclinical
  pregnancy
  puncture
  renal
  renal amino acid
  secondary
  starvation
  steroid
  steroidogenic
  subclinical
  thiazide
  type I insulin-dependent
  type II non-insulin-dependent
  uncontrolled
  vasopressin-resistant
  Young
diabetes innocens
diabetes insipidus (DI)
diabetes intermittens
diabetes mellitus (DM)
  adult-onset
  juvenile-onset
  type I, IDDM (insulin-dependent diabetes mellitus)
  type II, NIDDM (non-insulin-dependent diabetes mellitus)
  type II, NIDDM, non-obese
  type II, NIDDM, obese
diabetes mellitus classification
diabetes neonatorum
diabetic acidosis
diabetic amyotrophy
diabetic Charcot foot
diabetic colitis
diabetic coma
diabetic dermopathy
diabetic encephalopathy
diabetic foot
diabetic gangrene
diabetic gastroparesis
diabetic glomerulosclerosis
diabetic ketoacidosis
diabetic lipemia
diabetic microangiopathy
diabetic mother
diabetic myelopathy
diabetic nephropathy
diabetic neuroarthropathy of foot and ankle
diabetic neuropathy
diabetic peripheral neuropathy
diabetic polyneuropathy
diabetic polyradiculopathy
diabetic retinitis
diabetic retinopathy (DR)
diabeticogenic hormone
diabetic peripheral vascular insufficiency
diabetic third nerve palsy
diabetic ulcer
diabetogenic factor
diaceturia
diacetyl test for urea
diagnosis (pl. diagnoses)
  admitting
  antenatal
  clinical
  colposcopic
  cytologic
  definitive
  differential
  discharge
  empirical
  fetal
  final

diagnosis *(continued)*
  frozen section
  genetic
  gross
  histologic
  histopathological
  initial
  microscopic
  neonatal
  operative
  pathologic
  physical
  postoperative
  preliminary
  prenatal
  prenatal genetic
  preoperative
  presumptive
  principal
  provisional anatomic
  tentative
  ultrasound
  working
diagnosis by exclusion
diagnostic cascade
Diagnostic and Statistical Manual III—Revised (DSM-III-R)
diagnosis related group (DRG)
diagnostic imaging
diagnostic laparoscopy
diagnostic procedure
diagnostic radiation
diagnostic test
diagonal band of Broca
dialysis encephalopathy
diameter, anteroposterior
diaminobenzidine tetrahydrochloride
diamond-shaped conidia
diamond-shaped incision
Di antigen
diapedesis
diaper dermatitis
diaper rash dermatitis
diaphragm
  aponeurotic portion of
  arcuate ligaments of
  Bucky
  central tendon
  crus of
  dome of
  leaves of
  pelvic
  Potter-Bucky
  thoracoabdominal
  twigs to pelvic
  urogenital
diaphragmatic arch
diaphragmatic fascia
diaphragmatic hernia
diaphragmatic ligament
diaphragmatic node
diaphragmatic pleura
diaphragmatic pleurisy
diaphragmatic surface of liver
diaphragm of sella turcica
diaphyseal center
diaphyseal dysplasia
diaphysis (pl. diaphyses), curving of
diarrhea
  bacillary
  bloody
  chronic bacillary
  colliquative
  copious rice-water
  copious watery
  Dientamoeba
  dysenteric
  explosive
  lienteric
  mucous
  serous
  watery
diarrheal disease
diarrheal stool

diarthrodial cartilage
diarthrodial joint
diaspirin-cross-linked hemoglobin (CDLHb)
Dibothriocephalus latus
DIC (disseminated intravascular coagulation)
dichroic reflector
dichromate, potassium
dichuchwa
Dick intracutaneous test
Dick test for scarlet fever susceptibility
dicrotic notch
dicrotic pulse
dicrotic wave
didelphia, uterine
didelphic uterus
Diego blood group
Dientamoeba diarrhea
Dientamoeba fragilis
diener (morgue attendant)
Dientamoeba fragilis
dietary fat
Dieterle silver stain
dietetic neuritis
dietetic proteinuria
diethylstilbestrol (DES)
Dieulafoy lesion
Dieulafoy triad
Dieulafoy vascular malformation
differential count
    bone marrow
    leukocyte
    synovial fluid
    white blood cell
differential diagnosis
differential renal function test
differential sugars
differential test for infectious mononucleosis
differential threshold
differential ureteral catheterization test
differential white blood cell count
differentiated
differentiation, cluster of (CD)
diffuse abscess
diffuse dermal neutrophil infiltration
diffuse esophageal spasm
diffuse fibrotic reaction
diffuse ganglion
diffuse goiter
diffuse hair loss
diffuse idiopathic atrophy of skin
diffuse interstitial fibrosis
diffuse large cell lymphoma
diffuse lymphoma
diffuse meningoencephalitis
diffuse mixed small and large cell lymphoma
diffuse myelitis
diffuse necrosis
diffuse opacities
diffuse pleurisy
diffuse psoriasis
diffuse sclerosing osteomyelitis
diffuse septal cirrhosis
diffuse small cleaved cell lymphoma
diffuse toxic goiter
diffusely
diffusion capacity of lungs for carbon monoxide (DL_{CO})
diffusion capacity of lungs for oxygen (DLO_2)
diffusion capacity of lungs for single-breath ($DLCO_{SB}$)
diffusion capacity of lungs for steady state ($DLCO_{SS}$)
diffusion, double
digastric fossa
digastric groove
digastric impression
digastric muscle
digastric notch
digastric triangle

DiGeorge anomaly
digestive enzyme
digestive fluid
digestive tract
digestive tube
digit
  accessory
  webbed
digital artery
digital collateral artery
digital fossa
digital joint
digital process of fat
digital pulp
digital reflex
digital vein
digital web
digital whorl
digit, accessory
digit articulation
digitate dermatosis
digitation
dihydrotestosterone (DHT) test
1,25-dihydroxycholecalciferol assay (1,25-OH-D_3)
dihydroxyphenylalanine (DOPA)
dilatation
  cardiac
  cavitary
  gastric
  idiopathic
  post-stenotic
  prognathic
dilatation of duct or vessel
dilate
dilated
dilation, digital
dilator muscle
dilator pupillae
"dils" (dilutions)
diluent
diluted whole blood clot lysis
dilutional hyponatremia
dilution, serial
dimensions of specimen
diminution
dimorphic fungus
dineric interface
dinitrophenol poisoning
dinitrophenylhydrazine test
dioxide, carbon
DIP (desquamative interstitial pneumonia)
DIP (distal interphalangeal) joint
DiPAS-positive granule
diphtheria bacillus
diphtheria culture
diphtheria test
diphtheritic membrane
diphtheritic myocarditis
diphtheroids
diplococci, gram-negative intracellular (GNID)
diplococcus of Morax-Axenfeld
diplococcus of Neisser
Diplococcus pneumoniae
diploic artery
diploic canal
diploic vein
diploid nucleus
diplopia
dipslide, Uricult
dipstick
  Clinistix
  Combistix
  Glucostix
  Ketodiastix
  Labstix
  Multistix
  N-Multistix
  Uristix
direct antiglobulin test
direct bilirubin
direct Coombs test

direct embolism
direct fluorescent antibody–*Treponema pallidum* (DFA-TP) test
direct immunofluorescence
direct inguinal hernia
direct pyramidal tract
direct radioimmunoassay
direct-reacting bilirubin
direct transfusion
disarray
disc (from Latin *discus*) (see *disk*)
discernible
discharge
  cheesy
  copious
  curdlike
  foul
  frothy
  purulent
  serosanguineous
  scant
discharge diagnosis
discharging tubule
discission needle
discoid lupus erythematosus (LE)
discoidal cleavage
discoloration
discontinuation test
discrete objects
discrete tumor
discrete yellow masses in pus
disease
  Addison
  Albers-Schoenberg
  Alexander leukodystrophy
  allogeneic
  Alzheimer
  anhydride-induced immunologic respiratory
  anti-glomerular basement membrane (anti-GBM) antibody
  aorticorenal

disease *(continued)*
  Armanni-Ebstein
  autoimmune (collagen)
  Besnier-Boeck
  Besnier-Boeck-Schaumann
  Blount
  Boeck
  Bowman
  Bornholm
  bowel
  Bowen
  Brill-Zinsser
  Brinton
  Bruton
  Buerger
  Calvé-Perthes-Legg
  Canavan
  Canavan–van Bogaert–Bertrand
  cardiac
  cat-scratch
  celiac
  Chagas
  choked disk
  Christian-Hand-Schüller
  Christmas
  collagen
  combined system
  Creutzfeldt-Jakob
  Crohn
  Cushing
  cytomegalovirus
  Darier
  degenerative joint
  Degos
  demyelinating
  dengue-like
  de Quervain
  Devic
  diarrheal
  Duhring
  Ebola
  Ebstein-Armanni

disease *(continued)*
endocrine
Fabry
fibrocystic breast
fifth
foot, hand, and mouth
Freiberg
Gaucher
Gilchrist
Glanzmann
glycogen storage
Graves
Grover
Hailey-Hailey
Hallopeau
hand, foot, and mouth
Hand-Schüller-Christian
Hansen
Hartnup
Hashimoto
hemoglobin
hemolytic d. of newborn
hepatic
highly contagious sexually transmitted
Hirschsprung
Hodgkin
hyaline membrane
hydatid cyst
idiopathic
infectious
communicable
contagious
transmissible
inflammatory bowel
Jakob-Creutzfeldt
Jüngling
Kaposi
Kawasaki
Kienböck
Kimmelstiel-Wilson
Köhler (Koehler)

disease *(continued)*
Krabbe
Legg-Calvé-Perthes
legionnaire's
lethal
Letterer-Siwe
Lichtheim
life-threatening
linear IgA bullous
lumpy skin
Lyme
Majocchi
maple syrup urine
marble bone
Marburg
Marie-Strümpell
Merzbacher-Pelizaeus
metastatic
Mondor
Morquio
mouth, foot, and hand
myeloproliferative
neurodegenerative
Niemann-Pick
nonvenereal skin
Norwalk
Osgood-Schlatter
Osler-Weber-Rendu
osteochondritis dissecans
Paget
Panner
Parkinson
Pelizaeus-Merzbacher
pelvic inflammatory (PID)
Perthes-Legg-Calvé
Peyronie
Pick-Niemann
Pick
Pompe
Pott
primary
progressive

disease *(continued)*
- pulseless
- Quervain (also, de Quervain)
- reactive airways
- Recklinghausen (also, von Recklinghausen)
- renal
- Rendu-Osler-Weber
- respiratory syncytial
- Ritter
- Runeberg
- Sachs-Tay
- Scheuermann
- Schilder
- Schlatter-Osgood
- Schoenberg-Albers
- Schüller-Christian-Hand
- secondary
- Senear-Usher
- sexually transmitted (STD)
- sickle cell
- silo filler's
- Simmonds
- Siwe-Letterer
- smallpox-like
- Still
- storage
- streptococcal (of newborn)
- Strümpell-Marie
- Sweet
- systemic
- Takayasu
- Tay-Sachs
- thromboembolic
- Unna
- vascular
- von Gierke
- von Recklinghausen
- von Willebrand
- Weber-Rendu-Osler
- Weil
- Wilson-Kimmelstiel

disease *(continued)*
- Wilson
- woodworker lung's
- woolsorter's
- Zinsser-Brill

diseased kidney

dish, Petri

disk (Greek *diskus*) (also, *disc*)
- A
- acromioclavicular
- acromioclavicular joint
- anal
- anisotropic
- articular
- blastodermic
- Bowman
- cervical vertebral
- choked
- chorionic
- ciliary
- cone
- culture
- distal radioulnar joint
- embryonic
- emery
- germ
- germinal
- H
- hair
- Hensen
- herniated
- I
- intercalated
- intervertebral
- isotropic
- lumbar vertebral
- mandibular
- Merkel tactile
- noncontained
- optic
- placental
- Placido da Costa

disk *(continued)*
- protruded
- Q
- radioulnar
- Ranvier
- ruptured
- sequestered
- slipped intervertebral
- sternoclavicular joint
- temporomandibular joint
- thoracic vertebral
- transverse
- triangular
- vertebral

disk diffusion test for antibiotic sensitivity in bacteria
disk electrophoresis
disk kidney (disk-shaped)
disk sensitivity method
disorganization of connective tissue
disparity angle
disproportionately short limbs
disruption of nerve tracts
dissecans, osteochondritis
dissecting aneurysm of abdominal aorta
dissecting aneurysm of thoracic aorta
dissecting cellulitis of scalp
dissecting needle
dissection tubercle
disseminated condensing osteopathy
disseminated cutaneous gangrene
disseminated gonococcal infection
disseminated inflammation
disseminated intravascular coagulation (DIC)
disseminated lupus erythematosus (LE)
disseminated myelitis
disseminated tuberculosis
Disse space
dissociation
- albuminocytologic
- bacterial

distal bile duct
distal bulbar septum
distal clot
distal colon
distal convoluted tubule
distal duodenum
distal esophageal ring
distal interphalangeal (DIP) joint
distally
distal part
distal radioulnar articulation
distal radioulnar joint
distal surface
distal tibiofibular joint
distend
distended gallbladder
distention
distention of fibroblasts and macrophages by mucoid material
distinct
distortion of cells
distortion of fibrils within cell processes
distributing artery
disturbance
- metabolic
- respiratory

disuse atrophy
disuse osteoporosis
diurese
diuresis
diuretic agent
diuretic drug
diverging meniscus
diverticulitis
- colonic
- Meckel

diverticulum (pl. diverticula)
- bladder
- colonic
- cricopharyngeal
- esophageal

diverticulum *(continued)*
  Meckel
  metanephric
  pulsion
  traction
  urethral
  Zenker
diving goiter
division, mitotic
divisum, pancreas
DJD (degenerative joint disease)
dL (deciliter)
dm (decimeter)
DM (diabetes mellitus)
dmol (decimole)
DNA (deoxyribonucleic acid)
DNA analysis
DNA gap
DNA marker
DNA ploidy
DNA probe
DNA sequencing electrophoresis
DNA tumor virus
DNA tumor virus protein
DNA virus
DNA, wild-type
Döderlein bacillus (also, Doederlein)
dog-bite infections
Dogiel cells
Dogiel corpuscles
Döhle body (also, Doehle)
dolichopellic pelvis
dolorogenic zone
Dombrock blood group
dome cell
dome of diaphragm
dome of liver
dominance
dominant gene
dominant hemisphere
dominant trait
Donath-Landsteiner antibody
Donath-Landsteiner test for paroxysmal cold hemoglobinuria
donor blood
donor cells
donor kidney
donor organ
donor serum
donor sperm
Donovan bodies in monocytes
Donovania granulomatis
DOPA (dihydroxyphenylalanine) stain
d'orange, peau
Dorello canal
Dorothy Reed cell
dorsal (D)
dorsal antebrachial cutaneous nerve
dorsal aorta
dorsal arch, venous
dorsal artery
dorsal branch of posterior intercostal artery
dorsal calcaneocuboid ligament
dorsal carpal artery
dorsal carpal ligament
dorsal carpometacarpal ligament
dorsal cuboideonavicular ligament
dorsal cuneocuboid ligament
dorsal cuneonavicular ligament
dorsal interosseous artery
dorsal lingual vein
dorsal mesogastrium
dorsal metacarpal artery
dorsal metacarpal ligament
dorsal metatarsal ligament
dorsal nasal artery
dorsal nerve of penis
dorsal pancreatic bud
dorsal point
dorsal primary ramus
dorsal radiocarpal ligament
dorsal ramus (pl. rami) nerve
dorsal sacroiliac ligament

dorsal talonavicular bone
dorsal talonavicular ligament
dorsalis pedis
dorsal artery
dorsally
dorsi, latissimus
dorsispinal vein
dorsolateral fasciculus
dorsolateral placode
dorsolateral tract
dorsomedial hypothalamic nucleus
dorsomedial nucleus
dorsum of foot reflex
dorsum of penis
dorsum pedis reflex
dorsum sellae
dot-blot hybridization
dots
  Gunn
  Horner-Trantas
  Marcus Gunn
  Maurer
  Schüffner
  Trantas
  Ziemann
double-crush syndrome
double diffusion procedure
double gallbladder
double glucagon test
double-inlet left ventricle of heart
double-inlet right ventricle of heart
double-labeling immunocytochemistry
double-layered sheets of peritoneum
double-mouthed uterus
double-outlet left ventricle of heart
double-outlet right ventricle of heart
double penis
double pleurisy
double pneumonia
double-pointed needle
double tertian malaria
double uterus
double vagina
doughnut kidney
Douglas
  cul-de-sac of
  pouch of
Douglas abscess
Douglas fold
Douglas ligament
Douglas pouch suppuration
Douglas rectouterine pouch
Downey cell
Down syndrome
Doyne familial colloid degeneration
Doyne honeycomb degeneration
DR (diabetic retinopathy)
Drabkin solution
dracontiasis (Guinea worm)
Dracunculus medinensis
Dragendorff test for bile
drenching sweats
Dresbach syndrome
Dreulofoy lesion
dried-out material
dried smears of urine
drift, antigenic
dromedary kidney
droplet nucleus
droplet, respiratory
drop metastases
dropsy
drug, diuretic
drug fever
drug-induced diabetes
drug-induced hemolytic anemia
drugs of abuse, test on venous blood
  for
drum membrane
drusen
dry abscess
dry gangrene
dry joint
dry necrosis

dryness of mouth
dry pericarditis
dry pleurisy
dry scales (dandruff)
dry scaling
DSM-III-R (Diagnostic and Statistical Manual III—Revised)
DUB (dysfunctional uterine bleeding)
Dubin and Amelar varicocele classification
Dubin-Johnson syndrome
Dubois abscess
Duchenne-Aran muscular atrophy
Duchenne muscular dystrophy
Ducrey bacillus
Ducrey intradermal test
duct (see also *ductule*)
  aberrant
  aberrant bile
  accessory hepatic
  accessory pancreatic
  alveolar
  amniotic
  arterial
  Bartholin
  beaded hepatic
  bile
  biliary
  branchial
  bucconeural
  canalicular
  carotid
  choledochous
  cochlear
  common
  common bile (CBD)
  common gall
  common hepatic
  craniopharyngeal
  cystic
  cystic gall
  deferent

duct *(continued)*
  distal bile
  efferent
  ejaculatory
  endolymphatic
  excretory
  extrahepatic bile
  frontonasal
  galactophorous
  gall
  Gartner
  genital
  hepatic
  Hering
  His
  interlobular bile
  intrahepatic biliary
  lacrimal
  left hepatic
  lymph
  lymphatic
  main pancreatic
  middle extrahepatic bile
  müllerian
  obstruction of
  pancreatic
  paramesonephric
  paraurethral
  perilobular
  preampullary portion of bile
  prepapillary bile
  prostatic
  right hepatic
  Santorini
  Stensen
  subvesical
  terminal bile
  thoracic
  thyroglossal
  vitelline
  Wirsung
ductal aneurysm

ductal carcinoma
ductal carcinoma in situ (DCIS)
ductal cell
ductal duct
duct cell
duct cell carcinoma
duct ectasia
duct epithelial atypia
ductless gland
duct lumen
duct papilloma
duct system, intrahepatic
ductular element
ductule
  aberrant
  biliary
  excretory
ductule of testis, efferent
ductus arteriosus
  patent
  remnant of
ductus deferens
  ampulla of
  artery of
Duffy blood group
Duhring disease
Duke bleeding time test
Dukes classification of carcinoma
Dukes staging for colon carcinoma
Dulbecco modified Eagle medium
dullness, superficial cardiac
dumping syndrome
Duncan placenta
Duncan ventricle, fifth ventricle
duodenal ampulla
duodenal artery
duodenal bulb, apex of
duodenal C-loop
duodenal cap
duodenal contents examination
duodenal end of dorsal pancreatic duct
duodenal end of main pancreatic duct
duodenal fold
duodenal fossa
duodenal gland
duodenal impression on liver
duodenal ligament
duodenal loop
duodenal lumen
duodenal papilla
duodenal recess
duodenal sphincter, first
duodenal stump
duodenal sweep
duodenal ulcer
duodenal vein
duodenal villi
duodenal web
duodenojejunal angle
duodenojejunal flexure
duodenojejunal fold
duodenojejunal fossa
duodenojejunal junction
duodenojejunal recess
duodenojejunal sphincter
duodenomesocolic fold
duodenorenal ligament
duodenum
  C-loop of
  curve of
  descending
  distal
  supravaterian
  suspensory muscle of
duplex kidney
DuPont ACA analyzer
Dupuytren canal
dural septa
dural sheath
dural sinus
dura mater
Duran-Reynals permeability factor
Duran-Reynals spreading factor
Duret lesion

dust-borne infection
dust cell
dust corpuscle
Dutton relapsing fever
Duverney foramen
Duverney gland
D vitamin
dwarfism
  achondroplastic
  deprivation
  Lorain-Lévi
  pituitary
  renal
  Russell-Silver
  Walt Disney
dwarf pelvis
dwarf tapeworm
D-xylose absorption test
D-xylose tolerance test
dye
  blue aniline
  phenanthridium
  synthetic azo
  Taq
  vital
dye exclusion test
dye-tagged substrate
DynaBeads
dynamic aorta
dynamic/spastic ileus
dyschromic dermatosis
dyscrasia
dysenteric algid malaria
dysenteric diarrhea
dysentery
  amebic
  bacillary
dysfunctional uterine bleeding (DUB)
dysgerminoma
dysgranular cortex
dyshidrotic eczema
dyskeratoma
dyskeratosis
dyskeratotic cells with inclusions
dysmenorrheal membrane
dysmorphic
dysmotility
dysostosis, mandibulofacial
dysphagia
dysplasia
  bone
  bronchopulmonary
  cervical
  diaphyseal
  ectodermal
  epithelial
  fibromuscular
  fibrous
  low-grade
  mammary
  metaphyseal
  mild
  moderate
  retinal
  severe
  thymic
dysplastic epithelium
dysplastic nevus
dyspnea
dyssebacia (also, dyssebacea)
dystrophic calcification
dystrophic calcinosis
dystrophic degeneration
dystrophy
  Becker
  Dejerine-Landouzy
  Duchenne muscular
  Emery-Dreifuss muscular
  Erb muscular
  Fuchs
  Fukuyama
  Gowers muscular
  infantile neuroaxonal (INAD)
  Landouzy-Dejerine muscular

dystrophy *(continued)*
- muscular (MD)
- otic
- progressive muscular (PMD)
- thoracic-pelvic-phalangeal
- vulvar

dystrophy-dystocia syndrome (DDS)

E, e

ear
- artificial
- auricula dextra
- aviator's
- Aztec
- cauliflower
- cockleshell
- constricted
- cup
- darwinian
- diabetic
- external
- glue
- hairy
- inflammation of
- inner
- middle
- Morel
- Mozart
- ossicles of
- outer
- prizefighter's
- protruding
- swimmer's
- telephone
- tin
- tropical

ear canal
eardrum
earlobe adipose tissue
early pneumonitis
ear, nose, and throat (ENT) examination
earthy degeneration
easily compressible nodule
eastern equine encephalitis antibody
"eating cell" (phagocyte)
Eaton agent
Eaton agent pneumonia
Eberth bacillus
Eberth line
Ebner gland
Ebner line
Ebner reticulum
Ebola disease
Ebola hemorrhagic fever
Ebola virus
Ebstein-Armanni disease
Ebstein lesion
eburnated bone
eburnation
ECC (endocervical curettage)
eccentric atrophy
eccentric nuclei

eccentrically
ecchymosis (pl. ecchymoses)
eccrine gland
ecdysial gland
echinococcosis
Echinococcus granulosus
echinocyte
ECHO (enterocytopathogenic human orphan) virus
ECHO infection
Eck fistula
ECL cell (enterochromaffin-like)
ECLT (euglobulin clot lysis time)
ECM (extracellular matrix)
E. coli (Escherichia coli)
E. coli serotype O157:H7
ectasia, ductal (of breast)
ectatic aneurysm
ecthyma, contagious
ecthyma gangrenosum
ectoblast
ectocervical surface
ectoderm
ectodermal dysplasia
ectopia
ectopically
ectopic endometrium
ectopic pregnancy
ectopic testis
ectopic tissue
ectoplasm
ectropion
eczema
  allergic
  atopic
  baker's
  chronic
  dyshidrotic
  facial
  flexural
  hand
  infantile

eczema *(continued)*
  lichenoid
  seborrheic
  stasis
  tropical
  varicose
  vascular
  weeping
  winter
eczema craquelé ("marred with cracks")
eczema diabeticorum
eczema epilans (with hair loss)
eczema erythematosum
eczema herpeticum (herpesvirus type 1)
eczema hypertrophicum (lichenoid eczema)
eczema papulosum
eczema parasiticum
eczema pustulosum
eczema rubrum
eczema squamosum
eczema tyloticum
eczema vaccinatum
eczema verrucosum
eczema vesiculosum
eczematization
eczematoid
eczematous dermatitis
eczematous plaques
eddy (pl. eddies)
edema
  ambulant
  angioneurotic
  bronchiolar
  bronze
  cardiac
  cerebral
  dependent
  epithelial
  focal
  generalized

edema *(continued)*
gestational
heat
hereditary angioneurotic
ileocecal
inflammatory
laryngeal
local
lymphatic
lymphedema
malignant
massive pulmonary hemorrhagic
osmotic
patchy intercellular
periorbital
pitting
premenstrual
presacral
pretibial
pulmonary
Quincke
renal
visceral
edema neonatorum
edema of parotid glands
edematous brain
edematous kidneys
edge
ligament reflecting
ligament shelving
liver
Poupart ligament shelving
Edmondson grading system
EDRF (endothelium-derived relaxing factor)
EDTA (ethylenediaminetetraacetic acid)
Edwardsiella
Edwardsiella tarda
effect
estrogen
isomorphic
effect *(continued)*
mass
Somogyi
effector cell
effects of poisoning
efferent arteriole
efferent duct
efferent ductule of testis
efferent fiber
efferent glomerular arteriole
efferent limb
efferent loop
efferent lymph vessel
efferent lymphatic vessel
efferent nerve
efferent vessel
effluvium
effort proteinuria
effusion
bloodstained
hemorrhagic
pericardial
pleural
pleuropericardial
serous
subdural
EG (esophagogastric) junction
EGD (esophagogastroduodenoscopy)
EGFR (epidermal growth factor receptor)
egg cell
egg membrane
egg yolk agar
eggs in intestinal venules
Eglis gland
E hemoglobin
E hepatitis
Ehlers-Danlos syndrome
Ehrlich acid hematoxylin stain
Ehrlich granule
Ehrlichia canis
Ehrlichia chaffeensis

Ehrlichia sennetsu
Ehrlich neutral stain
ehrlichiosis, human granulocytic (HGE)
Ehrlich triacid stain
Eichhorst atrophy
Eichhorst neuritis
Eikenella corrodens (formerly *Bacteroides corrodens*, HB-1)
Eisenmenger complex
ejaculatory duct
ejection fraction
Ektachem analyzer
elastica–van Gieson stain
elastic artery
elastic cartilage
elastic fiber
elastic fibers stain (Weigert)
elasticity
elastic lamella
elastic lamina
elastic lattices
elastic layer
elastic ligature
elastic membrane
elastic skin
elastic stain
elastic tissue
elastic web
elastin
elastoid degeneration of arteries
elastosis
  nodular
  senile
  solar
elbow articulation
elbow bone
elbow joint
elbow reflex
electrical energy
electrical shock
electric coagulation
electrode pad
electrolyte
  serum
  sweat
  testing
  test on venous blood for
  urine
electrolyte balance
electrolyte metabolism
electrolyte panel
electrolytes, consisting of
  bicarbonate
  calcium
  chloride
  potassium
  sodium
electron microscope
electron microscopy
electrophoresis
  agarose gel
  capillary zone (CZE)
  carrier
  cellulose acetate
  disk
  DNA sequencing
  free
  gel
  hemoglobin
  isoenzyme
  lipoprotein
  paper
  polyacrylamide gel (PAGE)
  protein
  pulsed-field gel
  SDS-polyacrylamide gel (SDS-PAGE)
  serum protein
  thin-layer
  two-dimensional gel
  urinary protein
electrophoretically
electrotonic current

electrotonic junction
electrotonic synapse
element
  ductal
  ductular
  end-ductal
  epithelial
  lobular
  stromal
elementary body
elementary cell
elementary granule
elementary particle
elephantiasis
elephantoid fever
elevation, frontonasal
ELISA (enzyme-linked immunosorbent assay)
ELITE Analyzer flow cytometer
ellipse of skin
ellipsoid
ellipsoid joint
ellipsoidal articulation
elliptic
elliptical
elliptocyte
elliptocytosis, hereditary
Ellison-Zollinger syndrome
Ellsworth-Howard test
elongate pattern
elongated mass
elongated structure
eluate
eluent
elute
elution
EMA (epithelial membrane antigen)
emanation, actinium
embalm
embalmer
embalming fluid
embed
embedded
embedding medium
embedding of tissue specimen
emboli (pl. of embolus)
embolic phenomenon
embolic pneumonia
emboliform nucleus
embolism (also called *embolus*)
  air
  amniotic fluid
  arterial stenosis
  atheromatous
  bacillary
  bland
  bone marrow
  cancer
  capillary
  cardiogenic
  catheter-induced
  cellular
  cerebral
  cholesterol
  coronary artery
  cotton-fiber
  crossed
  direct
  fat
  fibrin platelet
  foam
  gas
  gas nitrogen
  hematogenous
  infective
  intraluminal
  lymphogenous
  massive
  miliary
  multiple
  obturating
  occluding spring
  oil
  pantaloon

embolism *(continued)*
- paradoxical
- peripheral
- plasmodium
- prosthetic valve
- pulmonary (PE)
- pulmonary venous–systemic air
- pyemic
- recurrent
- renal cholesterol
- retinal
- retrograde
- riding
- septic
- septic pulmonary
- straddling
- submassive pulmonary
- thrombus
- trichinous
- tumor
- venous
- visceral

embolus (pl. emboli)
embryo, frozen
embryonal area
embryonal carcinoma
embryonal cell carcinoma
embryonic area
embryonic axis
embryonic blastoderm
embryonic cell
embryonic development
embryonic disk
embryonic membrane
embryonic mesenchymal cell
embryonic ovary
embryonic sac
embryonic shield
embryonic thyroglossal duct
embryonic truncus arteriosus
embryonic umbilical vein
emery disk
emesis
emetic
eminence
- arcuate
- articular
- collateral
- cruciate
- cruciform
- deltoid
- facial
- frontal
- genital
- hypothenar
- iliopubic
- intercondylar
- median
- occipital
- pyramidal
- thenar
- thyroid

emiocytosis
emissary sphenoidal foramen
emissary vein
emphysema
- bullous
- centrilobular
- cutaneous
- interstitial
- panlobular
- pulmonary
- pulmonary subcutaneous

emphysematous bleb
emphysematous bulla
emphysematous lungs
empirical diagnosis
empty sella syndrome
empyema
emulsion proteinuria
en bloc
en cuirasse
en face
en masse

ENA (extractable nuclear antigen)
enamel cap
enamel cell
enamel cleavage
enamel crypt
enamel cuticle
enamel epithelium
enamel fiber
enamel fissure
enamel-forming cells
enamel lamella
enamel layer
enamel ledge
enamel membrane
enamel niche
enamel organ
enamel pearl
enamel projection
enamel pulp
enamel wall
enanthema
enarthrodial joint
encapsulated abscess
encapsulated subdural hematoma
encasing cell
encephalic vesicle
encephalitis
  acute necrotizing
  bunyavirus
  California
  cytomegalovirus
  Dawson
  Eastern equine
  hemorrhagic
  HIV
  Japanese B
  La Crosse
  measles
  mumps
  St. Louis
  Strümpell-Leichtenstern
  tick-borne

encephalitis *(continued)*
  Venezuela equine
  viral
  Western equine
encephalitogenic protein
encephalocele
encephalomalacia
encephalomyelonic axis
encephalomyelitis
encephalomyocarditis virus
encephalopathy
  AIDS
  boxer's
  dialysis
  hepatic
  HIV
  hypoxic
  Korsakoff
  metabolic
  myoclonic
  spongiform
  Wernicke
enchondral bone
enchondral ossification
encircle
encrusted
en cuirasse, carcinoma
encysted pleurisy
endarteritis, obliterative
end artery
end bud
end bulb, Krause
end-ductal element
endemic goiter
endemic hematuria
endemic typhus
endocardial fibrosis
endocardial tumor
endocarditis
  atypical verrucous
  fungal
  infective

endocarditis *(continued)*
- Libman-Sacks verrucous
- rheumatic
- Sacks-Libman
- subacute bacterial

endocardium
endocervical canal
endocervical cell
endocervical curettage
endocervical epithelium
endocervical gland
endocervical mucosa
endocervical smear
endocervical tissue
endochondral bone
endocranium
endocrine atrophy
endocrine gland
endocrine system
endoderm
endodermal cell
endodermal pouch
endoepithelial gland
endogenous fiber
endogenous infection
endogenous lipoid pneumonia
endogenous obesity
endogenous pigment
endolymphatic duct
endolymphatic sac
endometrial adenocarcinoma
endometrial atrophy
endometrial biopsy
endometrial cavity
endometrial curettage
endometrial cyst
endometrial gland
endometrial hyperplasia
endometrial polyp
endometrial sampling
endometrial smear
endometrial stroma
endometrial stromal sarcoma
endometriosis
endometritis
endometrium
- atrophic
- bland
- cystic hyperplasia of
- late secretory
- menstrual
- mixed phase
- progestational
- proliferative
- proliferative phase
- secretory

endomyocardial fibrosis
endomysial antibody
endomysium
endopelvic fascia
endoplasm
endoplasmic reticulum
end organ
endoscope
endosteum
endothelial cell
endothelial leukocyte
endothelial proliferation
endothelial relaxing factor
endothelial space
endothelial swelling
endothelial tissue
endothelin-1 peptide
endothelium
endothelium-derived relaxing factor (EDRF)
endothoracic fascia
endothoracic tube
endotoxin-induced mediator
endotracheal (ET) tube
end piece
end plate
end point
end-stage renal disease

energy
  electrical
  kinetic
  radiant
  thermal
en face
engorged
engorgement
  splenic
  vascular
engorgement of tissues with blood
enhanced polymer one-step method of labeling
enlarged marrow cavities
enlargement
  heart
  liver
  skull
  spleen
en masse
enolase, neuron-specific
ensheathing callus
ensiform appendix
ensiform cartilage
ensiform process
Entamoeba histolytica
enteric bacillus
enteric fever
enteric orphan viruses
enteric plexus
enteritis, regional
Enterobacter (formerly *Aerobacter*)
Enterobacter aerogenes
Enterobacter agglomerans
Enterobacter cloacae
Enterobacter gergoviae
Enterobacter hafniae
Enterobacter liquefaciens
Enterobacter sakazakii
enterobacterial common antigen (ECA)
enterobiasis
Enterobius vermicularis
enterochromaffin cell
Enterococcus (pl. *Enterococci*)
Enterococcus avium
Enterococcus faecalis
Enterococcus faecium
enterocolitis, pseudomembranous
enterocytopathogenic human orphan (ECHO) virus
enteroendocrine cell
enterogenic proteinuria
enterogenous methemoglobinemia
enteroinsular axis
enteropathy, asymptomatic gluten-sensitive
enterotome
enterotoxin
enterovaginal fistula
Enterovirus, enterovirus
entodermal canal
entodermal cell
entodermal cloaca
entodermal pouch
entoplasm (endoplasm)
entorhinal area
entry zone
enveloped virus
enzymatic
enzyme
  acetyl-activating
  acetylcholinesterase
  adaptive
  angiotensin converting (ACE)
  autolytic
  beta-carotene cleavage
  brancher
  branching
  CK
  D
  deamidizing
  debranching
  digestive
  extracellular

enzyme *(continued)*
  lactase
  lipase
  lipolytic
  liver (glucuronosyltransferase)
  muscle
  pancreatic
  proteinase
  proteolytic
  uroporphyrinogen-1-synthetase
enzyme activity
enzyme hyaluronidase, streptococcal
enzyme-linked immunosorbent assay (ELISA)
enzyme panel
"eo" (eosinophil)
eosin azure
eosin, hematoxylin and (H&E)
eosinopenia
eosinophil count
eosinophil granule
eosinophilia
eosinophilic crystalloid
eosinophilic cytoplasm
eosinophilic gastroenteritis
eosinophilic granuloma
eosinophilic homogeneous cytoplasm
eosinophilic hyaline
eosinophilic leukemia
eosinophilic leukocyte
eosinophilic meningitis
eosinophilic myocarditis
eosinophilic pneumonia
eosinophil leukocyte
eosinophil smear
eosin-phloxine
eosin stain
EP (erythrocyte protoporphyrin) test
epactal bone
epactal ossicle
epamniotic cavity
eparterial bronchus
ependyma
ependymal cell
ependymal layer
ependymal lining
ependymal zone
ephelides (freckles)
ephemeral fever
ephemeral pneumonia
epicanthal fold
epicardial
epicardium
epicolic lymph node
epicondyle
epicranial aponeurosis
epicranial muscle
epicranius
Epics Profile II flow cytometer
epidemic cerebrospinal meningitis
epidemic hemorrhagic fever
epidemic keratoconjunctivitis
epidemic keratoconjunctivitis virus
epidemic parotitis
epidemic pleurodynia
epidemic typhus
epidermal atrophy
epidermal carcinoma
epidermal cyst
epidermal growth factor
epidermal growth factor receptor (EGFR)
epidermal growth factor–urogastrone
epidermal hyperplasia
epidermal inclusion cyst
epidermal ridge
epidermal tissue
epidermal ulceration
epidermic cell
epidermidization
epidermis
  centrally slightly thickened
  pigmented
  superficial

epidermoid carcinoma
epidermolysis bullosa, acquired
Epidermophyton
Epidermophyton floccosum
Epidermophyton stockdaleae
epididymis
  appendix of
  body of
  edema of
  inflammation of
  interstitial congestion of
  ligament of
  lobule of
  sinus of
  tail of
epididymitis
epidural abscess
epidural cavity
epidural hemorrhage
epidural space
epifluorescence
epigastric angle
epigastric artery
epigastric fold
epigastric fossa
epigastric lymph node
epigastric reflex
epigastric region
epigastric vein
epiglottic cartilage
epiglottic tubercle
epiglottis
epiglottiditis
epihyal bone
epihyal ligament
epi-illumination
epilation
epileptogenic zone
epinephrine
epineurium
epiotic center
epipapillary membrane
epipericardial ridge
epiphyseal artery
epiphyseal cartilage
epiphyseal cartilage plate
epiphyseal cartilaginous zone
epiphyseal ischemic necrosis
epiphyseal line
epiphyseal plate
epiphysis (pl. epiphyses)
  annular
  atavistic
  capital
  hypertrophy of
  pressure
  slipped
  stippled
  traction
epiphysis cerebri
epiphysis of long bone
  bulky
  irregularly calcified
  knobby
epiploic abscess
epiploic appendage
epiploic appendices
epiploic foramen, node of
epipteric bone
episcleral artery
episcleral lamina
episcleral space
episcleral tissue
episcleral vein
epispadias
epistaxis
episternal bone
epistropheus
epithelial adenoma
epithelial body
epithelial bridging
epithelial cast
epithelial cell
epithelial choroid layer

epithelial cyst
epithelial dysplasia
epithelial edema
epithelial element
epithelial hyperplasia
epithelial keratinization
epithelial lamina
epithelial layer
epithelial lining
epithelial membrane antigen (EMA)
epithelial neoplasm
epithelial nests
epithelial plug
epithelial reticular cell
epithelial tissue
epithelial "pearls" of keratinous debris
epithelioid cell
epithelioid granulomas
epithelioma, basal cell
epitheliosis
epithelium
  acetowhite
  Barrett
  ciliated
  ciliated columnar
  ciliated respiratory-type
  columnar
  columnar metaplasia of
  crypt
  cuboidal
  cylindric
  dysplastic
  enamel
  endocervical
  germinal
  glandular
  junctional
  keratinizing squamous
  low columnar
  metaplastic squamous
  nonkeratinizing
  perineural

epithelium *(continued)*
  pseudostratified
  pseudostratified columnar
  respiratory
  secretory
  simple
  simple columnar
  simple cuboidal
  simple squamous
  squamous
  squamous cell
  stratified
  stratified columnar
  stratified cuboidal
  stratified squamous
  stratified transitional
  surface
  tall columnar
  transitional
epithelium adenocarcinoma
epithelium fluid
epithelium-lined mastoid air cell
epithelium-lined tubular structure
epitrichial layer
epitrochlear node
epituberculous infiltration
epitympanic recess
epitympanic space
epivaginal connective tissue
Epon embedding medium
Eppendorf tube
Epstein-Barr virus
Epstein nephrosis
epulis
Eq (equivalent)
equatorial cleavage
equatorial plate
equina, cauda
equine encephalitis
  Eastern
  Venezuelan
  Western

equivalent (Eq)
ERA (estrogen receptor assay)
Erb atrophy
Erdheim cystic medial necrosis
Erb muscular dystrophy
erectile nodule
erectile tissue
erector muscle of penis
erector muscle of spine
erector spinal reflex
Erlanger and Gasser peripheral nerve classification
Erlenmeyer flask deformity
erogenous zone
erosion
  cervical
  cutaneous
  tumor
erosion of epiphyseal bone
erosive
E-rosette test
erotogenic zone
eruption
  pruritic
  purpuric cutaneous
erysipelas
erysipeloid
Erysipelothrix rhusiopathiae
erythema
  cold
  Jacquet
  "slapped cheek"
erythema ab igne
erythema and scaling, papular
erythema chronicum migrans
erythema infectiosum (fifth disease)
erythema marginatum
erythema migrans
erythema multiforme
erythema nodosum
erythema nodosum leprosum
erythema simplex
erythematosus
  discoid lupus
  lupus (LE)
  systemic lupus (SLE)
erythematous lesion
erythematous patches, itchy
erythrasma, Baerensprung
erythroblast
erythroblastosis fetalis
erythrocyte
  broken-down
  incubation
  nucleated
  sickle-shaped
  teardrop-shaped
erythrocyte adherence test
erythrocyte agglutinin
erythrocyte antigen
erythrocyte fragility
erythrocyte index
erythrocyte maturation factor
erythrocyte progenitor cell
erythrocyte protoporphyrin (EP) test
erythrocyte sedimentation rate (ESR)
erythrocytopenia
erythrocytosis
erythroderma
erythrohepatic porphyria
erythroid cell
erythroid hyperplasia of bone marrow
erythroplasia of Queyrat
erythropoiesis
erythropoietic hormone
erythropoietic porphyria
erythropoietin
eschar at site of mite bite
Escherich bacillus
Escherichia coli (*E. coli*)
Escherichia fergusonii
Escherichia hermannii
Escherichia vulneris
esophageal A ring

esophageal acid infusion test
esophageal artery of aorta
esophageal artery of inferior thyroid
esophageal atresia
esophageal B ring
esophageal body
esophageal candidiasis
esophageal degeneration
esophageal diverticulum
esophageal gland
esophageal groove
esophageal hiatal hernia
esophageal hiatus
esophageal impression
esophageal inlet
esophageal lumen
esophageal mucosal ring
esophageal opening
esophageal plexus of nerves
esophageal ring, distal
esophageal spasm, diffuse
esophageal sphincter
  hypertensive
  inferior
esophageal stenosis
esophageal varix (pl. varices)
esophageal vein
esophageal web
esophagitis
esophagogastric (EG) junction
esophagogastric orifice
esophagogastric vestibule
esophagogastroduodenoscopy (EGD)
esophagosalivary reflex
esophagospasm
esophagostenosis
esophagotracheal (ET) junction
esophagus
  achalasia of
  Barrett
  B ring of
  nutcracker

espundia
ESR (erythrocyte sedimentation rate)
essential amino acid
essential fatty acid (EFA)
essential fever
essential hematuria
essential hypertension
essential proteinuria
essential pruritus
Essick cell band
established cell line
esterase
  alpha naphthol
  C1
  leukocyte (LE)
  naphthol-ASD chloroacetate
esthesiodic system
estradiol hormone
estradiol test
estriol (E_3) hormone
  free
  total
estrogen
  serum
  total
  urinary
estrogen effect
estrogen level, urine
estrogen receptor assay (ERA)
estrogenic hormone
estrogenic stimulation
estrone (E_1) test
ethanol intoxication
ethanolism
ethidium bromide
ethmoidal air cell
ethmoid, alae of
ethmoidal artery
ethmoidal bulla
ethmoidal cell
ethmoidal crest
ethmoidal foramen

ethmoidal groove
ethmoidal labyrinth
ethmoidal notch
ethmoidal process
ethmoidal roof of nasal cavity
ethmoidal sinus
ethmoidal vein
ethmoid angle
ethmoid bone
ethmoid canal
ethmoid infundibulum
ethmoidolacrimal suture
ethmoidomaxillary suture
ethmovomerine plate
ethyl alcohol
ethylenediaminetetraacetic acid
  (EDTA)
ET-NANB (enterically transmitted
  non-A, non-B) hepatitis
Eubacterium alactolyticum
Eubacterium lentum
Eubacterium limosum
euglobulin clot lysis
euglobulin clot lysis time (ECLT)
euglobulin lysis test
euglycemia
eukaryosis
euplastic lymph
European blastomycosis
eustachian canal
eustachian tube
eustachian valve
evanescent
eversion, cervical
Ewingella
Ewing sarcoma
Ewing tumor
ExacTech blood glucose meter
examination
  cursory
  darkfield
  duodenal contents
examination *(continued)*
  external
  gross
  internal
  microscopic
  physical
  postmortem
  urine
exanthem (also, exanthema)
  Boston
  maculopapular
  mosquito-borne febrile
  papular
  pustular
  vesicular
  viral
exanthema subitum
exanthematous fever
exanthematous necrosis
excavatum, pectus
excessive absorption and impaired
  excretion of copper
excessive intake of iron
excessive loss of water due to diuresis
excessive loss of water due to sweating
excessive loss of water due to vomiting
exchange transfusion
excise
excision
excisional biopsy
excitable area
excitable cell
excitor nerve
excitoreflex nerve
excoriation
excrescence
  curdlike
  nodular
excretion of 5-hydroxyindoleacetic acid
  (5-HIAA), urinary
excretion of carbon dioxide,
  pulmonary

excretion of coproporphyrin, urinary
excretion of delta-aminolevulinic acid
excretion of hydrogen ion, renal
excretion of water, increased renal
excretion, urinary 17-ketosteroid
excretory duct
excretory ductule
excretory gland
excretory system
executive profile
exercise bone
exfoliate
exfoliation
exfoliativa neonatorum, dermatitis
(staphylococcal scalded skin
syndrome)
exfoliative cytology
exfoliative dermatitis
exhaustion atrophy
exhaustive blood grouping
Exner-Call bodies
exoccipital bone
exocelomic membrane
exocervical tissue
exocrine gland
exocytosis
exodic nerve
exogenous fiber
exogenous obesity
exogenous pigment
exogenous pneumonia
Exophiala dermatitidis
Exophiala heteromorpha
Exophiala jeanselmei
Exophiala spinifera
exophthalmic goiter
exophthalmos-producing substance
exophytic
expansion arch
expansion of duct or vessel
expansion of the cerebral ventricles
expiration
expire
expired
exploratory biopsy
exploratory laparotomy
explosive diarrhea
exsanguination transfusion
Exserohilum rostratum
exstrophy of bladder
extension, gland neck
extensor aponeurosis
extensor carpi ulnaris sheath
extensor retinacular
externa muscularis
externa
otitis
theca
external acoustic meatus
external anal sphincter
external auditory canal
external auditory meatus
external biliary ductule
external carotid artery
external clot
external collateral ligament of wrist
external ear
external examination
external genitalia
external hemorrhoid
external iliac lymph node
external intercostal membrane
external intercostal muscle
external ligament
external maxillary artery
external oblique muscle
external oblique reflex
external os, cervical
external pillar cell
external pubic artery
external pudendal artery
external pudendal branches
of femoral artery
external pudendal vein

external ring, apex of
external spermatic artery
external urethral opening
external urethral orifice
extracapsular ligament
extracellular enzyme
extracellular fluid
extracellular matrix (ECM)
extracellular tissue
extrachromosomal gene
extracorporeal circulation
extractable nuclear antibody
extractable nuclear antigen (ENA)
extradural abscess
extradural hemorrhage
extraembryonic blastoderm
extraembryonic celom
extraembryonic mesoderm
extrahepatic bile duct
extrahepatic biliary duct
extrahepatic biliary system
extraintestinal
extramedullary hematopoiesis
  in liver and spleen
extranodal
extraosseous osteosarcoma
extraperitoneal fascia
extraperitoneal fat
extraperitoneal organ
extraperitoneal tissue
extrapyramidal motor system
extrauterine pregnancy
extravasate
extravasated blood
extravasation of erythrocytes
extravascular fluid
extravisual zone
extremity arteries
extrinsic allergic alveolitis
extrinsic factor
extrinsic sphincter
extruded disk

exuberant granulation tissue
exuberant hypertrophic granulation
  tissue
exudate
  fibrinous
  fibrin-rich
  foamy
  frothy
  hemorrhagic
  neutrophilic
  purulent
  purulent subarachnoid
  serous
  stringy mucous
  subarachnoid
  viscous greenish
exudate in alveoli, mucopurulent
exudation cell
exudation corpuscle
exudation of fibrin-rich fluid
exudative dermatitis
exudative discoid and lichenoid
  dermatitis
exudative inflammation
exudative inflammation of glomeruli
exudative nephritis
exudative pharyngitis
exudative pleurisy
exudative tuberculosis
exude
ex vivo
eye
  aphakic
  artificial
  black
  congenital malformation of
  crossed
  cystic
  deviating
  epiphyseal
  following
  inflammatory conditions of

eye *(continued)*
- innermost coat of
- lifeless
- neoplasm of
- pannus of
- parietal
- pink
- pseudophakic
- shrunken

eyeball

eye-closure reflex

eye-ear plane

eye fundus

eyelid
- inflammation of
- lower
- upper

eye tumor

F, f

F (Fahrenheit)
FA (fluorescent antibody) test
FAB (formalin ammonium bromide)
FAB (French, American, British) classification of acute nonlymphoid leukemia
fabella bone
Fabry disease
face
  en
  labial artery of
  moon
facet
  articular
  atlas
  capitate
  clavicular
  corneal
  costal
  flat
  hamate
  inferior articular
  inferior costal
  Lenoir
  locked
  lunate
  scaphoid

facet *(continued)*
  squatting
  superior articular
  superior costal
  transverse costal
facetectomy
facet for head of rib
facet for tubercle of rib
facet joint
facial angle
facial artery
facial atrophy
facial axis
facial bone
facial canal
facial cleft
facial colliculus
facial eczema
facial eminence
facial herpes simplex
facial hirsutism
facial lymph node
facial muscle
facial nerve
facial plane
facial plexus
facial reflex

facial root
facial surface
facial triangle
facial vein
facies, moon
FACS (fluorescence-activated cell sorter)
FACScan
FACScan flow cytometer
FACSGal assay system
FACSort flow cytometer
FACSprep automated staining system
FACStrak flow cytometer
FACSVantage cell sorter
factitial dermatitis (self-inflicted lesions)
factitious purpura
factor
 ABO
 accelerator
 adrenal weight
 adrenocorticotropic releasing
 angiogenesis
 antiacrodynia
 antialopecia
 antianemic
 antiberiberi
 anti-black-tongue
 anticomplementary
 antidermatitis
 antihemophilic
 antihemophilic globulin (AHG, factor VIII)
 antihemorrhagic
 antineuritic
 antinuclear
 antipellagra
 antisterility
 atrial natriuretic (ATF)
 augmenting
 B-cell differentiating
 B-cell stimulatory

factor *(continued)*
 beta
 blood (see *coagulation*)
 branching
 B_T
 C
 CAMP (Christie, Atkins, Munch-Petersen)
 capillary permeability
 Castle intrinsic
 Christmas (factor IX)
 citrovorum
 clearing
 clotting
 coagulation, blood
  I (fibrinogen)
  II (prothrombin)
  III (tissue thromboplastin)
  IV (calcium)
  V (labile; proaccelerin)
  VI (stable)
  VII (proconvertin)
  VIII (antihemophilic globulin, AHG)
  IX (Christmas; plasma thromboplastin component)
  X (Stuart-Prower)
  XI (plasma thromboplastin antecedent)
  XII (Hageman)
  XIII (fibrin stabilizing)
 coenzyme
 colon-stimulating (CSF)
 complement chemotactic
 corticotropin-releasing
 debranching
 diabeticogenic
 Duran-Reynals permeability
 Duran-Reynals spreading
 endothelial relaxing
 endothelium-derived relaxing (EDRF)

factor *(continued)*
- epidermal growth
- erythrocyte maturation (EMF)
- extrinsic
- fertility
- fibrin-stabilization (FSF)
- filtrate
- Fitzgerald
- Flaujeac
- Fletcher
- follicle-stimulating hormone releasing
- G
- galactagogue
- galactopoietic
- glass
- glucose tolerance
- glycotropic
- gonadotropin-releasing (GRF)
- granulocyte-macrophage colony-stimulating
- growth
- growth hormone-releasing (GH-RF)
- Hageman (HF)
- human antihemophilic
- hyperglycemic-glycogenolytic
- immunogenetic
- immunoglobulin-binding (IBF)
- inhibition
- initiation
- insulin-antagonizing
- insulin-like growth
- intrinsic
- ischemia-modifying
- labile (V)
- Laki-Lorand
- LE (lupus erythematosus)
- lethal
- leukocytosis-promoting
- leukopenic
- lipotropic
- L-L

factor *(continued)*
- luteinizing hormone/follicle-stimulating hormone-releasing (LH/FSH-RF)
- lymph node permeability
- macrophage-activating
- macrophage colony-stimulating
- mammotropic
- melanotropin-releasing
- mesodermal
- migration-inhibitory (MIF)
- monocyte derived neutrophil chemotactic (MDNCF)
- multi-colon-stimulating (multi-CSF)
- myocardial depressant
- natural killer cell stimulating (NKSF)
- nephritic
- nerve growth (NGF)
- neural
- neutrophil activating
- neutrophil chemotactant
- osteoclast activating
- pellagra-preventing
- plasma clotting
- plasma labile
- plasma thromboplastin antecedent (XI)
- plasma thromboplastin component (IX)
- platelet
- platelet-activating
- platelet-aggravating
- platelet-derived growth
- predisposing
- proaccelerin (V)
- proconvertin (VII)
- prolactin-inhibiting
- prolactin-releasing
- protein
- Prower-Stuart
- psi

factor *(continued)*
- relaxation
- releasing (RF)
- resistance
- resistance-inducing
- resistance-transfer
- Rh
- rheumatoid (RF)
- risk
- secretor
- sex
- sigma
- somatotropin-releasing (SRF)
- somatotropin releasing-inhibiting (SRIF, SIF)
- stable (VI)
- stringent
- Stuart
- Stuart-Prower (X)
- T cell growth
- termination
- testis-determining (TDF)
- thymic lymphopoietic
- thyroid-stimulating hormone-releasing (TSH-RF)
- thyrotoxic complement-fixation
- thyrotropin-releasing (TRF)
- tissue
- transfer
- transforming
- transforming growth
- tumor angiogenic (TAF)
- tumor necrosis (TNF)
- uterine relaxing (URF)
- von Willebrand
- Williams

Fahrenheit scale (F)

failure
- adrenal
- bone marrow
- cardiac
- hepatic

failure *(continued)*
- multiple organ
- multisystem
- pituitary
- renal
- respiratory

failure of long-bone growth
failure of skull closure in the midline
failure to thrive
fair-skinned person
falciform cartilage
falciform crest
falciform ligament
falciform lobe
falciform margin
falciform process
falciform retinal fold
falcine meningioma
falciparum malaria
fall-and-rise phenomenon
fallopian aqueduct
fallopian arch
fallopian artery
fallopian canal
fallopian hiatus
fallopian ligament
fallopian neuritis
fallopian pregnancy
fallopian tube
Fallot, tetralogy of
false aneurysm
false colonic obstruction
false coxa
false glottis
false hematuria
false joint
false macula
false membrane
false mole
false negative
false pelvis
false positive

false positive RPR
false pregnancy
false proteinuria
false rib
false ringbone
false suture
false vertebra
false vocal cord
falx cerebelli
falx cerebri
falx meningioma
familial adenomatous polyposis (FAP)
familial disorder
familial hepatitis
familial hypercatabolism
familial hypophosphatemic osteomalacia
familial lipodystrophy
familial nonhemolytic jaundice
familial polyposis
Fananás cell
Fanconi syndrome
fan-shaped mesentery
fan-shaped muscle
FAP (familial adenomatous polyposis)
Farber test
farmer's lung
Farr test
fascia (pl. fasciae)
  anal
  antebrachial
  anterior rectus
  axillary
  bicipital
  brachial
  broad
  buccopharyngeal
  Camper
  cervical
  clavipectoral
  Cloquet
  Colles
  cremasteric

fascia *(continued)*
  cribriform
  Cruveilhier
  deep
  Denonvilliers
  dentate
  diaphragmatic
  endopelvic
  endothoracic
  extraperitoneal
  Gerota
  iliac
  lateral oblique
  obturator
  obturator internus
  parietal pelvic
  pelvic
  perineal
  psoas
  renal
  rim of
  Scarpa
  subcutaneous
  superficial
  thoracolumbar
  visceral pelvic
  Waldeyer
fasciae latae, tensor
fascia iliaca
fascial covering
fascia lata (pl. fasciae latae)
fascial layer
fascial sheath
fascia of abdomen
fascia of arm
fascia of penis, deep
fascia transversalis
fascicle, interlacing
fascicular degeneration
fascicular sarcoma
fasciculata zona
fasciculation

fasciculus (pl. fasciculi)
  calcarine
  central tegmental
  cuneate
  dorsolateral
  fronto-occipital
  nerve
fasciitis, necrotizing
Fasciola gigantica
Fasciola hepatica
fasciolar gyrus
fascioliasis
fasciolopsiasis
Fasciolopsis buski
fashion, pagetoid
fast blue
fast green
fastidious
fastigiobulbar tract
fasting blood glucose
fasting blood sugar
fasting chemistry panel
fasting triglyceride level, normal
fast red
fast smear
fat
  brown
  corpse
  dietary
  digital process of
  extraperitoneal
  fecal
  free (FF)
  intracellular
  ischiorectal pad of
  microvesicular
  pericolonic
  perirectal
  perirenal
  preperitoneal
  properitoneal
  protective layer of

fat *(continued)*
  renal
  subcutaneous
fat body
fat cell
fat content
fat-containing chyme
fat-digesting enzyme
fat embolism
fat globule
fatigability
fatigue fever
fat-induced hyperlipidemia
fat in stool
fat lobule
fat marrow
fat necrosis
fat pad
  antimesenteric
  ischiorectal
fat stores, depletion of
fat-storing cell
fatty acid
  activated
  aliphatic
  essential
  free nonesterified
  medium chain
  nonesterified, free
  omega-3
  short chain
  straight-chain
  total
  unesterified free
  unsaturated
fatty acid profile
fatty acid synthase complex
fatty acid thiokinase
fatty areolar tissue, subperitoneal
fatty atrophy
fatty change
fatty cirrhosis

'atty degeneration of liver
'atty granule cell
'atty heart
'atty infiltration of liver
'atty kidney
'atty meal
'atty metamorphosis
'atty nevus
'atty pigment
'atty renal capsule
'atty stool
'atty superficial layer
'atty tissue
'atty vacuole
'auces (pl. of faux)
  anterior pillar of
  arch of
'aucial reflex
'aucial tonsil
'aux (pl. fauces)
'ava bean
'avism
'avus
Fazio-Londe atrophy
FBA (fecal bile acid)
FBD (fibrocystic breast disease)
Fe (iron)
'ebrifuge
'ebrile agglutinin panel
'ebrile agglutinins
'ebrile antigen
'ebrile proteinuria
'ecal abscess
'ecal bile acid (FBA)
'ecal concretion
'ecal fat test
'ecalith
'ecal material
'ecal urobilinogen
'eces, mass of inspissated
FeCO$_2$ (fraction of expired carbon dioxide)
Felix-Weil test
feltlike
female genital tract (FGT) cytologic smear
female hormone
female pattern alopecia
female pelvis
female, perimenopausal
female prostate
female reproductive system
feminization
femoral aneurysm
femoral arch
femoral artery
femoral articulation
femoral bone
femoral canal
femoral circumflex artery
femoral-femoral bypass graft
femoral fossa
femoral head
femoral hernia
femoral ligament
femoral muscle
femoral neck
femoral nerve
femoral opening
femoral plexus
femoral-popliteal bypass graft
femoral reflex
femoral region
femoral ring
femoral septum
femoral sheath
femoral triangle
femoral vein
femoroabdominal reflex
femoropatellar joint
femorotibial joint
femtogram (fg)
femtoliter (fL)
femtometer (fm)

femtomole (fmol)
femur (pl. femora)
  apex of
  body of
  greater trochanter of
  head of
  lesser trochanter of
  neck of
  nutrient artery of
fenestrated capillary
fenestrated membrane C
fenestrated sheath
fermentation test for sugar in urine
fern test
ferning
Ferrata cell
Ferrein canal
Ferrein ligament
ferric ammonium sulfate
ferric chloride
ferric chloride test
ferritin, serum
ferritin test
ferrocyanide salt
ferrohemoglobin solubility test
ferrozine
fertility factor
fertilization ex vivo
fertilization in vitro (IVF)
fertilization in vivo
fertilization membrane
fertilized ovum
fetal alcohol syndrome
fetal chromosome analysis
fetal death
  early
  intermediate
  late
fetal diagnosis
fetal hemoglobin (hemoglobin F)
fetal hypoxia
fetalis, erythroblastosis
fetal lobe
fetal maturity
fetal membrane
fetal placenta
fetal small parts
fetal tissue
fetal viability
fetal zone
fetoglobulin, alpha-
fetomaternal transfusion
fetoprotein
  $alpha_1$-
  fucosylated alpha
fetus
  aborted
  amorphous
  calcified
  growth-retarded
  harlequin
  HLA-compatible
  impacted
  macerated
  maturity of
  mummified
  nonstressed
  nonviable
  paper-doll
  parasitic
  placenta of
  presentation of
  previable
  retained dead
  small parts of
  stressed
  stunted
  tissue of
  umbilical artery in
  viable
fetus papyraceus
fetus sanguinolentus
Feulgen method of staining
Feulgen stain

fever
- absorption
- acute rheumatic (ARF)
- Aden
- aestivoautumnal
- African hemorrhagic
- African tick-borne
- algid pernicious
- ardent
- Argentinian hemorrhagic
- arthropod-borne relapsing
- artificial
- aseptic
- Australian Q
- black
- blackwater
- blue
- Bolivian hemorrhagic
- bouquet
- boutonneuse
- brass founder's
- Brazilian spotted
- breakbone
- bullous
- Bunyamwera
- Burdwan
- Bwamba
- cachectic
- camp
- canicola
- Carter
- catarrhal
- cat-bite
- cat-scratch
- catheter
- Central European tick-borne
- Charcot intermittent
- Colorado tick
- Congolian red
- cotton-mill
- Crimean-Congo hemorrhagic
- dehydration

fever *(continued)*
- dengue hemorrhagic
- drug
- Dutton relapsing
- Ebola hemorrhagic
- elephantoid
- enteric
- ephemeral
- epidemic hemorrhagic
- essential
- exanthematous
- fatigue
- Fort Bragg
- Gambian
- glandular
- harlequin
- Haverhill
- hay
- hemorrhagic
- herpetic
- icterohemorrhagic
- inanition
- jail
- jungle
- Katayama
- Kenya
- Kew Gardens
- Korean hemorrhagic
- Lassa
- Malta
- Manchurian
- meningotyphoid
- Mexican spotted
- miliary
- milk
- monoleptic
- nodal
- Omsk hemorrhagic
- Oroya
- papular
- parathyroid
- parenteric

fever *(continued)*
- parrot
- periodic
- petechial
- pharyngoconjunctival
- Philippine hemorrhagic
- phlebotomus
- pinta
- polymer fume
- Pontiac
- pretibial
- puerperal
- pyogenic
- Q
- quartan
- rat-bite
- redwater
- relapsing
- remittent
- rheumatic
- Rocky Mountain spotted
- Ross River
- San Joaquin Valley
- Saõ Paulo
- scarlet
- septic
- spirillary rat-bite (sodoku)
- steroid
- streptobacillary rat-bite
- syphilitic
- Texas
- Thai hemorrhagic
- tick-borne
- typhoid
- undulant
- uveoparotid
- valley
- viral hemorrhagic
- vivax
- yellow
- Zika

fever, chills, and circulatory collapse

fever of unknown origin (FUO)

fever-producing substance

fg (femtogram)

FGT (female genital tract) cytologic smear

F hemoglobin

fiber
- A
- accelerator
- afferent
- alpha
- anastomosing
- anastomotic
- arcuate
- argyrophilic
- association
- augmentor
- B
- beta
- C
- cardiac muscle
- cholinergic
- chromatic
- circular
- climbing
- collagen
- collagenous
- commissural
- cone
- connective-tissue
- corticobulbar
- corticonuclear
- corticopontine
- corticoreticular
- corticospinal
- dental
- dentinal
- depressor
- efferent
- elastic
- enamel
- endogenous

fiber *(continued)*
- exogenous
- intercrural
- interlacing
- interlacing tendinous
- matrix of collagenic
- motor
- muscle
- myocardial
- nerve
- pain
- postganglionic
- preganglionic
- preganglionic sympathetic
- Purkinje
- reticular
- sensory
- Sharpey
- skeletal muscle
- sling muscle
- unmyelinated postganglionic
- yellow elastic

fiber of Remak
fibril
- collagen
- connective tissue
- degeneration
- nerve

fibril distortion within cell processes
fibrillar protein
fibrillar structure, delicate
fibrillary bacteria
fibrillary degeneration
fibrin breakdown products
fibrin clot
fibrin debris
fibrin deposition
fibrin in bronchi
fibrin, insoluble
fibrinocartilaginous ring
fibrinogen, plasma protein
fibrinogen uptake
fibrinopurulent inflammation
fibrinoid degeneration
fibrinoid necrosis
fibrinoligase
fibrinolysin
fibrinolysis
fibrinolytic purpura
fibrinopeptide A
fibrinous debris
fibrinous degeneration
fibrinous exudate
fibrinous inflammation
fibrinous pericarditis
fibrinous pleurisy
fibrinous pleuritis
fibrinous pneumonia
fibrinous polyp
fibrin platelet embolism
fibrin-rich exudate
fibrin-rich fluid, exudation of
fibrin split products
fibrin-stabilizing factor
fibrin thrombus
fibroadenoma of breast
fibroadipose tissue
fibroareolar tissue
fibroblast
fibroblastic meningioma
fibroblastic osteosarcoma
fibrocartilage
- circumferential
- intra-articular plates of
- triangular

fibrocartilaginous joint
fibrocartilaginous pad
fibrocartilaginous ring
fibrocartilaginous tissue
fibrocollagenous
fibrocystic breast
fibrocystic breast disease (FBD)
fibrocyte
fibroelastic band

fibroelastic cartilage
fibroelastic septa
fibroepithelial papilloma
fibroepithelial polyp
fibrofatty connective tissue
fibrofatty layer
fibrofatty stroma, tissue
fibrohyaline tissue
fibroid (pl. fibroids)
  intramural
  pedunculated
  uterine
fibroid degeneration
fibroid myocarditis
fibroid uterus
fibrolipomatous nephritis
fibroma, ovarian
fibromatosis
fibromuscular band
fibromuscular dysplasia
fibromuscular pelvic floor
fibromuscular stroma
fibromuscular tissue
fibromyelinic plaque
fibromyoma, uterine
fibroplasia, retrolental
fibroplastic process
fibroplastic proliferation
fibrosa cystica, osteitis
fibrosarcoma
fibrosing granulation tissue
fibrosing inflammation
fibrosing osteochondroma
fibrosis
  cystic
  diffuse interstitial
  endocardial
  endomyocardial
  idiopathic interstitial
  interstitial
  interstitial pulmonary
  leptomeningeal

fibrosis *(continued)*
  mediastinal
  nodular subepidermal
  pericentral
  periductal
  perimuscular
  periportal
  pipestem
  pulmonary
  replacement
  retroperitoneal
  subadventitial
  subintimal
  subserosal
  Symmers
fibrosis in cornea
fibrosus, annulus
fibrotic band
fibrotic patches
fibrotic pattern
fibrotic reaction
fibrotic stricture of urethra
fibrous adhesion
fibrous ankylosis
fibrous apex
fibrous arch
fibrous articulation
fibrous band
fibrous capsule of kidney
fibrous cartilage
fibrous connective tissue
fibrous cortical defect
fibrous dysplasia
fibrous goiter
fibrous induration
fibrous joint
fibrous layer
fibrous matrix
fibrous mediastinitis
fibrous membrane
fibrous meningioma
fibrous myocarditis

fibrous nodules
fibrous obliteration
fibrous odontoma
fibrous pericardium
fibrous plaque
fibrous pneumonia
fibrous protein
fibrous reaction
fibrous renal capsule
fibrous ring
fibrous scar
fibrous scar tissue
fibrous septa
fibrous sheath
fibrous skeleton
fibrous stroma
fibrous tissue
fibrous tubercle
fibrovascular adhesion
fibrovascular stroma
fibrovascular tissue
fibula
  apex of
  nutrient artery of
fibular artery
fibular articular surface
fibular bone
fibular circumflex artery
fibular collateral ligament of ankle
fibular lymph node
fibular margin
fibular notch
fibular surface
fibular vein
Ficoll gradient
Ficoll-Hypaque separation
Fiedler myocarditis
field
  auditory
  dark
  Flechsig
  high-power

field *(continued)*
  low-power
  morphogenic
  myelinogenic
  visual
  Wernicke
field of Forel
fièvre boutonneuse
fifth disease (erythema infectiosum)
FIGLU excretion test
FIGO (International Federation of Gynecology and Obstetrics)
FIGO grade
FIGO grade of adenocarcinoma of endometrium
FIGO staging of adenocarcinoma of endometrium
FIGO staging of cervical carcinoma
figure, mitotic
filament
  actin
  branching
filamented neutrophil
filament-forming bacillus
filamentous mass
filariasis (elephantiasis)
filiform papilla (pl. papillae)
Filley method
filling defect
Filobasidiella neoformans
Filovirus, filovirus
filter
  band-pass
  LeukoNet
  Millipore
  Nuclepore
filtrate factor
filtration angle
filtration fraction
filtration, glomerular
filtration of fluid specimen
filtration space

fimbria (pl. fimbriae), ovarian
fimbriated fold
fimbriodentate sulcus
final diagnosis
fine needle
fine-needle aspiration (FNA)
fine-needle aspiration biopsy (FNAB)
finger
  base of
  bolster
  clubbed
  sausage
  spade
  speck
  trigger
  webbed
fingerlike dermal papillae
fingernail
fingerprint whorl
fingerstick puncture
fingerstick specimen
finger-thumb reflex
Finkeldey-Warthin giant cell
Finn chamber patch test
FiO_2 (fractional inspired oxygen concentration)
first cranial nerve
first cuneiform bone
first duodenal sphincter
first parallel pelvic plane
first permanent molar
first-set phenomenon
first-set rejection
first ventricle of cerebrum
first visceral cleft
first-voided specimen
first-voided urine specimen
FISH (fluorescence in situ hybridization)
Fishberg concentration test for renal function
fish-mouth cervix
Fishman-Doubilet test for diagnosis of pancreatitis
fishtank granuloma
fissure
  abdominal
  anal
  antitragohelicine
  brain
  calcarine
  callosomarginal
  cerebellar
  cerebral
  chronic
  collateral
  cutaneous
  decidual
  dentate
  glaserian
  horizontal
  oblique
  oral
  palpebral
  short palpebral
fissure of lung
Fissuricella filamenta
fistula
  abdominal
  arteriovenous
  biliary
  branchial
  bronchobiliary
  bronchocavitary
  bronchoesophageal
  bronchopleural
  cholecystoduodenal
  colonic
  colovaginal
  colovesical
  congenital pulmonary arteriovenous
  cystic
  Eck
  enterovaginal

fistula *(continued)*
- fecal
- gastric
- gastrocolic
- gastroduodenal
- genitourinary
- hepatopleural
- H-type
- orofacial
- parietal
- perineovaginal
- pilonidal
- rectovaginal
- rectovesical
- sigmoidovesical
- tracheoesophageal
- urethrovaginal
- vesical
- vesicouterine
- vitelline

fistulous tracts

Fite-Faraco stain

Fitzgerald factor

Fitz-Hugh–Curtis syndrome

fixation, complement (CF)

fixative (see also *fluid*, *solution*, *stain*)
- absolute alcohol
- acetic acid
- acetone
- Altmann solution
- B5
- Bouin picroformol-acetic
- buffered formalin
- Carnoy solution
- Champy
- chlorpalladium
- chromic acid
- Delafield solution
- Flemming solution
- formaldehyde
- formalin
- formalin-alcohol

fixative *(continued)*
- formalin-ammonium bromide
- formol-calcium
- formol-Müller solution
- formol-saline
- formol-Zenker
- FU-48 Zenker solution
- Gendre solution
- glacial acetic acid
- glutaraldehyde
- Golgi osmiobichromate
- Helly
- Helly Zenker-formalin solution
- Hermann
- Jores solution
- Kaiserling solution
- Karnowsky
- Luft potassium permanganate
- Marchi
- Maximow solution
- methanol
- Michel transport
- Millonig phosphate-buffered formalin
- Müller solution
- neutral (buffered) formalin
- Orth
- osmic acid
- osmium tetroxide
- Park-Williams
- periodate-lysing-paraformaldehyde
- picric acid
- picroformol
- potassium bichromate (or dichromate)
- Regaud
- Schaudinn
- Tellyesniczky solution
- Thoma
- Zamboni
- Zenker-formol
- Zenker solution

fixator muscle
fixed interval of time
fixed macrophage
fixed time interval
fL (femtoliter)
flabby myocardium
flabby tissue
flaccid
flaccid membrane
flaccid paralysis, irreversible
flagellate cell
flagellum
flail joint
flame cell
flammeus nevus
flange, buccal
flank bone
flank scar
flank stripe, properitoneal
flap, raised
flask-shaped phialides
flask-shaped ulcer of colonic mucosa
flat abdominal muscles
flat bone
flat cell
flat condyloma
flat facet
flat genital wart
flat muscle
flat pelvis
flat plaque
flattened stool
flattening of gyri of brain
flatus
Flaujeac factor
flavivirus
Flavobacterium meningosepticum
flea-bitten kidney
flea-borne typhus
Flechsig field
Flechsig primordial zone
fleecy masses
Fleischer-Kayser ring
Flemming solution
fleshy mole
fleshy texture
Fletcher factor
Flexner bacillus
flexor canal
flexor reflex
flexural eczema
flexure
  caudal
  cephalic
  cerebral
  cervical
  cranial
  duodenojejunal
  hepatic
  left colic
  left colonic
  right colic
  right colonic
  sigmoid
  splenic
floating cartilage
floating gallbladder
floating kidney
floating organ
floating patella
floating protein
floating rib
floating section
floating spleen
floating stool
floating villus
floccular fossa
flocculation
flocculonodular lobe
flocculus, accessory
Flood ligament
floor
  bladder
  fibromuscular pelvic

floor *(continued)*
  inguinal
  pelvic
floor cell
floor of inguinal region
floor of nasal cavity
floor of thorax
flora
  bacterial
  normal
florid
florid cirrhosis
flotation bath
flow cytometer (see *cytometer*)
flow cytometry
flow microfluorimetry
Flower bone
Floyd peripheral nerve classification
fluid
  amniotic
  articular
  ascitic
  bloody
  body
  Bouin
  cavitary
  cerebrospinal
  clear
  cystic
  Delafield
  dentinal
  digestive
  edema
  embalming
  extracellular
  extravascular
  frothy
  gelatinous
  intercellular
  interstitial
  intracellular
  joint

fluid *(continued)*
  loculated
  low-viscosity
  lymphatic
  meconium-stained amniotic
  natural body
  pericardial
  pericardial effusion
  peritoneal
  peritoneal effusion
  pleural
  pleural effusion
  prostatic
  protein-rich
  seminal
  serosanguineous
  serous
  spinal
  straw-colored
  synovial
  testing
  thoracentesis
  transcellular
  turbid
  viscous
  Zenker
fluid-filled cleft
fluid-filled cyst
fluid-filled papule
fluid-filled sac
fluid-filled vacuole within lens
fluid material
fluid protein
fluid specimen, filtration of
fluid wave
fluke (trematode)
  liver
  lung
fluorescein isothiocyanate (FITC)
fluorescence
  homogeneous
  nuclear rim

fluorescence *(continued)*
  nucleolar
  speckled
fluorescence-activated cell sorter (FACS)
fluorescence in situ hybridization (FISH)
fluorescence microscope
fluorescent antibody (FA) test
fluorescent antibody technique
fluorescent antinuclear antibody test (FANA)
fluorescent cytoprint assay
fluorescent dye
fluorescent lighting
fluorescent microscopy
fluorescent polarization
fluorescent-tagged antibody
fluorescent *Treponema pallidum* absorption test
fluorescent treponemal antibody (FTA) test
fluorescent treponemal antibody absorption test (FTA-ABS)
fluoride intoxication
fluoride poisoning
fluoride test
fluorochrome
fm (femtometer)
F method of staining
fmol (femtomole)
FNA (fine-needle aspiration)
FNAB (fine-needle aspiration biopsy)
foam cell
foam embolism
foamy cytoplasm
foamy exudate
foamy fluid
foamy histiocyte
foamy stool
focal edema
focal fibrotic reaction
focal glomerular sclerosis
focal hemorrhage
focal hepatic necrosis
focal hepatocellular necrosis with hemorrhagic cyst
focal inflammation
focal myocytolysis of heart
focal necrosis
focal osteolysis
focal pneumonitis
focal sclerosing osteomyelitis
focal ulceration and hemorrhage
focally puckered pleura
focus (pl. foci)
folate absorption test
fold
  adipose
  alar
  amniotic
  aryepiglottic
  axillary
  caval
  cecal
  cholecystoduodenocolic
  ciliary
  circular
  circulator
  costocolic
  Douglas
  duodenojejunal
  duodenomesocolic
  epigastric
  falciform retinal
  fibriated
  gastric
  gastropancreatic
  genital
  glossopalatine
  gluteal
  Guérin
  haustral
  hepatopancreatic

fold *(continued)*
  ileocecal
  ileocolic
  inferior duodenal
  inferior transverse rectal
  inguinal
  interureteric
  Kerckring
  labioscrotal
  latcral umbilical
  medial umbilical
  mucosal
  Nélaton
  palatopharyngeal
  paraduodenal
  peritoneal
  rectal
  rectouterine
  sacrogenital
  semilunar
  sentinel
  sigmoid
  spiral
  superior duodenal
  superior transverse rectal
  vestigial
folded fundus gallbladder
folded gallbladder
fold pattern
foliaceus, pemphigus
foliate papilla
folic acid
follicle
  aggregated lymphatic
  agminated
  anovular ovarian
  atretic ovarian
  gastric
  gastric lymphatic
  graafian
  hair
  lash

follicle *(continued)*
  lymphoid
  malpighian
  nabothian
  ovarian
  pilosebaceous
  primordial
  ruptured
  thyroid
  unruptured
follicle cell
follicle-stimulating hormone (FSH)
follicle-stimulating hormone-releasing factor
follicular abscess
follicular adenocarcinoma
follicular adenoiditis
follicular carcinoma
follicular cell
follicular center cell lymphoma
follicular cyst
follicular epithelial cell
follicular gland
follicular goiter
follicular hormone
follicular hyperkeratosis
follicular hyperplasia
follicular lymphoma
follicular mixed small cleaved and large cell lymphoma
follicular mucinosis
follicular ovarian cell
follicular phase
follicular plugging
follicular predominantly large cell lymphoma
follicular predominantly small cleaved cell lymphoma
follicular tonsillitis
folliculi, liquor
folliculitis decalvans
folliculitis, keloidal

following eye
follow up (verb)
follow-up (adj.)
followup, follow-up (noun, adj.)
fomites
Fonsecaea compacta
Fonsecaea dermatitidis
Fonsecaea pedrosoi
Fontana canal
Fontana-Masson stain
Fontana methenamine-silver stain
Fontana space
fontanelle (also, fontanel)
  anterior
  anterolateral
  bregmatic
  cranial
  frontal
  Gerdy
  mastoid
  occipital
  posterior
  posterolateral
  sagittal
  sphenoid
  triangular
fonticulus (pl. fonticuli)
food-borne gastroenteritis
food faddist
food poisoning
foot
  arch of
  arcuate artery of
  articulations of
  athlete's
  Charcot
  diabetic
  digital artery of
  Madura
  perforating artery of
  phalanges of
  trench
football knee
foot fungus
foot, hand, and mouth disease
Foot reticulum stain
foramen (pl. foramina)
  alveolar
  anterior condyloid
  aortic
  apical
  arachnoidal
  blind
  carotid
  cecal
  conjugate
  costotransverse
  cranial
  emissary sphenoidal
  epiploic
  ethmoidal
  greater palatine
  greater sciatic
  intervertebral
  lesser sciatic
  node of epiploic
  nutrient (of bone)
  obturator
  pelvic sacral
  sciatic
  vertebral
foramen cecum of tongue
foramen lacerum
foramen magnum
foramen of Bochdalek
foramen of Luschka
foramen of Magendie
foramen of Winslow
foramen ovale
foramen rotundum
foramen spinosum
foramen transversarium
foramide
forced grasping reflex

forced vital capacity (FVC)
foregut
foregut artery
foreign body
foreign body giant cell
foreign body granuloma
foreign body reaction
foreign material, retained
foreign protein
Forel, field of
forensic pathology
foreskin, inflammation of
Formad kidney
formaldehyde
formaldehyde solution
formalin-alcohol
formalin ammonium bromide (FAB)
formalin, buffered neutral
formalin solution
formation
  adipocere
  callus
  capsid
  coffin
  horn cyst
  horn pearl
  keloid
  keratin pearl
  palisade
  pearl
  pseudopalisade
  rosette
  rouleaux
  syncytium
formation of abnormal hemoglobin S
formation of excessive porphyrin in marrow
formation of red nodules beneath skin
formative cell
formed stool
forme fruste (pl. formes frustes)
forme tardive
formol-calcium fixative
formol-Mueller solution
formol-saline fixative
formol-Zenker fixative
formol-Zenker solution
formyl-methionyl-leucryl-phenylalamine
fornix of vagina
Forssman antigen
Forssman reaction
Fort Bragg fever
forward light scatter
Foshay test for tularemia
fossa (pl. fossae)
  acetabular
  adipose
  amygdaloid
  anconeal
  anterior recess of ischiorectal
  articular
  axillary
  bony
  condylar
  crural
  cubital
  digastric
  digital
  duodenal
  duodenojejunal
  epigastric
  femoral
  floccular
  gallbladder
  glenoid
  hypochondriac
  iliac
  infrasternal
  ischiorectal
  navicular
  olecranon
  ovarian
  pararectal

fossa *(continued)*
  paravesical
  valve of navicular
fossa ovalis (pl. fossae ovalis)
fossa plane, ischiorectal
Fouchet reagent
Fouchet test for bilirubin in urine
foul discharge
foul-smelling
fourchette
Fourier transformation
foveated chest
foveola
foveolar cell
foveolar cells of stomach
foveolar gastric mucosa
F plasmid
fraction
  beta
  beta lipoprotein
  blood plasma
  depressed ejection
  ejection
  filtration
  growth
  heparin-precipitable (HPF)
  linear
  MB
  plasma
  plasma protein (PPF)
  regurgitant
  S phase
fractional inspired oxygen concentration (FiO_2)
fraction of expired carbon dioxide ($FeCO_2$)
fracture of bone
fracture repair
fracture site
Fraenkel typhus nodule
fragile bones
fragile X chromosome
fragile X syndrome
fragility
  capillary
  capillary hereditary
  erythrocyte
  hereditary (of bone)
  osmotic
  red blood cell
fragility test, osmotic
fragmentation myocarditis
fragmentation of cell into particles
fragmentation of cell nuclei
fragmentation of fibers
fragmented axons and dendrites
fragmented tissue
frambesia (yaws)
Francisella tularensis (formerly *Pasteurella tularensis*)
Francis test for bile acids in urine
frank blood in stool
Frankfort horizontal plane
Frankfort-mandibular incisor angle
Frankfort plane
frank blood
Frank capillary toxicosis
frank cyanosis from hypoxemia
frank hemorrhage
frank necrosis
frank perforation
frank pulmonary edema
frank pus
frank rigors
Frank-Starling curve
Frank-Starling mechanism
frank suppuration
Franseen needle
fraught with error
freckle, Hutchinson melanotic
freckle-like lesion
freckles (ephelides)
freckling, myxoma syndrome with facial

free band of colon
free electrophoresis
free erythrocyte protoporphyrin
free fluid
free hemoglobin
free macrophage
free radical
free thyroxine index (FTI)
free triiodothyronine test
free wall
freeze-dried
freezing microtome
Freiberg disease
Frei intracutaneous diagnostic test
fremitus, bronchial
French scale
frenulum (pl. frenula)
frenulum of clitoris
frenulum of ileocecal valve
frenulum of labia minora
frenulum of valve
frequency of stool
fresh frozen plasma
fresh frozen section
fresh normal plasma
friable clot
friable mass
friable papilloma
friction rub in knee
Friderichsen-Waterhouse syndrome
Friedländer bacillus
Friedländer pneumonia
Friedreich ataxia
fringe, costal
Frisch bacillus
Frommann line
frond
fronding sign
frondlike pattern
frontal abscess
frontal air sinus
frontal angle
frontal area
frontal artery
frontal axis
frontal bone
frontal bossing
frontal convolution
frontal cortex
frontal crest
frontal eminence
frontal fontanel
frontal horn
frontal lobe
frontal margin
frontal nerve
frontal notch
frontal plane
frontal plate
frontal pole
frontal process
frontal region
frontal section
frontal sinus
frontal suture
frontal triangle
frontal tuber
frontal vein
frontobasal artery
frontoethmoidal suture
frontolacrimal suture
frontomaxillary suture
frontonasal duct
frontonasal elevation
frontonasal process
frontonasal roof of nasal cavity
frontonasal suture
fronto-occipital fasciculus
fronto-orbital area
frontopontine tract
frontosphenoidal process
frontotemporal tract
frontozygomatic suture
Froriep induration

frostbite (dermatitis congelationis)
frosted liver
frost itch
frothy discharge
frothy exudate
frothy fluid
frozen embryo
frozen pelvis
frozen section diagnosis
frozen section, fresh
frozen sperm
fructosamine
fructose
fructose challenge test
fructose loading test
fructose tolerance test
Frykman classification of hand fractures
FSH (follicle-stimulating hormone)
FSH-HR (follicle-stimulating hormone-releasing hormone)
FTA (fluorescent treponemal antibody) test
FTA-ABS (fluorescent treponemal antibody absorption) test
FTI (free thyroxine index)
fuchsin body
fuchsinophil cell
fuchsinophil granule
fuchsinophilic granule
fucosylated alpha fetoprotein
FU-48 Zenker solution
fulgurate
fulguration
full-thickness tear
fulminant hepatitis
fulminant tuberculosis
functional congestion
functional hematuria
functional hypertrophy
functional ovarian cyst
functional proteinuria
functional residual capacity (FRC)
functioning neoplasm
functioning tumor
function, platelet
function test
fundal placenta
fundic-antral junction
fundic gland
fundic metaplasia
fundiform ligament
fundus (pl. fundi)
  bladder
  eye
  gallbladder
  gastric
  stomach
  urinary bladder
  uterine
  vaginal
fundus reflex
fundus uteri
fungal antibody
fungal body
fungal culture
fungal endocarditis
fungal infection
fungal myocarditis
fungal pneumonia
fungal scrapings
fungal smear
fungating mass
fungating neoplasm
fungemia
fungiform papillae
fungoides, mycosis
fungus (pl. fungi) (see also *pathogen*)
  dimorphic
  foot
  mold
  mosaic
  mycelial
  pathogenic

fungus *(continued)*
- slime
- yeast
- yeastlike
- zygomycetous

funguslike bacteria
fungus testis
funicular artery
funiculus, cuneate
funis
funisitis
funnel-like deformity
funnel-shaped cavity
funnel-shaped pelvis
funnel-shaped portion of hair follicle
FUO (fever of unknown origin)
furcal nerve
furuncle
furuncular
furunculoid
furunculosis
fusariotoxicosis
Fusarium moniliforme
Fusarium oxysporum
Fusarium solani
fused kidney
fused rib
fusiform aneurysm
fusiform bacillus
fusiform cell
fusiform gyrus
fusiform layer
fusiform muscle
fusion, labial
fusion of the stapes
Fusobacterium, fusobacterium
Fusobacterium gonidiaformans
Fusobacterium mortiferum
Fusobacterium mucleatum
Fusobacterium natiforme
Fusobacterium necrophorum
Fusobacterium nucleatum
Fusobacterium plauti-vincenti
Fusobacterium russii
Fusobacterium varium
fusocellular
fusospirillary
fusospirillosis
fusospirochetal
fusospirochetosis
FVC (forced vital capacity)

G, g

g (gram)
GABHS (Group A beta-hemolytic streptococcus)
Gaddum and Schild test
gag reflex
galactagogue factor
galactocele
galactokinase deficiency
galactophorous canal
galactophorous duct
galactopoietic factor
galactopoietic hormone
galactorrhea
galactose in tissues
galactose-1-phosphate uridyl transferase deficiency
galactosemia
galactose tolerance test
galactosylceramidase, congenital deficiency of
galea aponeurotica
Galeati gland
Galen ventricle
gallbladder
    bilobed
    body of
    Courvoisier

gallbladder *(continued)*
    dilated
    distended
    double
    fish-scale
    floating
    folded fundus
    fundus of
    hourglass
    mobile
    multiseptate
    neck of
    sandpaper
    stasis
    strawberry
    thick-walled
    thin-walled
    wandering
gallbladder bed
gallbladder bile
gallbladder calculi
gallbladder fossa
gallbladder fundus
gallbladder hydrops
gallbladder mucosa
gallbladder sludge
gallbladder stone

gallbladder villi
gallbladder wall
gall duct
Gallego method
gallstone
  cholesterol
  opacifying
  silent
Gallyas method
GALT (gut-associated lymphoid tissue)
galvanic cell
galvanic threshold
Gambian fever
gamete intrafallopian transfer (GIFT)
gametoid cell
gametokinetic hormone
Gamgee tissue
gamma angle
gamma cell
gamma counter
gamma globulins
gamma-glutamyl transferase (GGT)
gamma-glutamyl transpeptidase (GGTP)
gamma granule
gamma-hemolytic streptococcus
gamma loop
gamma motor neuron
gammopathy, monoclonal
Gandy-Gamma nodule
ganglia (pl. of ganglion)
gangliated cord
gangliated nerve
ganglion (pl. ganglia)
  aberrant
  acousticofacial
  aorticorenal
  auditory
  auricular
  autonomic
  basal
  cardiac
ganglion *(continued)*
  carotid
  celiac
  cervicothoracic
  ciliary
  coccygeal
  diffuse
  gasserian
  geniculate
  otic
  paravertebral
  prevertebral
  sensory
  sphenopalatine
  submandibular
  spinal
  stromal
  superior mesenteric
  sympathetic
  uterine cervical
  vestibular
ganglion artery, semilunar
ganglion cell
ganglion cyst
ganglion of Arnold
ganglion of Auerbach
ganglion of nerve
ganglion of tendon sheath
ganglion ridge
ganglionic blockade
ganglionic canal
ganglionic crest
ganglionic layer
ganglioside
gangrene
  diabetic
  dry
  gas
  wet
gangrenous granuloma
gangrenous necrosis
gangrenous pneumonia

gap
  air-bone
  anion
  anteromedian
  auscultatory
  Bochdalek
  chromatid
  isochromatid
gaping wound
Gardnerella vaginalis (formerly *Haemophilus vaginalis* or *Corynebacterium vaginale*)
Gardnerella vaginitis
gargantuan mastitis
gargoylism
Garré osteomyelitis
Gärtner bacillus
Gartner canal
Gartner cyst
Gartner duct
Gärtner phenomenon
gas
  arterial blood
  bowel
  carbon dioxide
  colorless
  formaldehyde
  nitrogen
  odorless
  pulmonary
gas abscess
gas chromatography
gas embolism
gas exchange in lungs, normal
gas exchange, pulmonary
gas gangrene
gas liquefaction
gas nitrogen embolism
gas pattern
gaseous
gases of putrefaction
gasophil granule
gasserian ganglion
gastral mesoderm
gastric achlorhydria
gastric acid secretion
gastric acid test
gastric algid malaria
gastric analysis
gastric antrum
gastric artery
gastric atrophy
gastric calculus
gastric canal
gastric carcinoma
gastric cardia
gastric channel
gastric contents
gastric fistula
gastric fold
gastric follicle
gastric function test
gastric fundus
gastric gland
gastric groove
gastric impression
gastric inhibitory polypeptide (GIP)
gastric juice
gastric lavage
gastric lymph nodes
gastric lymphatic follicle
gastric mucin
gastric mucosa
gastric mucosa atrophy
gastric obstruction
gastric omentum
gastric pacemaker region
gastric partition
gastric pit
gastric plexus
gastric polyp
gastric polyposis
gastric pouch
gastric remnant

gastric sclerosis
gastric secretion rate
gastric stump
gastric surface
gastric ulcer
gastric vein
gastric washing
gastrin hormone
gastrinoma
gastrin-secreting cell
gastrin-secretin stimulation test
gastrin test
gastritis
  acute
  antral
  atrophic
  chronic
  cirrhotic
  hemorrhagic
  hypertrophic
  necrotizing
  pseudomembranous radiation
gastrocolic fistula
gastrocolic ligament
gastrocolic omentum
gastrocolic reflex
gastrodiaphragmatic ligament
gastroduodenal artery complex
gastroduodenal fistula
gastroduodenal lumen
gastroduodenal lymph node
gastroduodenal orifice
gastroenteritis
  acute infectious
  bacterial
  Campylobacter
  eosinophilic
  food-borne
  infantile
  Norwalk
  viral
  water-borne
gastroepiploic arcade
gastroepiploic artery
gastroepiploic gland
gastroepiploic vein
gastroepiploic vessel
gastroesophageal junction
gastroesophageal laceration
gastroesophageal variceal plexus
gastroesophageal vestibule
gastrohepatic bare area
gastrohepatic ligament
gastrohepatic omentum
gastroileac reflex
gastrointestinal (GI)
gastrointestinal hormone
gastrointestinal mucosal hemorrhage
gastrointestinal plaque
gastrointestinal stoma
gastrointestinal tract
gastrointestinal tumor
gastrointestinal ulceration
gastrolienal ligament
gastro-omental artery
gastropancreatic fold
gastropancreatic ligament
gastroparesis
gastrophrenic ligament
gastrosplenic ligament
gastrosplenic omentum
Gaucher cell
Gaucher disease
gauge
gauze
Gay gland
GBIA (Guthrie bacterial inhibition assay)
GBS (Group beta-hemolytic *Streptococcus*) (also, Group B)
GC (gonorrhea)
G cell
g/dL (grams per deciliter)
GE (gastroesophageal) junction

Gegenbaur cell
gel
  acrylamide/urea
  agarose
  colloidal
  polyacrylamide
gelatiginous tissue
gelatin-chrome slide
gelatiniform degeneration
gelatinized marrow
gelatinous ascites
gelatinous infiltration
gelatinous material
gelatinous otolithic membrane
gelatinous polyp
gel diffusion precipitin test
gel diffusion reaction
gel diffusion test
gel electrophoresis
Gell and Coombs hypersentivity reactions
gel-like consistency
gel-like envelope
gel-like fluid
gel-like material
gel medium
gel slab
Gelvatol
gemastete cell
Gemella morbillorum
gemistocyte
gemistocytic astrocytoma
gemistocytic cell
genal gland
Gendre fixative
Gendre solution
gene (pl. genes)
  allelic
  APC (adenomatous polyposis coli) tumor suppressor
  antioncogene
  autosomal

gene *(continued)*
  bcl-2
  codominant
  control
  DCC (deleted in colon carcinoma) tumor suppressor
  dominant
  extrachromosomal
  H
  histocompatibility
  holandric
  homeobox
  homeotic
  housekeeping
  immune response
  jumping
  lethal
  mitochondrial
  modifier
  mutant
  NF (neurofibromatosis)
  NF1 tumor suppressor
  NF2 tumor suppressor
  operator
  p53 tumor suppressor
  pleiotropic
  polyphrenic
  RB1 tumor suppressor
  recessive
  regulator
  repressor
  SOS
  split
  transforming
  tumor suppressor
  V
  X-linked
  Y-linked
  Z
gene mapping
general sensory cortex
generalized morphea

generalized pustular psoriasis of Zambusch
generalized reticular to maculopapular rash
genetic amniocentesis
genetic counseling
genetic death
genetic diagnosis
genetic marker
genetic material
genetic sex of individual
genetically induced overdevelopment
Gengou phenomenon
genial (chin) tubercle
genicular artery
geniculate body
geniculate ganglion
geniculocalcarine tract
genioglossus muscle
genital branch of genitofemoral nerve
genital canal
genital carcinoma
genital cord
genital corpuscle
genital duct
genital eminence
genital fold
genital gland
genital groove
genital herpes
genital herpes simplex
genitalia
  ambiguous external
  virilization of
genital ligament
genital neoplasm
genital organ
genital ridge
genital swelling
genital system
genital tract
genital tubercle
genital ulcer
genital wart, flat
genitocrural nerve
genitofemoral nerve, genital branch of
genitoinguinal ligament
genitourinary fistula
genitourinary system
genitourinary tuberculosis
Gennari band
genoblast
genomic mutation
genotype
gentamicin
gentian orange stain
gentian violet
gentian violet stain
genu of pancreatic duct
genus (pl. genera)
geotrichosis
Geotrichum capitatum
Geotrichum fermentans
Geotrichum penicillatum
Geraghty test
Gerdy fontanelle
Gerdy interatrial loop
Gerdy ligament
Gerhardt test for acetoacetic acid in urine
Gerhardt test for bile pigments in urine
Gerlach tendon
germ cell, primordial
germ disk
germinal area
germinal cell
germinal center in lymphoid tissue
germinal cord
germinal disk
germinal epithelium
germinal inclusion cyst
germinal infection
germinal membrane

germinal pole
germinal rod
germinal spot
germinal vesicle
germination
germinative layer
germinoma
germ layer
germ membrane
germ nucleus
germ tube test
Gerota fascia
Gerrard test for glucose in urine
gestational age (GA)
gestational diabetes
gestational edema
gestational proteinuria
gestational sac
GFAP (glial fibrillary acidic protein)
GFAP antibody
GFR (glomerular filtration rate)
GGT (gamma-glutamyl transpeptidase)
GGTP liver function test
GH (growth hormone)
Ghon primary lesion
Ghon-Sachs bacillus
Ghon tubercle
ghost cell
ghost corpuscle
Giacomini, band of
Giannuzzi cell
giant Betz cell
giant cell
giant cell arteritis
giant cell carcinoma
giant cell hepatitis
giant cell monstrocellular sarcoma
giant cell myeloma
giant cell myocarditis
giant cell of bone tumor
giant cell pneumonia
giant cell sarcoma
giant cell tumor
giant chromosome
giant follicle lymphoma
giant follicular hyperplasia
giant hairy nevus
giant neutrophil
giant osteoid osteoma
giant pigmented nevus
Giardia lamblia
giardiasis
Gibberella fujikuroi
gibbous deformity
Giemsa stain
Giemsa-Wright stain
Gierke cell
Gies biuret test for proteins
GIFT (gamete intrafallopian transfer)
gigantism, pituitary
Gilchrist disease
Gilchrist skin test
gill arch skeleton
gill cleft
Gillette suspensory ligament
Gilson solution
Gimbernat ligament
Gimenez stain
gingivobuccal groove
gingiva (pl. gingivae)
gingival abscess
gingival crest
gingival curvature
gingival gland
gingival margin
gingival mucosa
gingival septum
gingival space
gingival sulcus
gingival trough
gingival zone
gingiva proper
gingivitis, necrotizing
gingivobuccal sulcus

gingivodental ligament
gingivolabial groove
gingivolabial sulcus
gingivolingual groove
gingivolingual sulcus
ginglymoid joint
ginglymus
Giordano sphincter
GIP (gastric inhibitory polypeptide)
GIP (glucose-dependent insulinotropic polypeptide)
GI (gastrointestinal) tract
gitter cell
glabrous
glacial acetic acid
glancing wound
gland
  absorbent
  accessory
  accessory lacrimal
  accessory parotid
  accessory suprarenal
  accessory thyroid
  acid
  acinar
  acinotubular
  acinous
  admaxillary
  adrenal
  aggregate
  agminate
  agminated
  Albarrán
  albuminous
  alveolar
  anal
  anteprostatic
  aortic
  apical (of tongue)
  apocrine
  aporic
  areolar

gland *(continued)*
  arterial
  arteriococcygeal
  arytenoid
  Aselli
  axillary
  axillary sweat
  Bartholin
  Bauhin
  biliary
  Blandin
  Blandin and Nuhn
  blood
  blood vessel
  Boerhaave
  Bonnot
  Bowman
  brachial
  bronchial
  Bruch
  Brunner
  buccal
  bulbocavernous
  bulbourethral
  cardiac
  carotid
  celiac
  ceruminous
  cervical (of uterus)
  cheek
  Ciaccio
  ciliary
  circumanal
  Cloquet
  closed
  Cobelli
  coccygeal
  coil
  compound
  compound tubuloalveolar
  conglobate
  conjunctival

gland *(continued)*
convoluted
Cowper
cutaneous
ductless
duodenal
Duverney
Ebner
eccrine
ecdysial
Eglis
endocervical
endocrine
endoepithelial
endometrial
esophageal
excretory
exocrine
follicular (of tongue)
fundic
fundus
Galeati
gastric
gastroepiploic
Gay
genal
genital
gingival
Gley
globate
glomiform
glossopalatine
greater vestibular
Guérin
gustatory
guttural
Harder
Havers
haversian
hemal
hemal lymph
hemolymph

gland *(continued)*
Henle
hepatic
heterocrine
hibernating
holocrine
incretory
intercarotid
intermediate
interscapular
interstitial
intestinal
intraepithelial
intramuscular
jugular
Knoll
Krause
labial
lacrimal
lactiferous
large intestine
large sweat
laryngeal
lenticular
Lieberkühn
Littré
Luschka
lymph
lymphatic
major salivary
malpighian
mammary
mandibular
master
meibomian
merocrine
Méry
mesenteric
mesocolic
mixed
molar
Moll

gland *(continued)*
- monoptychic
- Montgomery
- Morgagni
- mucous (lingual)
- mucus-secreting
- multicellular
- myometrial
- nabothian
- Naboth
- nasal
- Nuhn
- oil
- olfactory
- oxyntic
- palatine
- palpebral
- pancreaticosplenic
- parafrenal
- parathyroid
- paraurethral
- parotid
- pectoral
- peptic
- Peyer
- pharyngeal
- Philip
- pineal
- pituitary
- Poirier
- polyptychic
- pregnancy
- prehyoid
- preputial
- prostate
- pyloric
- racemose
- retromolar
- Rivinus
- Rosenmüller
- saccular
- salivary

gland *(continued)*
- Sandström
- saw-toothed
- Schüller
- sebaceous
- seminal
- sentinel
- seromucous
- serous
- Serres
- sexual
- Sigmund
- simple
- Skene
- small intestine (solitary)
- splenoid
- Stahr
- staphyline
- subauricular
- sublingual
- submandibular
- submaxillary
- sudoriferous
- suprarenal
- Suzanne
- sweat
- synovial
- target
- tarsal
- tarsoconjunctival
- Terson
- Theile
- thymus
- thyroid
- Tiedemann
- tongue
- tracheal
- trachoma
- triangular suprarenal
- tubular
- tubuloacinar
- tubuloalveolar

gland *(continued)*
- tympanic
- Tyson
- ultimobranchial
- unicellular
- urethral
- uropygial
- uterine
- utricular
- vaginal
- vascular
- vestibular
- Virchow
- vitelline
- vulvovaginal
- Waldeyer
- Wasmann
- Weber
- Wepfer
- Wölfer
- Wolfring
- Zeis
- Zuckerkandl

glanders
glanders bacillus
glandes (pl. of glans)
gland neck extension
gland of neck
glands of biliary mucosa
glands of Haller
glands of mouth
glands of prepuce, odoriferous
glands of Wolfring
glandular alveolus
glandular artery
glandular epithelium
glandular fever
glandular mastitis
glandular system
glandular tissue
glandulopreputial lamella
glans (pl. glandes)
glans clitoridis
glans, corona of
glans penis, inflammation of
Glanzmann disease
glaserian artery
glaserian fissure
glass factor
glass-rod phenomenon
glassy degeneration in muscle
glassy swelling
glaucoma
- chronic
- congenital
- narrow-angle
- open-angle
- posttraumatic
- wide-angle

Gleason grade
Gleason score
Gleason tumor grade
glenohumeral articulation
glenohumeral ligament
glenoid cavity
glenoid fossa
glenoid ligament
glenoid surface
glenoidal labrum
Glerke cell
Gley cell
Gley gland
glia
glia cell
glial cytoplasmic inclusion
glial fibrillary acidic protein (GFAP)
glial proliferation
glial reaction
gliding joint
glioblast
glioblastoma multiforme
glioma
gliosis
Glisson capsule

glistening degeneration
glistening masses
glitter cell
globate gland
globoid cell
globoid cell leukodystrophy
globoid material
globose
globotriaosylceramide deposition in arterial intima and media
globotriaosylceramide deposition in kidney
globotriaosylceramide deposition in myocardium
globular cytoplasmic inclusions
globular protein
globular proteinuria
globular valve
globule, dentin
globulin
  accelerator (AcG, ac-g)
  alpha
  alpha antitrypsin
  antihemophilic
  beta
  chickenpox immune
  copper-containing plasma
  corticosteroid-binding
  gamma
  hepatitis B hyperimmune
  thyroxine-binding (TBG)
globulin test
glomerular artery
glomerular basement membrane antibody
glomerular capillary membrane
glomerular filtrate (also, filtration)
glomerular filtration rate (GFR)
glomerular nephritis
glomerular selectivity test
glomerular tufts
glomerulocapsular nephritis
glomerulonephritis
  acute
  acute poststreptococcal
  chronic
  membranoproliferative
  membranous
  necrotizing
  proliferative
  segmental necrotizing
glomerulosa cell
glomerulosa zona
glomerulosclerosis
glomerulus (pl. glomeruli)
glomiform gland
glomus body
glomus cell
glossitis
glossoepiglottic ligament
glossopalatine arch
glossopalatine fold
glossopalatine gland
glottis, false
glucagon hormone
glucagon stimulation test
glucocerebrosidase deficiency
Glucocheck glucose monitoring machine
glucogenic storage
Glucola screen
Glucometer II
glucosamine
glucose
  blood
  body fluid
  cerebrospinal fluid (CSF)
  fasting blood
  random blood
  rapid absorption of dietary
  spinal fluid
  test
  2-hour postprandial blood
  urine

glucose-dependent insulinotropic
polypeptide (GIP)
glucose in urine
glucose level of spinal fluid
glucose oxidase method
glucose oxidase paper strip test
glucose-6-phosphatase
glucose-6-phosphatase deficiency
glucose-6-phosphate dehydrogenase
deficiency (G-6-PD, G6PD)
glucose test
glucose tolerance curve
glucose tolerance factor
glucose tolerance test (GTT)
glucose tolerance test with cortisone
Glucostix
glucuronic acid
glucuronosyltransferase (liver enzyme)
glucuronyl transferase, deficiency of
glue ear
glutamic oxaloacetic transaminase
(GOT)
glutamic pyruvic transaminase (GPT)
glutamine, cerebrospinal fluid
glutamyltransferase (GGT) test
glutaraldehyde
glutathione reductase in erythrocytes
test
gluteal aponeurosis
gluteal artery
gluteal fold
gluteal nerve
gluteal region
gluteal vessel
gluten-sensitive enteropathy
gluteofemoral
gluteoinguinal
glutethimide
gluteus maximus
glycated hemoglobin
glycerol test, free
glycerophosphate test for renal function
glycine test
glycogen
glycogen deposits in muscle
glycogenic degeneration
glycogen infiltration
glycogen nephrosis
glycogen phosphorylase kinase
glycogen starch synthase
glycogen storage disease
glycogen vacuolation
glycogen vacuoles in cytoplasm and
nuclei of hepatocytes
glycogen vacuoles in renal tubule cells
glycogenolytic
glycogenosis
glycogeusia
glycohemia
glycohemoglobin
glycolic acid test
glycolipid pattern
glycol methacrylate
glycoprotein
alpha acid
CA-125
histidine-rich (HRGP)
glycosuria
alimentary
renal
glycosylated hemoglobin (hemoglobin
A_{1c})
glycosylated hemoglobin test
glycotropic factor
glycyltryptophan test for carcinoma of
stomach
glygenolysis
glyoxylic acid test
GM activator protein
Gmelin test for bile pigments
GNID (gram-negative intracellular
diplococci)
GMS (Gomori's methenamine-silver)
stain

Gn-RH (gonadotropin-releasing
hormone)
Goa antigen (Gonzales blood antigen)
goblet cell
Goethe bone
Gofman test
Gogli cell
goiter
aberrant
adenomatous
Basedow
colloid
congenital
cystic
diffuse
diving
endemic
exophthalmic
fibrous
follicular
intrathoracic
iodide
lingual
lymphadenoid
multinodular
nodular
nontoxic
parenchymatous
perivascular
plunging
retrovascular
simple
soft
substernal
suffocative
thyroid
toxic (diffuse)
vascular
wandering
gold (Au)
Goldblatt hypertension
Goldblatt kidney
gold chloride
gold stain
gold test
golf-hole ureteral orifice
Golgi apparatus
Golgi epithelial cell
Golgi method of staining
Golgi osmiobichromate fixative
Golgi stain
Golgi zone
Gombault degeneration
Gombault neuritis
Gomori aldehyde fuchsin
Gomori methenamine-silver (GMS)
Gomori stain
Gomori-Takamatsu stain
gomphosis articulation
gomphosis, dentoalveolar
gomphosis joint
gonadal neoplasm
gonadotropic hormone (GTH)
gonadotropic-releasing factor (GRF)
gonadotropin
chorionic
human chorionic (HCG, hCG)
gonococcal ophthalmia of newborn
gonococcal perihepatitis
gonococcal salpingitis
gonococcal stomatitis
gonococcal urethritis
gonococcus (pl. gonococci)
gonorrhea (GC)
gonorrheal stomatitis
Gonzales blood antigen (Goa)
Goodpasture syndrome
Goormaghtigh cell
gooseflesh
Gordon test for globulin-albumin in
spinal fluid
Gosset, spiral band of
GOT (glutamic oxaloacetic
transaminase)

Gothic arch formation
Gothlin capillary fragility test
Gougerot-Blum syndrome
gout, uric acid crystals in
gouty arthritis
gouty proteinuria
Gowers muscular dystrophy
Gowers solution
G protein
GPT (glutamic pyruvic transaminase)
graafian follicle
grade (see also *classification*, *stage*)
  FIGO (International Federation of
    Gynecology and Obstetrics)
    adenocarcinoma of endometrium
  Gleason tumor
  Hyams esthesioneuroblastoma
  murmur
  osteoarthritis
  placental
grade of malignant neoplasm
gradient
  atrioventricular
  Ficoll
grading neoplasm
grading of malignancy
grading of tumor
graft, chorioallantoic
Gregerson and Boas test
Graham-Cole cholecystography
grainy texture
gram (g)
Gram iodine
Gram method
gram-negative bacilli
gram-negative bacteria
gram-negative coccus
gram-negative diplococci
gram-negative intracellular diplococci
  (GNID)
gram-negative rod
gram-positive
gram-positive bacteria
Gram solution
grams per deciliter (g/dL)
Gram stain
granular appearance
granular atrophy
granular casts in urine
granular cell
granular cell layer
granular cytoplasm
granular endoplasmic reticulum
granular induration
granular kidney
granular leukocyte
granular pneumonocyte
granular texture
granulation tissue
granulation tissue of mucous
  membrane
granulation tissue of skin
granulation, toxic
granule
  acidophil
  acidophilic
  acrosomal
  albuminous
  Alder-Reilly
  alpha
  Altmann
  amphophil
  argentaffin
  azure
  azurophil
  basal
  basophil
  basophilic cytoplasmic
  beta
  Birbeck
  Bollinger
  Chédiak-Higashi
  chromatic
  chromophil

granule *(continued)*
- chromophobe
- coarse
- coarse azurophilic
- cone
- cytoplasmic
- delta
- DiPAS-positive
- Ehrlich
- elementary
- eosinophil
- fuchsinophil
- gamma
- granule
- hemosiderin
- iodophil
- kappa
- keratohyalin
- Langerhans
- matrix
- Much
- Neusser
- Nissl
- rod-shaped
- secretory
- sulfur
- toxic
- vermiform
- Weibel-Palade
- zymogen

granule cell of connective tissue
granules of cornstarch
granuloadipose
granulocyte
granulocyte colony–stimulating factor
granulocyte–macrophage colony–stimulating factor
granulocytic leukemia
granulocytic sarcoma
granulocytic white cell
granulocytopenia
granulocytosis

granuloma (pl. granulomata)
- amebic
- apical
- beryllium
- candidal
- cholesterol
- coccidioidal
- coli
- eosinophilic
- epithelioid
- fishtank
- foreign-body
- gangrenous
- Hodgkin
- infectious
- inguinal
- laryngeal
- lipoid
- lipophagic
- Majocchi
- malarial
- midline
- Mignon eosinophilic
- miliary
- paracoccidioidal
- plasma cell
- pseudopyogenic
- pyogenic
- reticulohistiocytic
- rheumatic
- silicotic
- stellate
- swimming pool
- trichophytic
- umbilicus
- xanthomatous

granuloma annulare
granuloma formation
granuloma inguinale
granuloma multiforme
granuloma telangiectaticum
granuloma-theca cell tumor

granulomatosis
  allergic
  Wegener
granulomatous conjunctivitis
granulomatous hepatitis
granulomatous infection
granulomatous inflammation
granulomatous lymphoma
granulomatous myocarditis
granulomatous pannus invading cartilage
granulomatous pneumonia
granulomatous pneumonitis
granulomatous ulcer
granulomatous vasculitis
granulopenia
granulopoiesis
granulosa cell
granulosa cell tumor
granulosa-lutein cells
granulovacuolar degeneration
grape cell
grape-cluster shape
grapelike clusters of cysts
grass bacillus
grass dermatitis
grave prognosis
gravel particle
Graves disease
gravida
gravid uterus
Gravindex pregnancy test
gravis, myasthenia
gravitation abscess
gravity, specific (of urine)
gray (Gy) (radiation dose equal to 100 rads)
gray hepatization stage of pneumonia
gray induration
graying of the hair
gray matter, degeneration of
gray scale
gray tumor
greasy scaling
greasy texture
great alveolar cells
great auricular nerve
great cardiac vein
great saphenous vein
great vein
great vessels, transposition of
greater curvature
greater curvature of stomach
greater multangular bone
greater omentum
greater palatine artery
greater palatine canal
greater palatine foramen
greater palatine nerve
greater peritoneal sac
greater sac of peritoneal cavity
greater trochanter of femur
greater tubercle
greater vestibular gland
green liver
Greene biopsy needle
green pus
green stool
Gregerson and Boas test for blood in feces
grenz zone
Gridley stain
Grigg test for proteins
grinder tissue
Griscelli syndrome
gritty material
Grocott-Gomori methenamine-silver nitrate stain
Grocott-Gomori stain
Grocott methenamine-silver
groove (pl. grooves)
  abomasal
  alveolingual
  alveolobuccal

groove *(continued)*
- alveololabial
- anal intersphincteric
- anterolateral
- anteromedian
- arterial
- atrioventricular (AV)
- auriculoventricular
- basilar
- bicipital
- branchial
- buccal
- carotid
- carpal
- cavernous
- central
- coronary
- costal
- dental
- developmental
- digastric
- esophageal
- ethmoidal
- gastric
- genital
- gingivobuccal
- gingivolabial
- Harrison
- infraorbital
- interatrial
- intertubercular
- interventricular
- labial
- lacrimal
- Liebermeister
- neural
- paravertebral
- radial
- radial neck
- Sibson
- spindle colonic
- ulnar

groove *(continued)*
- urethral
- venous
- Verga lacrimal
- vertebral

gross architecture
gross cystic disease
gross description of specimen
gross diagnosis
gross examination
gross examination of tissue
gross hematuria
gross lesion
grossly intact architecture
gross report
Gross test for trypsin in feces
ground-glass appearance
ground-glass-appearing cytoplasm
ground-glass cell
ground-glass pattern
ground itch (pruritus at site of skin invasion)
ground substance
Group A beta-hemolytic *Streptococcus*
Group B beta-hemolytic *Streptococcus* (GBS)
group, blood (also, blood type)
grouping, blood
group-specific
Grover disease
growth center
growth factor
growth, failure of long-bone
growth hormone
- deficiency of
- excess of
- somatotropin

growth hormone antibody
growth hormone–arginine stimulation test
growth hormone–glucagon stimulation test

growth hormone–L-dopa stimulation test
growth hormone–releasing hormone (GH-RH)
growth-onset diabetes
growth plate
growth, stunting of
Gruber fossa
grumose
grumous material
grumous tissue
Grynfeltt triangle
G-6-PD (G6PD) test
GTC (guanidine isothiocyanate)
GTC/silica beads protocol
GTH (gonadotropic hormone)
GU (genitourinary)
guaiac-negative stool
guaiac-negative test for occult blood in stool
guaiac-positive stool
guaiac-positive test for occult blood in stool
guaiac test for occult blood
Guama virus
guanidine isothiocyanate (GTC)
guanine cell
guanyl cyclase
guanyl-nucleotide-binding protein
guanylins
Guarnieri body
Guaroa virus
gubernacular canal
gubernaculum
Guérin fold
Guérin gland
Guérin sinus
Guidi canal
Guillain-Barré syndrome
guinea worm
gullet
gum, mucilaginous
gumma (pl. gummas or gummata)
gummata (pl. of gumma), tuberculous
gummatous abscess
gummatous meningitis
gums
  bleeding
  swollen
Gunn dots
Gunning-Lieben test
Gunning test for acetone in urine
gunshot wound
gunstock deformity
Günzberg test (Guenzberg)
Günz ligament (Guenz)
gustatory cell
gustatory gland
gut (intestine)
  blind
  large
  small
gut-associated lymphoid tissue (GALT)
Guthrie bacterial inhibition assay (GBIA)
Guthrie test for phenylketonuria
guttate
guttate morphea (white spot disease)
gutter
  lateral
  left
  paracolic
  peritoneal
  right
guttural gland
gutter wound
Gutzeit test for arsenic
Guyon canal
Gy (gray) (radiation dose equal to 100 rads)
gynatresia
gynecoid pelvis
gynecomastia
gynecophoric canal

gyrochrome cell
gyrus (pl. gyri)
  angular
  callosal
  dentate
  fasciolar
  fusiform
  middle temporal
gyrus rectus

H, h

HAA (hepatitis associated antigen)
habitual abortion
HACEK (*Haemophilus, Actinobacillus actinomycetemcomitans, Cardiobacterium hominis, Eikenella corrodens, Kingella kingae*) gram-negative bacilli
Haemophilus
Haemophilus aegyptius
Haemophilus aphrophilus
Haemophilus ducreyi
Haemophilus haemolyticus
Haemophilus influenzae
Haemophilus influenzae meningitis
Haemophilus influenzae pneumonia
Haemophilus influenzae type b (Hib)
Haemophilus parahaemolyticus
Haemophilus parainfluenzae
Haemophilus paraphrophilus
Haemophilus segnis
Haemophilus vaginalis
Hafnia
Hafnia alvei (formerly *Enterobacter hafniae*)
Hagedorn needle
Hageman factor
Haglund deformity
HAI, HI (hemagglutination inhibition) test
HAI (hepatic arterial infusion)
Hailey-Hailey disease
hair
  auditory
  bamboo
  catagen
  color and distribution of head and body
  ingrown
  scalp
  telogen
  vellus
hair bulb
hair canal
hair cell
hair disk
hair follicle
hairlike process
hairline crack in bone cortex
hair loss
hairy cell
hairy-cell leukemia (HCL)
hairy mole
hairy nevus
Haldane apparatus

Hale iron stain
half-normal solution
halisteresis phenomenon
Haller ansa
Haller cell
Haller, glands of
Hallopeau disease
halo melanoma
halo nevus
Ham acidified serum test
Ham F-10 solution
hamartoma
hamartoma of glial tissue
hamartomatous
hamate bone
hamate, capitate
hamate facet
hamatein test
Hamburger phenomenon
Hamdi solution
Hamel test for jaundice
Hammarsten test for globulin
hammock ligament
hamster egg penetration assay
hamstring tendon
hand
 articulations of
 digital artery of
 phalanges of
H&E (hematoxylin and eosin) stain
hand eczema
hand, foot, and mouth disease
H&H (hemoglobin and hematocrit)
hand muscle
hand, phalanges of joints of
Hand-Schüller-Christian disease
hanging drop preparation
Hanks buffer
Hanks stain
Hannover canal
Hansel stain
Hansen bacillus
Hansen disease
Hantaan virus
Hantavirus
Hantavirus pulmonary syndrome (HPS)
hapten inhibition test
haptoglobin (Hp)
hardened pelvis
hardening of arteries
Harder gland
Harding and Ruttan test for acetoacetic acid
hardness scale
hard palate
hard stool
harelip
Hargraves cell
harlequin fetus
Harris and Ray test
Harris band
Harrison spot test for bilirubin in urine
Hartmann point
Hartmann pouch
Hartnup disease
Hart test for oxybutyric acid in urine
Hashimoto disease
Hashimoto thyroiditis
Hassall corpuscle
HAT (hypoxanthine, aminopterin, thymidine) medium
HATTS (hemagglutination treponemal test for syphilis) test
haunch bone
haustra
haustral fold
haustral markings
haustral pattern
haustral pouch
haustrum (pl. haustra)
HAV (hepatitis A virus)
Haverhill fever
Havers gland

haversian canal
haversian gland
haversian system
Hayem solution
hay fever
Hay test for bile salts
Hb, Hgb (hemoglobin)
HbAg (hepatitis B antigen)
H band
HB_cAb (hepatitis B core antibody)
HB_cAg (hepatitis B core antigen)
HB_eAb (hepatitis B "e" antibody)
HB_eAg (hepatitis B "e" antigen)
HBIg (hepatitis B immunoglobulin)
HB_sAb (hepatitis B surface antibody)
HB_sAg (hepatitis B surface antigen)
HBV (hepatitis B virus)
HbF (fetal hemoglobin)
HCG, hCG (human chorionic gonadotropin)
HCl (hydrochloric acid)
HCO_3 (bicarbonate)
HCT (hematocrit)
H disk
HDL (high density lipoprotein)
HDL cholesterol (HDLC)
HDVAg (hepatitis D virus antigen)
head
head louse (pl. lice)
head of femur
head of pancreas
head of rib
"head post" (examination of brain)
Heaf test
healing ulcer
hearing loss
heart
- aortic opening of
- apex of
- artificial
- coronary artery of
- degeneration of

heart *(continued)*
- diaphragmatic surface of
- enlargement of
- fatty
- horizontal
- inferior border of
- inflammation of
- left
- left border of
- left ventricle of
- myxedema of
- right
- right border of
- right ventricle of
- sternocostal surface of
- superior border of
- vertical

heart clot
heart disease cell
heart failure cells
heart failure classification
heart lesion cell
heart-lung transplant
heart muscle
heart-shaped pelvis
heart transplant
heat capacity
heat coagulation test
heat edema
heat, injury due to
heat instability test
heat labile
heat-labile protein
heat shock protein
heat-stable
heavy chain disease, alpha
heavy metal poisoning
heavy metal screening test
Hebra prurigo
Hecht pneumonia
heckle cell
hectogram (hg)

hectoliter (hL)
hectomole (hmol)
Hector, tendon of (heel tendon)
Hedley technique of tissue preparation
heel bone
heel tendon
heelstick
Heidenhain cell
Heidenhain iron hematoxylin
Heidenhain pouch
Heidenhain stain
Heinz body stain
Heinz cytoplasmic inclusion bodies
Hektoen, Kretschmer, and Welker protein
Hektoen phenomenon
HeLa cell
helical bacterium
helicine artery
Helicobacter pylori
Helicobacter pylori urease test
Heller test for albumin in urine
Heller test for blood in urine
Helly fixative
Helly Zenker-formalin solution
helmet cell
Helmholtz axis ligament
helminthic abscess
helper (T4) cell
helper/inducer T cell
helper lymphocytes
helper/suppressor cell ratio
helper T cell
helper virus
hemadsorbing virus
hemadsorption
hemadsorption test
hemadsorption virus
  type 1 (HA1 v.)
  type 2 (HA2 v.)
hemagglutination inhibition (HAI, HI) test
hemagglutination treponemal test for syphilis (HATTS)
hemal canal
hemal gland
hemal lymph gland
hemalum
hemalum stain
hemangioendothelioma
hemangioma
  capillary
  cavernous
  racemose
  sclerosing
  senile
  spider
  strawberry
  verrucous
hemangioma planum extensum
hemangiomatous nodule
hemapoiesis (hematopoiesis)
hemarthrosis
hematin test for blood
hematemesis
Hematest
hemarthrosis
hematocrit ("crit") (HCT, Hct)
hematogenous abscess
hematogenous embolism
hematogenous jaundice
hematogenous metastasis
hematogenous osteomyelitis
hematogenous pigment
hematogenous proteinuria
hematogenous pyelonephritis
hematogenous tuberculosis
hematohyaloid degeneration
hematoidin
hematologic malignancy
hematology
hematoma
  chronic subdural
  corpus luteum

hematoma *(continued)*
  encapsulated subdural
  epidural
  intramural
  organized
  subdural
  wound
hematoma formation
hematopoiesis, extramedullary
hematopoietic malignancy
hematopoietic tissue
hematoxylin
  Boehmer
  Delafield
  Gill
  Harris
  iron
  phosphotungstic acid (PTAH)
hematoxylin and eosin (H&E) stain
hematoxylin–malachite green–basic fuchsin stain
hematoxylin–phloxine B stain
hematuria
  acute onset
  benign recurrent
  endemic
  essential
  false
  functional
  gross
  macroscopic
  microscopic
  painful
  painless
  persistent
  primary
  renal
  terminal
  total
  urethral
  vesical
heme iron
heme-negative stool
heme-positive stool
hemiazygos vein, accessory
hemicolon
hemidiaphragm
hemin test for blood
hemisphere
  cerebellar
  cerebral
  dominant
  left
  right
hemivertebra
hemoaccess
hemoagglutination
hemobilia
hemobilinuria
hemocatheresis
hemocatheretic
Hemoccult guaiac test for occult blood
hemocholecyst
hemocholecystitis
hemochromatosis
hemoconcentration
hemoculture
hemocytometer
hemoglobin (Hb, Hgb)
  aberrant
  Bart abnormal
  defective synthesis of
  fetal
  free
  glycated
  glycosylated
  mean corpuscular
  oxygenated
  plasma
  pyridoxilated stroma-free (SFHb)
  reduced
  serial
  serum
  sickle cell

hemoglobin *(continued)*
  target cell
  unstable
  urinary
hemoglobin A
hemoglobin A_{lc}
hemoglobin A_2
hemoglobin and hematocrit (H&H)
hemoglobin anti-Lepore
hemoglobin-binding capacity
hemoglobin breakdown
hemoglobin C
hemoglobin Chesapeake
hemoglobin Constant Spring
hemoglobin D
hemoglobin disease
hemoglobin E
hemoglobin electrophoresis
hemoglobin F (fetal hemoglobin)
hemoglobin Gower-1
hemoglobin Gower-2
hemoglobin H (HbH)
hemoblobin I
hemoglobin J
hemoglobin Kansas
hemoglobin Lepore
hemoglobin M
hemoglobinometer
hemoglobinopathy, hereditary
hemoglobin Portland
hemoglobin Rainier
hemoglobin S
hemoglobin test
hemoglobinuria
  bacillary
  paroxysmal cold
  paroxysmal nocturnal
hemoglobin Yakima
hemogram
hemolymph gland
hemolymphatic cells
hemolymphatic system
hemolymphatic tissue
hemolysin
  beta
  cold
hemolysis
hemolytic anemia
hemolytic disease of newborn
hemolytic malaria
hemolytic reaction
hemolytic-uremic syndrome
hemolyze
hemolyzed blood
hemolyzed red blood cells
hemolyzing antibody
hemopericardium
hemoperitoneum
hemophilia A
hemophilia B
hemophilia, classical
hemophilic joint
hemoptysis
hemorrhage
  epidural
  extradural
  focal
  frank
  interstitial
  intra-alveolar
  punctate
  salmon-patch
  severe
  stromal
  subarachnoid
  subdural
  subserosal
hemorrhagic colitis
hemorrhagic consolidation of lung
hemorrhagic cyst
hemorrhagic cystitis
hemorrhagic dengue
hemorrhagic effusion
hemorrhagic encephalitis

hemorrhagic fever
hemorrhagic gastritis
hemorrhagic infarct
hemorrhagic malaria
hemorrhagic myelitis
hemorrhagic necrosis
hemorrhagic necrosis of alveolar septa
hemorrhagic nephritis
hemorrhagic pericarditis
hemorrhagic plague
hemorrhagic pleurisy
hemorrhagic salpingitis
hemorrhagic shock
hemorrhagic telangiectasia
hemorrhagic tendency
hemorrhoidal artery
hemorrhoidal plexus
hemorrhoid
  external
  internal
  thrombosed
hemosiderin granule
hemosiderin in hepatocytes
hemosiderin-laden macrophage
hemosiderin test
hemosiderosis
hemothorax
HEMPAS cell
Henderson-Hasselbach equation
Henke space
Henke triangle
Henke trigone
Henle, ampulla of
Henle ansa
Henle canal
Henle gland
Henle loop
Henoch-Schönlein purpura
Henoch-Schönlein syndrome
Hensen canal
Hensen cell
Hensen disk
Hensing ligament
heparin anticoagulant
heparin lock flush solution
heparin therapy, monitoring of
hepatic abscess
hepatic architecture
hepatic arterial infusion (HAI)
hepatic artery
hepatic atrophy
hepatic bed
hepatic calculus
hepatic capsule
hepatic carcinoma
hepatic cirrhosis
hepatic coma
hepatic cord
hepatic degeneration
hepatic duct
hepatic encephalopathy
hepatic failure
hepatic flexure
hepatic function test
hepatic gland
hepatic glycogen storage
hepatic hilum
hepatic ligament
hepatic lobular parenchyma
hepatic lobule
hepatic lymph node
hepatic necrosis
hepatic nerve plexus
hepatic obstruction
hepatic osteomalacia
hepatic outflow tract
hepatic parenchyma
hepatic parenchymal cell
hepatic porphyria
hepatic-renal angle
hepatic segment of liver
hepatic sinusoid
hepatic triad
hepatic vein

hepatic venous outflow
hepatic web
hepatitis
  acute parenchymatous
  alcoholic
  autoimmune
  chronic active
  chronic persisting
  coinfection with
  enterically transmitted, non-A, non-B (ET-NANB)
  familial
  fulminant
  giant cell
  infectious
  neonatal
  non-A, non-B (NANB)
  plasma cell
  post-transfusion
  serum
  subacute
  testing
  toxic
  transfusion
  viral
hepatitis A
hepatitis associated antigen (HAA)
hepatitis A virus (HAV)
hepatitis B
hepatitis B antigen (HBAg)
hepatitis B core antibody (HB_cAb)
hepatitis B core antigen (HB_cAg)
hepatitis B e antibody (HB_eAb)
hepatitis B e antigen (HB_eAg)
hepatitis B hyperimmune globulin
hepatitis B immunoglobulin (HBIg)
hepatitis B surface antibody (HB_sAb)
hepatitis B surface antigen (HB_sAg)
hepatitis B virus (HBV)
hepatitis C
hepatitis C virus
hepatitis D (delta) virus (HDV)
hepatitis D virus antigen (HDVAg)
hepatitis E
hepatitis E virus
hepatization
hepatobiliary
hepatobiliary tree
hepatocarcinoma
hepatocellular carcinoma
hepatocellular jaundice
hepatocolic ligament
hepatocystocolic ligament
hepatocyte
hepatoduodenal ligament
hepatoduodenal-peritoneal reflection
hepatoerythropoietic porphyria (HEP)
hepatoesophageal ligament
hepatogastric duodenal ligament
hepatogastric ligament
hepatogenous jaundice
hepatogenous pigment
hepatoiminodiacetic acid (HIDA)
hepatolenticular degeneration
hepatomegaly
hepatopancreatic ampulla, sphincter of
hepatopancreatic fold
hepatophrenic ligament
hepatopleural fistula
hepatorenal angle
hepatorenal pouch
hepatorenal recess
hepatosplenomegaly
hepatoumbilical ligament
HEp-Z cell culture preparation
hereditary abetalipoproteinemia
hereditary adult-onset leukodystrophy
hereditary alopecia
hereditary angioneurotic edema
hereditary cerebral leukodystrophy
hereditary elliptocytosis
hereditary factor
hereditary hemoglobinopathy
hereditary hemolytic anemia

hereditary hemorrhagic telangiectasia
hereditary methemoglobinemia
hereditary optic neuritis
hereditary spherocytosis
hereditary telangiectasia
Herellea vaginicola (now
  Acinetobacter calcoaceticus)
Hering, canal of
Hering duct
Hermann fixative
hermaphroditism, true
hernia
  diaphragmatic
  direct inguinal
  esophageal
  femoral
  hiatal
  incarcerated
  incarceration of
  indirect inguinal
  inguinal
  peritoneal
  strangulated
  strangulation of
  umbilical
  ventral
hernial aneurysm
hernial canal
hernia sac
herniated disk
herniated nucleus pulposus
herpangina virus
herpes
  genital
  orofacial
  traumatic
  wrestler's
herpes circinatus bullosus
herpes genitalis
herpes gestationis
herpes simplex
herpes simplex virus (HSV)
herpes ulcer
herpesvirus
  type 1
  type 2
  type 3
  type 4 (Epstein-Barr virus)
  type 5 (cytomegalovirus)
  type 6
herpes whitlow
herpes zoster
herpes zoster auricularis
herpes zoster virus (HZV)
herpetic fever
herpetic stomatitis
herpetiform
Herzberg test
Hess capillary test
Hesselbach ligament
Hesselbach triangle
heterocrine gland
heteroduplex
heterogeneous
heterologous protein
heterologous tissue
heteromeric cell
heterophil
heterophile agglutination
heterophile agglutination test
heterophile antibodies
heterophile titer
heterophilic leukocyte
heterotopic pancreas
heterotopic pregnancy
heterotopic tissue
heterozygosity
hexagonal cell
hexamer
hexosaminidase A
hexosaminidase A deficiency
Hey ligament
hg (hectogram)
H gene

hGH (human growth hormone)
HI, HAI (hemagglutination inhibition) test
5-HIAA (5-hydroxyindoleacetic acid)
hiatal (or hiatus) hernia
hiatus
  aortic
  esophageal
  fallopian
  semilunar
  sternocostal
Hib (*H. influenzae* type b)
hibernating gland
Hickey-Hare test for diabetes insipidus
hidradenitis suppurativa
hidradenoma
high density lipoprotein (HDL)
highest genicular artery
highest intercostal artery
highest thoracic artery
highest turbinated bone
high frequency blood group
high-grade malignancy
high-grade surface osteosarcoma
Highmore, antrum cardiacum of
high normal
high normal test result
high-performance liquid chromatography
high power
high-power field (hpf)
high-pressure liquid chromatography (HPLC)
hilar cells
hilar cell tumor of ovary
hilar lymph node
hilar plate
hilar vessel
hila (pl. of hilum)
hila of kidneys
hila of lung
Hildebrandt test for urobilin in urine
Hill-Sachs lesion
hilum (pl. hila) (formerly hilus)
  hepatic
  lips of
  renal
  splenic
hilum of kidney
hilum of lung
hilus cell
hindgut
Hines-Brown cold pressor test
hinge joint
Hinton test
hip articulation
hip joint
hippocampus, Hirano bodies in the
Hirano bodies in the hippocampus
Hirschfeld canal
Hirsch-Peiffer stain
Hirschsprung disease
hirsutism
His
  angle of
  atrioventricular node of
  atrioventricular opening of
  bundle of
His band
His bundle
His canal
His duct
His space
Hiss capsule stain
Histalog test
histamine flare test
histidine loading test
histidine-rich glycoproteins (HRGP)
histidyl-tRNA synthetase
histiocyte
  cardiac
  hyperplasia of
  sea-blue
  wandering

histiocytes in neurons
histiocytic lymphoma
histiocytoma
  benign fibrous
  malignant fibrous
histiocytosis
  nonlipid
  sinus
histochemistry
histochromatosis
histoclastic
histoclinical evaluation
histocompatibility gene
histocompatible
histocyte (histiocyte)
histodiagnosis
histodialysis
histodifferentiation
Histofine SAB-PO kit
histogenesis
histogenous
histohematogenous
histohydria
histohypoxia
histokinesis
histologic diagnosis
histologic lesion
histologic specimen
histology
Histopaque
Histopaque-1077 isolation reagent
histopathological diagnosis
histopathology
Histoplasma capsulatum
Histoplasma capsulatum antigen (HPA)
Histoplasma myocarditis
histoplasmin-latex test
histoplasmosis
His zone
HIV (human immunodeficiency virus)
HIVAGEN test
HIV antibody
HIV antibody test on blood
HIV Blot 2•2 test
HIV classification of children
HIV encephalitis
HIV encephalopathy
HIV-negative
HIV-positive
HIV proteins
hives
hL (hectoliter)
HLA (human lymphocyte antigen)
hmol (hectomole)
hobnail cell
hobnailed appearance of liver surface
Hoboken nodule
hockey stick
Hodgkin cell
Hodgkin disease
Hodgkin granuloma
Hodgkin lymphoma
Hoehn and Yahr staging of Parkinson disease
Hofbauer cell
Hoffmann atrophy
Hoffmann duct
Hoffmann test for tyrosine
Hofmann bacillus
Hofmeister test for leucine
holandric gene
Hollander gastric function test
Hollande solution
Hollenhorst plaque
Holl ligament
hollow bone
hollow needle
hollow structure
hollow viscus
Holmes silver nitrate
Holmgrén-Golgi canal
holocrine gland
holoprotein

Holz phlegmon
Holzer method
homeobox gene
homeotic gene
Homer-Wright rosette
homocystine test
homogenate
homogeneity
homogeneous casts in urine
homogeneous composition
homogeneous fluorescence
homogeneous material
homogeneous medium
homogentisic acid
homogentisic acid oxidase
homogentisic acid oxidase deficiency
homogentisuria
homoglandular
homologous protein
homologous tissue
homologue
homovanillic acid (HVA)
homozygous typing cell (HTC)
honeycombed appearance
honeycomb pattern
honeymoon cystitis
hood of cervix
hooked bone
Hooker-Forbes test
hookworm disease
Hopkins-Cole test for protein
Hopkins thiophene test for lactic acid
Hopman criteria for counting nuclei
Hopmann polyp
Hoppe-Seyler test
hordeolum
horizontal cells of Cajal
horizontal cells of retina
horizontal fissure
horizontal fissure of lung
horizontal heart
horizontal plane, Frankfort
Hormiscium dermatitidis
Hormodendrum dermatitidis
hormonal factors
hormone
  adipokinetic
  adrenocorticotropic (ACTH)
  adrenotropic
  aldosterone
  aldosterone steroid
  androgenic
  angiotensin II
  anterior pituitary-like
  antidiuretic (ADH)
  antigonadotropic
  atrial natriuretic (ANH)
  cardiac
  chemotactic sexual
  chorionic gonadotropic
  chorionic growth
  chromatophorotropic
  cortical
  corticotropic
  corticotropin-releasing
  cortisol
  cortisol steroid
  deoxycortisol
  diabeticogenic
  erythropoietic
  estradiol
  estriol
  estrogenic
  female
  follicle-stimulating (FSH)
  follicle-stimulating hormone-releasing (FSH-HR)
  follicular
  galactopoietic
  gametokinetic
  gastrin
  gastrointestinal
  glucagon
  gonadotropin-releasing (Gn-RH)

hormone *(continued)*
growth
growth hormone-releasing (GH-RH)
human placental lactogen
inappropriate antidiuretic
inhibiting
insulin
interstitial cell-stimulating
lactation
lactogenic
lipid-mobilizing
lipotropic
local
luteinizing (LH)
luteinizing hormone-releasing (LH-RH, LRH)
luteotropic
mammotropic
melanocyte-stimulating
melanotropin release-inhibiting (MIH)
melanotropin-releasing (MRH)
neurotropic
ovarian
pancreatic
parathormone
parathyroid (PTH)
pineal
pituitary
pituitary gonadotropic
placental lactogen
progestational
progesterone
progesterone steroid
prolactin
prolactin anterior pituitary
prolactin-inhibiting
prolactin-releasing
prolactoliberin
proparathyroid
releasing (RH)

hormone *(continued)*
renin
salivary gland
sex
somatomedin-C polypeptide
somatotropic (STH)
somatotropin release-inhibiting (SIH)
somatotropin-releasing (SRH)
steroid
sympathetic
testicular
test on venous blood for
testosterone
testosterone steroid
thyroid
thyroid-stimulating (TSH)
thyrotropic
thyrotropin-releasing (TRH)
thyroxine (T_4)
tissue
triiodothyronine (T_3)
tropic
vasopressin
hormone assay
hormone-dependent neoplasm
hormone levels
hormonelike substances
hormone receptor protein analysis
hormonosis
horn
cicatricial
cutaneous
frontal
lateral
meniscal
projectile
uterine
ventral
horn cell
horn cyst formation
Horner-Trantas dots

hornification
horn of Ammon
horn of uterus
horn pearl
horn pearl formation
horny cell
horseradish peroxidase
horseshoe crab (*Limulus polyphemus*)
horseshoe kidney
horseshoe placenta
horseshoe-shaped nucleus
horseshoe-shaped syncytium
Horsley test for glucose
Hortega cell
Hortega neuroglia stain
host cell
hot abscess
hot nodule
hour (hr)
hourglass gallbladder
hourglass pattern
hourglass stomach
House-Brackmann facial weakness
housekeeping gene
housemaid's knee
Houston, valve of
Howard test for renal function
Howell-Jolly body
Howell test for prothrombin
Howship lacuna
Hoyer canal
HPA (*Histoplasma capsulatum* antigen)
hpf (high power field)
HPV (human papillomavirus)
HPV genotyping procedure
hr. (hour)
H_2 (histamine 2)
H_2 receptor antagonist
HRGP (histidine-rich glycoproteins)
HTLV I and II (human T cell lymphoma virus)
H-type fistula
Hucker-Conn stain
Huddleson agglutination test for brucellosis
Hueck ligament
Hugh-Curtis-Fitz syndrome
Huguier canal
Huhner test
human antihemophilic factor
human chorionic gonadotropin (HCG, hCG)
human herpesvirus 3 (and 4)
human immunodeficiency virus (HIV)
human intestinal roundworm
human lymphocyte antigen (HLA)
human papillomavirus (HPV) infection
human parvovirus B19
human placental lactogen hormone
human T cell leukemia virus (HTLV)
human T cell lymphotropic virus type I (HTLV-I)
human T cell lymphotropic virus type II (HTLV-II)
humeral articulation
humeral circumflex artery
humeral joint
humeral mechanism
humeroradial joint
humeroulnar articulation
humeroulnar joint
humerus
humerus varus
humor
  aqueous
  plasmoid
  vitreous
humoral immunity
Humphry ligament
hunger osteopathy
hunger swelling
Hunner ulcer
Hunt and Hess neurological classification

Hunter canal
Hunter ligament
Hunter line
Hunter-Schreger band
Huntington chorea
Huppert-Cole test for bile pigments
Huppert test for bile pigments
Hurler syndrome
Hürthle cell
Hürthle cell adenoma
Hürthle cell carcinoma
Hürthle cell metaplasia
Hürthle cell tumor
Hurtley test for acetoacetic acid
Huschke, auditory teeth of
Huschke canal
Huschke ligament
Hutchinson plaque
Hutchinson melanotic freckle
Hutchinson teeth
HV (herpesvirus)
HVA (homovanillic acid)
hyalin
  alcoholic
  eosinophilic
  hematogenous
  Mallory
  protein
hyaline articular cartilage
hyaline body, Mallory
hyaline cartilage
hyaline casts in urine
hyaline change in renal glomeruli
hyaline degeneration
hyaline membrane
hyaline membrane disease (HMD)
hyaline necrosis
hyalinization
hyalocapsular ligament
hyaloid artery
hyaloid canal
hyaloid corpuscle
Hyams grade of esthesioneuroblastoma
hybridization
  blot-dot
  chromosome in situ
  dot-blot
  fluorescence in situ (FISH)
  Northern
hydatid
  alveolar
  sessile
  Virchow
hydatid cyst
hydatid cyst disease
hydatid disease of liver
hydatid of Morgagni
hydatid polyp
hydatid pregnancy
hydatidiform
hydatidiform mole
hydroa herpetiforme
hydrocele
hydrocelectomy
hydrocephalus
hydrochloric acid (HCl)
hydrochloric acid test
hydrogen breath test
hydrogen ion
hydrogen peroxide test for blood
hydrogen sulfide poisoning
hydrolysate, protein
hydronephrosis
hydropericardium
hydrophilic gel
hydropic degeneration
hydropic degeneration of chorionic tissues
hydropic degeneration of myocardial fibers
hydrops
hydrothorax
hydroureter
hydroxybutyric acid test

hydroxycorticoid (HC, HOC)
17-hydroxycorticosteroids (17-OHCS)
5-hydroxyindole acetic acid (5-HIAA) test
hydroxylamine modification
hydroxylamine test for glucose
17-hydroxyprogesterone (17-OHP)
hydroxyproline
25-hydroxyvitamin D assay (25-OH-D)
hymen
  denticulate
  imperforate
hymenal caruncles
Hymenolepis nana
hyoepiglottic ligament
hyoglossus muscle
hyoid arch
hyoid artery
hyoid bone
hyparterial bronchus
hyperadrenocorticism
hyperaldosteronism
hyperazotemia
hyperbetalipoproteinemia
hyperbilirubinemia
hypercalcemia
hypercapnia
hypercarbia
hypercatabolism
hypercellular
hyperchloremia
hypercholesterolemia
hyperchromasia
hyperchromatic cell
hyperchromatic nuclei
hyperchromatism
hyperchromia
hypercoagulable state
hyperelastosis cutis
hyperemia
  active
  passive
hyperemic
hyperferremia
hypergammaglobulinemia
hyperglobulinemia
hyperglobulinemic purpura
hyperglycemia
hyperglycemic-glycogenolytic factor
hyperglycosuria
hypergranulosis
hyper-IgE syndrome
hyperimmune
hyperinflated
hyperinsulinar obesity
hyperinsulinism
hyperinterrenal obesity
hyperkalemia
hyperkeratosis
  epidermolytic
  follicular
hyperkeratotic papilloma
hyperkeratotic plaque
hyperketonemia
hyperketonuria
hyperlipidemia
  carbohydrate-induced
  combined fat- and carbohydrate-induced
  endogenous
  exogenous
  essential familial
  familial
  fat-induced
  mixed
hypermagnesemia
hypermelanosis
hypermenorrhea
hypermobile kidney
hypernatremia
hypernephroma
hyperosmolality
hyperosmolar nonketotic coma
hyperostosis

hyperparathyroidism (HPT)
hyperphenylalaninemia
  malignant
  transient
hyperphosphatemia
hyperpigmentation, blotchy facial
hyperpituitarism
hyperplasia
  adaptive
  adenomatous
  adrenocortical
  angiolymphoid
  basal epithelial
  benign prostatic
  bile duct epithelium
  C-cell
  compensatory
  congenital adrenal (CAH)
  cutaneous lymphoid
  endometrial
  epidermal
  epithelial
  fibrous tissue
  focal nodular (FNH)
  follicular
  giant follicular
  histiocytes
  intravascular papillary endothelial
  lipoid adrenal
  lymphoid
  marrow
  microglandular
  mucosal
  neoplastic
  nodular adrenal
  nodular lymphoid
  nodular regenerative
  parathyroid
  pituitary
  prostatic
  pseudoepitheliomatous
  reactive

hyperplasia *(continued)*
  sebaceous
  sinus
  splenic
  Swiss-cheese
  thymus
  thyroid
  verrucous
hyperplasmic obesity
hyperplastic-appearing synovium
hyperplastic arteriolar nephrosclerosis
hyperplastic-hypertrophic obesity
hyperplastic inflammation
hyperplastic marrow
hyperplastic polyp
hyperplastic pulpitis
hyperplastic tissue
hyperpotassemia
hyperreflexia
hypersegmented neutrophil
hypersensitivity myocarditis
hypersensitivity pneumonia
hypersensitivity reaction
hypertension (HT)
  accelerated
  adrenal
  arterial (AH)
  benign intracranial (BIH)
  borderline
  essential (EH)
  Goldblatt
  idiopathic
  intracranial
  labile
  malignant
  ocular
  portal
  postpartum
  primary
  pulmonary
  renal
  renovascular

hypertension *(continued)*
  secondary
  splenovascular
  vascular
hypertensive lower esophageal sphincter
hypertonic
hypertonicity
hypertrichosis
hypertriglyceridemia
hypertrophic cardiomyopathy
hypertrophic gastritis
hypertrophic obesity
hypertrophic osteoarthropathy
hypertrophic pulmonary osteoarthropathy
hypertrophic scar
hypertrophic scarring
hypertrophic villi
hypertrophy
  bladder
  biventricular
  clitoral
  compensatory
  complementary
  epiphyseal
  functional
  myocardial
  physiologic
  smooth-muscle
  ventricular
  villous
  virginal
hyperuricemia
hyperventilation
hypesthesia
hypha (pl. hyphae)
  aseptate
  brown distorted
  multiseptate
  sterile
hyphae in bronchi
hyphae in nail
hyphae in scrapings
hyphae in stratum corneum
hyphae in tissues
hypoalbuminemia
hypocalcemia
hypocapnia
hypocellular
hypochloremia
hypochloremic alkalosis
hypochondriac fossa
hypochondriac region
hypochromia
hypochromic anemia
hypochromic microcytic anemia
hypodermic needle
hypodermis
hypoferremia
hypofibrinolysis
hypogammaglobulinemia
hypogastric artery
hypogastric nerve
hypogastric plexus
hypogastric region
hypogastrium
hypoglossal canal
hypoglossal nerve
hypoglossal nerve of tongue
hypoglossal trigone
hypoglycemia
hypogonad obesity
hypogonadism
hypokalemia
hypokalemic alkalosis
hypokalemic nephrosis
hypomagnesemia
hyponatremia, dilutional
hypo-osmolality
hypoparathyroidism
hypophamine, alpha-
hypopharynx
hypophosphatasia

hypophosphatemia
hypophysial (also, hypophyseal)
hypophysial artery
hypophysial fossa
hypophysial pouch
hypophysis
hypophysis cerebri
hypopigmentation
hypopituitarism
hypoplasia
hypoplasia of dental enamel
hypoplasmic obesity
hypoplastic anemia
hypoplastic lip
hypoplastic lung
hypopotassemia
hypoprothrombinemia
hypopyon
hyporeninemia
hyporrhea
hyposalemia
hyposecretion
hyposmolarity
hyposomatotropism
hypospadias
hypostasis, postmortem
hypostatic abscess
hypostatic bronchopneumonia
hypostatic congestion
hypostatic pneumonia
hyposthenuria
hypotension
hypotensive
hypothalamus
hypothenar eminence
hypothyroidism
hypothyroid obesity
hypotonic bladder
hypotonicity
hypotrichiasis
hypovolemia
hypovolemic shock
hypoxemia
hypoxia, fetal
hypoxic encephalopathy
hypsiloid ligament
Hyrtl loop
Hyrtl sphincter
hysterectomy
hysterical joint
hysteric pregnancy
HZV (herpes zoster virus)

I, i

IAPP (islet amyloid polypeptide)
iatrogenic disease
iatrogenic hyperthyroidism
iatrogenic infection
iatrogenic injury
I band
IBAS 1&2 image analyzer system
I blood group
ICA (islet cell antibody screening)
I cell (inclusion cell)
ice water calorics
ichorous pleurisy
ichorous pus
ichthyosis
icing liver
ICP (intracranial pressure) catheter
icteric
icterohemorrhagic fever
icterus index
ID (immunodiffusion)
identification of specimen
idiocy, amaurotic familial
idiogenesis
idioheteroagglutinin
idioheterolysin
idioisoagglutinin
idiopathic abnormality
idiopathic abortion
idiopathic disease
idiopathic hypertension
idiopathic hypertrophic osteo-arthropathy
idiopathic interstitial fibrosis
idiopathic myocarditis
idiopathic thrombocytopenic purpura (ITP)
idiotypic antibodies
I disk
Ig (immunoglobulin)
IgA immunoglobulin
IgD immunoglobulin
IgE immunoglobulin
IgG immunoglobulin
IgM anti-HAV antibody
IgM anti-HBc antibody
IgM antibody
IgM antibody capture enzyme immunoassay (MAC EIA)
IgM immunoglobulin
Ig2b kappa monoclonal antibody
ileal artery
ileal crypt
ileal inflow tract
ileal margin

ileal mucosa
ileal spout
ileitis, regional
ileoanal pouch
ileocecal edema
ileocecal fold
ileocecal junction
ileocecal orifice
ileocecal pouch
ileocecal recess
ileocecal valve
ileocolic artery
ileocolic cecal artery
ileocolic fold
ileocolic vein
ileum
  antimesenteric border of distal
  mesentery of
  terminal
ileus
  adynamic
  adynamic/paralytic
  dynamic
  dynamic/spastic
  paralytic
  spastic
iliac artery
iliac bone
iliac canal
iliac circumflex artery
iliac colon
iliac crest
iliac fascia
iliac fossa
iliac lymph node
iliac node
iliac plaque
iliac spine
iliac tubercle
iliacus muscle
iliococcygeal muscle
iliofemoral articulation
iliofemoral ligament
iliopectineal ligament
iliopsoas muscle
iliopsoas muscle abscess
iliopsoas ring
iliopubic eminence
iliosacral articulation
iliotibial band
iliotibial ligament of Maissiat
iliotrochanteric ligament
ilium bone
illumination
Ilosvay test for nitrites
IMA (inferior mesenteric artery)
imaging, diagnostic
ImM citrate buffer
immature bone
immature cell
  red blood
  white blood
immature neutrophils
immature red blood cells
immediate transfusion
immersion
imminent abortion
immobilization of bone by casting
immobilization of bone by splinting
immobilization test
immovable articulation
immovable joint
immune adhesion test
immune complex
immune complex assay
immune deficiency
immune protein
immune response gene
immune thrombocytopenic purpura
immunity
  cellular
  humoral
immunoassay, IgM antibody capture
  enzyme (MAC EIA)

immunoblastic sarcoma
immunoblot
immunoblot procedure
immunoblotting
immunocheck fluorosphere
immunocyte
immunocytochemical
immunocytochemistry
immunodeficiency disorder
immunodiffusion (ID), radial
immunoelectrophoresis
immunofixation
immunofluorescence
  direct
  indirect
immunofluorescent stain
immunogenetic factors
immunoglobulin (Ig)
  anti-D
  chickenpox
  failure to form
  IgA
  IgD
  IgE
  IgM
  monoclonal
immunoglobulin A (IgA)
immunoglobulin D (IgD)
immunoglobulin G (IgG)
immunoglobulin G/albumin ratio
immunoglobulin G synthesis rate
immunoglobulin M (IgM)
immunogold technique
immunohistochemical staining
immunohistochemistry
immunologically activated cell
immunologically competent cell
immunologic diffusion procedure
immunologic pregnancy test
immunology
immunopanning parallel method of cell separation
immunoperoxidase
immunoperoxidase stain
immunoperoxidase test
immunophenotypic analysis
immunoreactivity
impacted fetus
impacted fracture
impacted stool
impaction lesion
impaired excretion of conjugated bilirubin
impaired platelet function
impaired wound healing
imperfecta, osteogenesis
imperforate anus
imperforate hymen
impetigo, Bockhart
impetigo neonatorum
impetigo of newborn, bullous
impetiginization
IMViC metabolic tests
inadequate luteal phase
inanition
inanition fever
inapparent infection
inappropriate antidiuretic hormone
incarcerated placenta
incarceration of hernia
incarceration of loop of intestine
incasing cell (also encasing)
incise
incised ulcer
incised wound
incision
  diamond-shaped
  recently healed surgical
  spindle-shaped
  thoracoabdominal
  Y-shaped
incisional biopsy
incisive bone
incisive canal

incisive foramen
incisive papilla
incisor angle, Frankfort-mandibular
incisor canal
incisor, central
incisor teeth
incisor tissue
inclusion
  cytoplasmic
  globular cytoplasmic
  mulberry-shaped intracytoplasmic
inclusion blennorrhea
inclusion body, cytoplasmic
inclusion body myositis
inclusion cell
inclusion conjunctivitis
inclusion cyst
  epidermal
  epithelial
  germinal
  germinal epithelial
incompetence, cervical
incompetent cervix
incompetent valve
incomplete abortion
incomplete protein
incomplete resolution of pneumonia
incontinence, melanin
increased blood flow
increased renal excretion of water
incremental line
incretory gland
incubation
incubation with erythrocytes
incubator
incudomalleolar articulation
incudostapedial articulation
incus bone
indeterminate leprosy
index (pl. indices)
  Ameth
  Ayala
index *(continued)*
  cardiac
  centromeric
  erythrocyte
  free thyroxine
  icterus
  karyopyknotic
  leukopenic
  maturation
  mitotic
  nucleoplasmic
  opsonic
  phagocytic
  red blood cell
  red cell
  Robinson
  saturation
  sensitivity
  volume-corrected mitotic
India ink
India ink capsule stain
India ink preparation
Indian childhood cirrhosis
indicator
indices (pl. of index)
indifferent cell
indigo carmine
indigo carmine test for renal permeability
indigo red test
indirect antiglobulin test
indirect bilirubin
indirect Coombs test
indirect fluorescent antibody test
indirect hemagglutination test
indirect immunofluorescence
indirect inguinal hernia
indirect radioimmunoassay
indirect-reacting bilirubin
indirect transfusion
indiscrete nodule
indiscriminate lesion

indistinct
indole test
indolent myeloma
indophenol test
induced abortion
induced labor
induced malaria
inducer cell
indurated zone of inflammation
indurated zone of necrosis
induration
  black
  brawny
  brown
  cyanotic
  fibrous
  Froriep
  granular
  gray
  laminate
  parchment
  phlebitic
  plastic
  red
indurative mediastinitis
indurative necrosis
indurative pleurisy
indurative pneumonia
industrial dermatitis
industrial dermatosis
inevitable abortion
infantile eczema
infantile gastroenteritis
infantile pneumonia
infantum, roseola
infarction (also, infarct)
  anemic
  bilirubin
  bone
  Brewer
  calcareous
  cerebral

infarction *(continued)*
  hemorrhagic
  myocardial
  pituitary
  pulmonary
  renal
  septic
  thrombotic
  uric acid
infarcted bowel
infected abortion
infected tissue
infection
  agonal
  airborne
  animal bite
  apical
  bacterial
  candidal
  chronic
  chronic Epstein-Barr virus
  colonization
  community-acquired
  cross
  cryptogenic
  disseminated gonococcal
  dog-bite
  droplet
  dust-borne
  ECHO (enterocytopathogenic
    human orphan) virus
  endogenous
  exogenous
  focal
  fungal
  genital
  germinal
  granulomatous
  human papillomavirus (HPV)
  iatrogenic
  inapparent
  latent

infection *(continued)*
- local
- mass
- mixed
- nosocomial
- ocular
- opportunistic
- postoperative
- preexisting
- pyogenic
- recurrent upper respiratory tract (RURTI)
- regional spread of
- rickettsial
- Salinem
- scalp
- secondary
- secondary bacterial
- skin
- subclinical
- suppurative
- systemic
- systemic fungal
- terminal
- TORCH (toxoplasmosis, rubella, cytomegalovirus, herpes simplex)
- tunnel
- upper respiratory infection (URI
- upper respiratory tract infection (URTI)
- urinary tract (UTI)
- vector-borne
- Vincent
- viral
- viral respiratory (VRI)
- water-borne
- wound

infection due to gram-positive bacteria
infection due to rickettsias
infection due to RNA virus
infection due to spirochetes
infectiosum, erythema
infectious arthritis
infectious avian nephrosis
infectious disease
- communicable
- contagious
- transmissible

infectious eczematous dermatitis
infectious granuloma
infectious hepatitis
infectious jaundice
infectious mononucleosis (IM)
infectious myocarditis
infectious myositis
infectious pancreatic necrosis
infectious pancreatic necrosis virus
infectious stomatitis
infectious wart virus
infective embolism
infective endocarditis
infective myocarditis
inferior alveolar artery
inferior artery
inferior border
inferior calcaneonavicular ligament
inferior cardiac branch
inferior cerebellar artery
inferior costal cartilage
inferior deep cervical lymph node
inferior demifacet
inferior dental artery
inferior dental canal
inferior duodenal fold
inferior duodenal recess
inferior epigastric artery
inferior esophageal sphincter
inferior frontal gyrus
inferior gastroduodenal artery
inferior genicular artery
inferior gluteal artery
inferior gluteal nerve
inferior hemorrhoidal artery

- inferior hypogastric nerve
- inferior labial artery
- inferior laryngeal artery
- inferior ligament of epididymis
- inferior lobe
- inferior lobe bronchus
- inferior longitudinal muscle of tongue
- inferior margin of superior rib
- inferior meatus
- inferior mesenteric artery (IMA)
- inferior mesenteric plexus
- inferior nasal concha
- inferior orbital fissure
- inferior pancreaticoduodenal artery
- inferior pelvic aperture
- inferior phrenic artery
- inferior poles
- inferior profunda artery
- inferior pubic ligament
- inferior pubic rami
- inferior pulmonary vein
- inferior radioulnar joint
- inferior rectal nerve
- inferior rectal vein
- inferior rib, superior margin of
- inferior sagittal sinus
- inferior six ribs
- inferior surface of pancreas
- inferior thoracic aperture
- inferior thyroid artery
- inferior thyroid, esophageal artery of
- inferior tibiofibular joint
- inferior tibiofibular ligament, anterior
- inferior transverse rectal fold
- inferior transverse scapular ligament
- inferior turbinated bone
- inferior tympanic artery
- inferior ulnar collateral artery
- inferior vena cava
- inferior vesical artery
- inferior wall
- inferolateral surfaces of prostate
- infertility
- infiltrating ductal carcinoma
- infiltrating plaque
- infiltration (also, infiltrate)
  - adipose
  - calcareous
  - calcium
  - cellular
  - epituberculous
  - fatty
  - gelatinous
  - glycogen
  - inflammatory
  - lymphocytic
  - lymphohistiocytic
  - mononuclear cell
  - neutrophilic
  - paraneural
  - parasitic
  - perivascular
  - perivascular round-cell
  - plasmacytic
  - punctate
  - sanguineous
  - serous
  - small round cell
  - tuberculous
  - urinous
- infiltration medium
- infiltration of calcareous materials into tissues
- infiltration of tissue specimen
- inflame
- inflamed tissue
- inflammation
  - acute phase of
  - adhesive
  - allergic
  - atrophic
  - catarrhal
  - chronic
  - cirrhotic

inflammation *(continued)*
  croupous
  diffuse
  disseminated
  ear
  exudative
  fibrinopurulent
  fibrinous
  fibrosing
  focal
  granulomatous
  hyperplastic
  hypertrophic
  interstitial
  local cutaneous
  metastatic
  necrotic
  obliterative
  parenchymatous
  proliferative
  pseudomembranous
  purulent
  repair phase of
  sclerosing
  serofibrinous
  seroplastic
  serous
  severe
  simple
  skin
  specific
  spleen
  subacute
  suppurative
  thyroid gland
  toxic
  tracheobronchial mucosal
  traumatic
  ulcerative
inflammation artery
inflammation about follicles
inflammation, causes of:

inflammation *(continued)*
  antigen-antibody reaction
  bacteria
  chemical agent
  disease-causing microorganism
  foreign body
  fungus
  parasite
  physical force
  virus
  pathogenic microorganism
  physical injury
  physical or chemical injury
    burning
    crushing
    cutting
    electrical shock
    foreign body
    freezing
    radiation
inflammation esophagus
inflammation features
  heat
  pain
  redness
  swelling
inflammatory atrophy
inflammatory bowel disease
inflammatory carcinoma
inflammatory cells
inflammatory change
inflammatory conditions
  allergic
  infectious
  toxic
  traumatic
inflammatory edema
inflammatory infiltration
inflammatory lymph
inflammatory macrophage
inflammatory myocarditis
inflammatory polyp

inflammatory pseudotumor
inflammatory reaction, smoldering
inflammatory response from living tissue
inflammatory response of cell
inflammatory response, self-limited
influenza
influenza virus
influenzal myocarditis
influenzal virus pneumonia
infolding
infraclavicular
infraclinoid aneurysm
infracolic compartment
infracostal artery
infraglottic
infrahepatic vena cava
infrahyoid artery
infraorbital artery
infraorbital canal
infraorbital cheek
infraorbital foramen
infraorbital groove
infrared light
infrascapular artery
infrasternal angle
infrasternal fossa
infratemporal crest
infratemporal fossa
infraumbilical mound
infundibulo-ovarian ligament
infundibulopelvic ligament
infundibulum (pl. infundibula)
infundibulum, ethmoid
infundibulum of bile duct
infundibulum of sebaceous gland
infusion
  brain-heart (BHI)
  hepatic arterial (HAI)
  saline
ingrown hair
inguinal artery
inguinal canal
inguinal crease
inguinal floor
inguinal fold
inguinal granuloma
inguinal hernia
inguinal ligament
inguinal ligament arch
inguinal lymph node
inguinal region
inguinal ring
inguinal triangle
inhalant antigen
inhalational anthrax
inhalation pneumonia
inhalation tuberculosis
inherited malformation syndromes
inhibiting antibody
inhibition factor
inhibition, hemagglutination (HI, HAI)
inhibition reaction
inhibition test
inhibitor
  alpha-trypsin
  plasminogen activator (PAI)
  platelet aggregation
  protein C (PCI)
inhibitory
initial cell
initial diagnosis
initiation factor
injection mass
injection, mucosal
injury, irreversible
inlet of esophagus
inlet, thoracic
inner cell mass
inner ear
inner membrane
innermost coat of the eye
innermost intercostal membrane
inner neural layer

inner table of skull
innocent bystander cell
innominate artery
innominate bone
innominate canaliculus
inoculation
inoculum
inorganic salt
inpacted fracture
INR (international normalized ratio)
insect dermatitis
insertion
 circum-marginate
 eccentric
 velamentous
insipidus, diabetes
in situ, carcinoma
insoluble fibrin
insoluble protein
inspiration, muscle of
inspiratory capacity
inspissated bile in hepatic canaliculi
inspissated feces, mass of
inspissated material
inspissation of semisolid material in tubular structure
insufficiency, renal
insula
insular artery
insulin and glucose suppression test
insulin-antagonizing factor
insulin antibody
insulin clearance test
insulin hormone
insulin hypoglycemia test
insulin-like growth factor
insulinoma
insulinopenic diabetes
insulin reaction
insulin tolerance test
insulin, 12-hour-fasting
insulin with oral glucose tolerance test
insult
 metabolic
 toxic
intact membranes
integral protein
integumentary
interalveolar septum
interarticular joint
interatrial groove
interatrial septum
interauricular arch
intercalary cell
intercalated disk
intercapillary cell
intercapital ligament
intercarotid gland
intercarpal articulation
intercarpal joint
intercarpal ligament
intercavernous sinus
intercellular bridge
intercellular canaliculus
intercellular fluid
intercellular lymph
intercellular space
interchondral articulation
interchondral joint
interclavicular ligament
interclinoid ligament
intercondylar eminence
intercornual ligament
intercostal artery
intercostal articulation
intercostal ligaments
intercostal membrane
intercostal muscle
intercostal nerve
intercostal space
intercostal vein
intercostal vessel
intercostobrachial nerve
intercrural fibers

intercuneiform articulation
intercuneiform joint
intercuneiform ligament
interdental canal
interdigitating cells
interface dermatitis
interface, dermoepidermal
interfacial canal
interferon, antiviral
interfollicular cell
interfoveolar ligament
interlacing bundles
interlacing fascicle
interlacing fibers
interlacing tendinous fibers
interlobar artery
interlobular artery of kidney
interlobular artery of liver
interlobular bile duct
interlobular biliary canal
interlobular pleurisy
intermaxillary bone
intermediary metabolism
intermediate atrial artery
intermediate bronchus
intermediate cell
intermediate cuneiform bone
intermediate gland
intermediate leprosy
intermediate lymphocytic lymphoma
intermediate tendon of diaphragm
intermesenteric plexus
intermetacarpal artery
intermetacarpal articulation
intermetacarpal joint
intermetatarsal articulation
intermetatarsal jont
intermittent malaria
intermittent proteinuria
intermixed
intermuscular septum, anal
internal abdominal ring
internal acoustic meatus
internal adhesive pericarditis
internal auditory artery
internal capsule
internal carotid artery
internal clot
internal collateral ligament of wrist
internal elastic membrane
internal hemorrhoid
internal iliac artery
internal iliac lymph node
internal iliac node
internal inguinal ring
internal intercostal membrane
internal intercostal muscle
internal jugular vein
internal malleolar artery
internal mammary artery
internal mammary
internal maxillary artery
internal oblique muscle, aponeurosis of
internal occipital crest
internal occipital protuberance
internal os, cervical
internal palpebral artery
internal pillar cells
internal plantar artery
internal pubic artery
internal pudendal artery
internal pudendal vessel
internal spermatic artery
internal thoracic artery
internal thoracic vessel
internal urethral orifice
internal vertebral plexus
International Classification of Diseases for Oncology (ICD-O)
international units (IU)
interosseous artery
interosseous border
interosseous cuneocuboid ligament
interosseous cuneometatarsal ligament

interosseous ligament
interosseous lunotriquetral ligament
interosseous membrane
interosseous metacarpal ligament
interosseous metatarsal ligament
interosseous nerve
interosseous sacroiliac ligament
interosseous talocalcaneal ligament
interosseous tibiofibular ligament
interparietal bone
interpeduncular cistern
interpeduncular fossa
interphalangeal articulation
interphalangeal joint
interscapular gland
intersection, tendinous
intersegmental artery
intersexuality
intersigmoid recess
interspace, dineric
interspersed
interspinous ligament
interspinous plane
intersternebral joint
interstitial atrophy
interstitial cell-stimulating hormone
interstitial cells of Cajal
interstitial cells of Leydig
interstitial cystitis
interstitial deletion
interstitial emphysema
interstitial fibrosis, diffuse
interstitial fluid
interstitial gland
interstitial hemorrhage
interstitial hypertrophic neuritis
interstitial inflammation
interstitial keratitis
interstitial mastitis
interstitial myocarditis
interstitial myositis
interstitial nephritis
interstitial pancreatitis
interstitial pattern
interstitial plasma cell pneumonia
interstitial pneumonia
interstitial pneumonitis
interstitial pregnancy
interstitial pulmonary fibrosis
interstitial salpingitis
interstitial tissue
intertarsal articulation
intertarsal joint
interterritorial matrix
intertrabecular
intertransverse ligament
intertubercular bursitis
intertubercular groove
interureteric fold
interval, fixed time
interval scale
interventricular artery
interventricular foramina
interventricular groove
interventricular septal area
interventricular septum
intervertebral articulation
intervertebral disk, slipped
intervertebral foramen (pl. foramina)
intervertebral joint
intervillous space
intestinal artery
intestinal calculus
intestinal canal
intestinal contents
intestinal gland
intestinal juice
intestinal loop
intestinal lumen
intestinal metaplasia
intestinal mucosa
intestinal obstruction
intestinal parasitism
intestinal ulcer

intestinal villi
intestinal web
intestine
  coils of
  kink in
  large
  malrotation of
  small
intima tunica
intimal
in toto
intoxication
  alcohol
  ethanol
  fluoride
  vitamin D
intra-alveolar hemorrhage
intra-articular ligament
intra-articular plates of fibrocartilage
intra-articular sternocostal ligament
intracartilaginous bone
intracartilaginous ossification
intracavernous aneurysm
intracellular bacteria
intracellular fat in cells of amniotic fluid
intracellular fluid
intracellular metabolism
intrachondrial bone
intracortical osteosarcoma
intracranial aneurysm
intracranial hypertension
intracranial pressure (ICP) catheter
intracranial tumor
intracutaneous test
intracutaneous tuberculin test
intracytoplasmic canal
intradermal nevus
intradermal test
intraductal papilloma
intraductal papillomatosis/epitheliosis
intradural abscess
intraepidermal carcinoma of glans
intraepidermal neutrophilic IgA dermatosis
intraepithelial gland
intrafollicular space
intrahaustral contraction ring
intrahepatic duct system
intrahepatic biliary duct
intrahepatic radicle
intraligamentary pregnancy
intralobular biliary canal
intraluminal acid mucin
intraluminal embolism
intramastoid abscess
intramembranous bone
intramembranous ossification
intramural fibroid
intramural portion
intramuscular gland of tongue
intraocular malignancy
intraocular melanoma
intraocular neuritis
intraosseous low-grade osteosarcoma
intraperitoneal pregnancy
intraperitoneal transfusion
intrascapular ligament
intrathoracic goiter
intrathoracic pressure
intrauterine pneumonia
intrauterine transfusion
intravascular congestion
intravascular lymph
intravascular thrombosis
intravenous (IV, I.V.)
intravenous drug abuse
intravenous narcotism
intravital microscopy
intravital stain
intrinsic factor antibody
intrinsic factor, vitamin B_{12} test
intrinsic muscle
intrinsic protein

introitus, vaginal
intubation
intussuscepted bowel
intussusception
in utero
invagination
invasion, stromal
invasive carcinoma
invasive mole
inversion
  chromosomal abnormality of
  nipple
  paracentric
  pericentric
inversion of A/G ratio
inversion of ratio
inversus, situs
inverted pelvis
in vitro
Invitrogen CDNA synthesis system
in vivo
involucrin
involucrum
involuntary muscle
involuntary reflex
involuntary sphincter of anal canal
involutional
Iodamoeba buetschlii
iodide goiter
iodinated I 125 (^{125}I) serum albumin
iodinated I 131 (^{131}I) serum albumin
iodine, Gram
iodine stain
iodine test
iodine topical solution
iodized protein
iodoform test for acetone
iodophil granule
ion
  bicarbonate
  hydrogen
  phosphate
ion-exchange chromatography
ionized calcium
ionizing radiation
iridescent virus
iridis, coloboma
iridocorneal angle
iridocyclitis
iridovirus
iris (pl. irises, irides)
iritis
  acute
  chronic
iron (Fe)
  excessive intake of
  heme
  increased absorption of
  non-heme
  reduced stainable
  stainable
iron-binding capacity of blood
iron-binding cacacity, total (TIBC)
iron-deficiency anemia
iron deposition
iron hematoxylin
iron hematoxylin stain
iron saturation
iron stain
iron stain of bone marrow
iron store
iron-sulfur protein
irradiation pneumonia
irradiation, solar
irregular bone
irregular enchondral ossification
irregular knots or clumps of degenerating fibrils within neurons
irregularly distributed
irregularly shaped
irreparable damage
irreversible brain damage
irreversible coma
irreversible flaccid paralysis

irreversible injury
irritability of nerve cell
irritant dermatitis
irritation cell
irritative lesion
Isamine blue stain
ischemia-modifying factor
ischemia secondary to vascular
  occlusion
ischemic bowel
ischemic kidney
ischemic muscular atrophy
ischemic necrosis
ischemic zones
ischial bone
ischial spine
ischial tuberosity
ischiocapsular ligament
ischiocavernosus muscle
ischiofemoral ligament
ischiopubic ramus
ischiorectal abscess
ischiorectal fat pad
ischiorectal fossa
  anterior recess of
  apex of
  base of
  posterior recess of
ischiorectal fossa plane
ischiorectal pad of fat
ischiospongiosus muscle of penis
ischium
  ascending ramus of
  ramus of
island
  lipid
  mucosal
islet amyloid polypeptide (IAPP)
islet cell
islet cell antibody screening (ICA)
islet, pancreatic
islets of Langerhans
isoantibody
isochromosome
isocitrate dehydrogenase (ICD)
isoenzyme
  cardiac
  CK (creatine kinase)
  CK-BB (CK_1)
  CK-MB (CK_2)
  CK-MM (CK_3)
  CPK (creatine phosphokinase)
  LDH_1 (LDH1)
  LDH_2 (LDH2)
  Regan
  serial cardiac
isoenzyme electrophoresis
isoenzyme fractionation, CPK or C-K
isoenzyme of creatine kinase (CK)
  CK_1 (BB, brain)
  CK_2 (MB, cardiac muscle)
  CK_3 (MM, skeletal muscle)
isoenzyme, serum LDH (1 through 5)
isoform
isogenous nests
isolated diffuse myocarditis
isolated proteinuria
isoleucine test
isomorphic effect
isopropanol precipitation test
IsoQuick DNA isolation kit
Isosensitest agar
Isospora belli
isosthenuria
isothiocyanate, fluorescein (FITC)
isotopically tagged allergen
isotropic disk
isthmus, aortic
isthmus of auditory tube
isthmus of uterus
itch
  frost
  ground
  jock

itch *(continued)*
- lumberman's
- straw
- swimmer's
- water
- winter

itching
itchy erythematous patches
Ito cell
Ito, nevus of
Ito-Reenstierna test
ITP (idiopathic thrombocytopenic purpura)
^{131}I uptake (thyroid function) test
I.V. or IV (intravenous)
ivory bone
ivorylike bone
ivory osteoma
Ivy bleeding time
Ixodes dammini
Ixodes pacificus

J, j

Jackson and Parker classification of Hodgkin disease
Jacobson canal
Jacquemin test
Jacquet dermatitis
Jacquet erythema
Jadassohn nevus
Jadassohn-Tieche nevus
Jaffe test for creatinine and glucose
jagged bone fragments
jail fever
Jakob-Creutzfeldt disease
Jamestown Canyon virus
Jamshidi biopsy needle
Jamshidi needle
Janeway lesion
Jansky human blood group
Janus green B
Japanese B encephalitis
Japanese encephalitis virus
Jarjavay ligament
jars, Coplin
jaundice
- acholuric
- anhepatic
- breast milk
- choleric

jaundice *(continued)*
- cholestatic
- chronic acholuric
- chronic familial
- chronic idiopathic
- congenital hemolytic
- familial nonhemolytic
- hematogenous
- hepatocellular
- hepatogenous
- infectious
- neonatal
- obstructive
- physiologic
- yellow

jaw bone
jaw joint
JCV (JC virus)
jejunal artery
jejunal limb
jejunal loop
jejunal pouch
jejunum
- arterial arcades of
- coils of
- mesentery of
- windows of

jelly, Wharton
Jenner method (staining)
Jensen sarcoma
JEOL 100 CX electron microscope
Jewett classification of bladder
  carcinoma
Job syndrome
jock itch (tinea cruris)
Johne bacillus
Johnson-Dubin syndrome
Johnson test for albumin
joint (see also *articulation*)
  acromioclavicular
  amphiarthroses
  ankle
  antebrachiocarpal
  anterior intraoccipital
  arthrodial
  atlanto-occipital
  atlantoaxial
  ball-and-socket
  biaxial
  bicondylar
  bilocular
  bleeding into a
  Budin obstetrical
  calcaneocuboid
  capitate-hamate
  capitolunate
  capitular
  carpal
  carpometacarpal
  cartilaginous
  centrodistal
  Charcot
  Chopart
  Clutton
  coccygeal
  cochlear
  coffin
  composite
  compound

joint *(continued)*
  condylar
  condyloid
  costocentral
  costochondral
  costosternal
  costotransverse
  costovertebral
  cotyloid
  coxal
  cricoarytenoid
  cricothyroid
  Cruveilhier
  cubital
  cuboideonavicular
  cuneocuboid
  cuneometatarsal
  cuneonavicular
  dentoalveolar
  diarthroidial
  diarthrosis
  digit
  digital
  DIP (distal interphalangeal)
  distal radioulnar
  distal tibiofibular
  dry
  elbow
  ellipsoid
  enarthrodial
  facet
  false
  femoropatellar
  femorotibial
  fibrous
  flail
  ginglymoid
  gliding
  gomphosis
  hemophilic
  hinge
  hip

joint *(continued)*
- humeral
- humeroradial
- humeroulnar
- hysterical
- immovable
- incudomalleolar
- incudostapedial
- inferior radioulnar
- inferior tibiofibular
- interarticular
- intercarpal
- interchondral
- intercuneiform
- intermetacarpal
- intermetatarsal
- interphalangeal
- intersternebral
- intertarsal
- intervertebral
- jaw
- knee
- knuckle
- lateral atlantoaxial
- Lisfranc
- lower extremity
- lumbosacral
- lunotriquetral
- Luschka
- mandible
- manubriosternal
- median atlantoaxial
- metacarpophalangeal
- metatarsophalangeal
- midcarpal (middle carpal)
- middle radioulnar
- midtarsal
- mortise
- movable
- multiaxial
- neurocentral
- neuropathic

joint *(continued)*
- peg-and-socket
- petrobasilar
- petro-occipital
- phalangeal
- PIP (proximal interphalangeal)
- pisiform
- pisotriquetral
- pivot
- plane
- polyaxial
- posterior intraoccipital
- primary cartilaginous
- proximal interphalangeal
- proximal radioulnar
- proximal tibiofibular
- radiocarpal
- radiohumeral
- radioulnar
- rotary
- sacrococcygeal
- sacrococcygeal symphysis
- sacroiliac
- saddle
- scapholunate
- scaphotrapezoid trapezial (STT)
- scapuloclavicular
- schindyletic
- screw
- secondary cartilaginous
- shoulder
- simple
- skull-type
- socket
- spheno-occipital
- spheroid
- spiral
- sternal
- sternoclavicular
- sternocostal
- sternum
- stifle

joint *(continued)*
  STT (scaphotrapezoid trapezial)
  subtalar
  superior radioulnar
  superior tibiofibular
  suture
  symphysis cartilaginous
  synarthroses
  synchondrosis
  syndesmosis
  synovial
  talocalcaneal
  talocalcaneonavicular
  talocrural
  talonavicular
  tarsometatarsal
  tarsus
  temporomandibular
  tibiofibular
  tibiotarsal
  transverse tarsal
  triquetrohamate
  uncovertebral
  uniaxial
  unilocular
  wedge-and-groove
  weightbearing
  wrist
  xiphisternal
  zygapophyseal (zygoapophysial)
joint capsule
joint cavity
joint cyst
joint fluid
joint mice
joint tissues
Jolles test for bile pigments in urine
Jolly body
Jolly-Howell body
Jones and Cantarow urea concentration test
Jones fluorescein instillation test
Jones kidney stain
Jores solution
Jorissen test for formaldehyde
J-sella deformity
Judet epiphyseal fracture classification
jugal bone
jugal ligament
jugular arch
jugular foramen (pl. foramina)
jugular gland
jugular notch
jugular vein
juice
  acid-peptic
  appetite
  gastric
  intestinal
  pancreatic
jumper's knee
jumping gene
junction
  amnioembryonic
  anorectal
  cardioesophageal (CE)
  cementodentinal
  choledochoduodenal
  choledochopancreatic ductal
  corticomedullary
  costochondral
  costovertebral
  cystic-choledochal
  cystocholedochal
  dentinocemental
  dentinoenamel
  dermoepidermal
  desmosomal
  duodenojejunal
  EG (esophagogastric)
  electrotonic
  esophagogastric (EG)
  esophagotracheal (ET)
  fundoantral

junction *(continued)*
gastroesophageal (GE)
ileocecal
neurocentral
neuromuscular
pancreaticobiliary ductal
pyloroduodenal
rectosigmoid
sacrococcygeal
sclerocorneal
squamocolumnar
squamocolumnar mucosal
sternocostal
sternomanubrial
tracheoesophageal (TE)
tympanostapedial
ureteropelvic
ureterovesical (UVJ)
uterotubal
uterovesical
junctional complex
junctional epithelium
junctional nevus
jungle fever
Jüngling disease
juvenile cell
juvenile deforming metatarso-phalangeal osteochondritis
juvenile melanoma
juvenile muscular atrophy
juvenile neutrophil
juvenile nevus
juvenile-onset diabetes mellitus
juvenile pattern
juvenile pelvis
juvenile polyp
juvenile rheumatoid arthritis
juxtacortical osteogenic sarcoma
juxtacortical osteosarcoma
juxtacrine interaction
juxtaglomerular apparatus
juxtaglomerular cell

K, k

K (potassium)
Kaes-Bechterew, band of
Kaes line
Kaiserling fixative
Kaiserling solution
kala-azar (visceral leishmaniasis)
Kamerun swelling
Kantor and Gies test for proteins
Kaplan test for globulin-albumin
  in spinal fluid
Kaposi disease
Kaposi sarcoma
kappa chain
kappa granule
Kapsinow test for bile pigments
karatan sulfate
Karnowsky fixative
Karnovsky scale
Karnovsky status classification
karyochrome cell
karyocyte
karyokinesis
karyolysis
karyopyknotic index
karyorrhectic polymorphonuclear
  leukocyte
karyorrhexis
karyotype
karyotyping
Kasten fluorescent Feulgen stain
katal
Katayama fever
Katayama test
Kawasaki disease
Kayser-Fleischer ring in cornea
K (killer) cell
Keith-Wagener classification
  of retinopathy
Kell blood group
keloid, acne
keloidal folliculitis
keloid scar
keloid scarring
kelvin
Kelvin scale
Kemerovo virus
Kentmann test for formaldehyde
Kenya fever
kerasin
kerasin deposits in adrenal
kerasin deposits in kidney
kerasin deposits in lung
kerasin deposits in thyroid
keratan sulfate

keratic precipitates (KPs)
keratin debris
keratinization
keratinized cell
keratinized epithelial cell
keratinizing squamous epithelium
keratinizing stratified squamous
  epithelium
keratinocyte
keratinolytic
keratin pearl formation
keratin plug
keratin whorl
keratitis
  actinic
  dendritic
  interstitial
keratoacanthoma
keratocele
keratoconjunctivitis, epidemic
keratoconjunctivitis sicca
keratoconus
keratocyte
keratogenous zone
keratohyalin granule
keratomycosis
keratoprecipitates (KPs)
keratosis (pl. keratoses)
  actinic
  seborrheic
  senile
  solar
keratotic
Kerckring fold
Kerckring, valve of
keritonocyte
Kernechtrot
Kerner test for creatinine
kernicterus
ketoacidosis, diabetic
ketoaciduria
Ketodiastix
17-ketogenic steroids (17-KGS) test
ketoglutarate dehydrogenase, alpha-
ketone bodies (ketones)
ketones in urine
ketonuria
ketosis
ketosis-prone diabetes
ketosis-resistant diabetes
17-ketosteroid (17 KS) fractions
  (also, ketosteroid-17)
Ketostix
Kew Gardens fever
Keyes punch biopsy
keyhole deformity
K562 target cell
kg (kilogram)
Kidd blood group
kidney
  abdominal
  afferent vessels of
  amyloid
  arcuate artery of
  Armanni-Ebstein
  arteriosclerotic
  artificial
  Ask-Upmark
  atrophic
  biopsy of
  cake
  cicatricial
  congested
  contracted
  cow
  crush
  cyanotic
  cystic
  disk
  donor
  doughnut
  dromedary
  duplex
  edematous

kidney *(continued)*
- fatty
- fibrous capsule of
- flea-bitten
- floating
- Formad
- fused
- Goldblatt
- granular
- hila of
- horseshoe
- hypermobile
- interlobular artery of
- ischemic
- large red
- medullary sponge
- mortar
- movable
- mural
- myelin
- myeloma
- pancake
- pelvic
- polycystic
- putty
- pyelonephritic
- Rose-Bradford
- sacciform
- sclerotic
- sigmoid
- sponge
- supernumerary
- thoracic
- wandering
- waxy

kidney abscess
kidney calculus
kidney function test
kidney-shaped
kidney-shaped placenta
kidney transplant
kidney tumor
Kiel classification of non-Hodgkin lymphoma
Kienböck's disease
Kiernan space
killer T-cell
Killian test for carbohydrate tolerance
kilogram (kg)
kiloliter (kL)
kilometer (km)
kilomole (kmol)
Kimmelstiel-Wilson disease
kinetic energy
King-Armstrong unit
Kingella denitrificans
Kingella indologenes
Kingella kingae
kinked aorta
kinked intestine
kinked ureter
kink in bowel
Kinyoun acid-fast stain
Kinyoun carbolfuchsin stain
Kirby-Bauer test
Kirchner liquid medium
Kitasato bacillus
Kjeldahl test for nitrogen
kL (kiloliter)
Klatskin tumor classification
Klebs-Loeffler bacillus
Klebsiella
Klebsiella friedländeri
Klebsiella oxytoca
Klebsiella ozaenae
Klebsiella planticola
Klebsiella pneumoniae
Klebsiella pneumoniae ozaenae
Klebsiella pneumoniae rhinoscleromatis
Klebsiella rhinoscleromatis
Klebsiella terrigena
Kleihauer acid elution test
Kleihauer-Betke acid elution test
Kleihauer-Betke stain

Kleihauer-Betke test
Klieg eye
Klimow test for blood in urine
Klinefelter syndrome
Klumpp & Bieth method
Kluver-Barrera stain
Kluyvera
Kluyvera ascorbata
Kluyvera cryocrescens
km (kilometer)
kmol (kilomole)
Knapp test for glucose in urine
knee
  anterior cruciate deficit
  breaststroker's
  dislocated
  floating
  friction rub in
  game
  gimpy
  hamstrung
  housemaid's
  internal derangement of (IDK)
  jumper's
  locked
  Miller-Galante
  motorcyclist's
  runner's
  septic
  surfer's
  trick
  wrenched
knee articulation
knee-joint, anastomosis around
knob, aortic
knockknee
Knoll gland
knot
  net
  surfer's
  syncytial
Knott test for microfilariae in blood
knuckle
  aortic
  cervical aortic
knuckle joint
Kober test for estrogens (*not* Kobert)
Kobert test for hemoglobin (*not* Kober)
Koch bacillus
Koch phenomenon
Koch-Weeks bacillus
Kock pouch
Koebner phenomenon
Koehler disease
Koeppe nodule
KOH (potassium hydroxide)
KOH mount
KOH prep
KOH stain
KOH test
koilocytotic atypia
koilocytotic cellular change
Kokoskin modified Weber method
Kolmer test
Kondo test for indole
Koplik spots
Korean hemorrhagic fever
Korean hemorrhagic fever virus
Korotkoff test
Korsakoff encephalopathy
Koserella trabulsii
Kossa (von Kossa) stain
Kossel test for hypoxanthine
Kostmann infantile agranulocytosis
Kovalevsky canal
Kowarsky test for urine glucose
Krabbe disease
Krabbe leukodystrophy
Krause bone
Krause end bulb
Krause gland
Krause ligament
Kretschmann space
Krokiewicz urine test for bile pigment

Kronecker stain
Krukenberg tumor
Kuersteiner canal
Kühne methylene blue
Kuhnt space
Kulchitsky cell
Külz test for beta-hydroxybutyric acid
Kupffer cell
Kurthia zopfii
kuru
Kurzrok-Miller test
Kurzrok-Ratner test
Kussmaul coma
Kveim intradermal test
Kveim reaction
Kveim test for sarcoidosis
K vitamin
kwashiorkor
Kyasanur Forest hemorrhagic fever virus
kyphoscoliosis
kyphoscoliotic pelvis
kyphotic pelvis

L, l

L (liter)
L (lumbar)
LA (latex agglutination)
LAA (leukocyte ascorbic acid)
La autoantibody (SS-B)
Labbe triangle
Lab Tek chamber
labial artery
labial commissure
labial dysarthria
labial fusion
labial gland of mouth
labial groove
labial salivary gland
labial swelling
labial vein
labia majora
labia minora
labile factor (Factor V)
labile, heat
labile hypertension
labioglossolaryngeal paralysis
labioglossopharyngeal paralysis
labioscrotal fold
labioscrotal swelling
labium (pl. labia)
labium majus (pl. labia majora)
labium minus (pl. labia minora)
laboratory (lab) test
    precision of
    sensitivity of
labrum
    acetabular
    articular
    glenoidal
Labstix
labyrinth
    artery of
    bony
    cochlear
    ethmoidal
    Ludwig
    membranous
    osseous
    renal
    Santorini
    vestibular
labyrinthine
labyrinthitis
lacerated wound
laceration
    gastroesophageal
    V-shaped
    wound

laciniate ligament
lacis (meshwork) cell
lacrimal abscess
lacrimal apparatus
lacrimal artery
lacrimal bone
lacrimal canal
lacrimal caruncle
lacrimal crest
lacrimal duct
lacrimal fluid
lacrimal gland
lacrimal gland atrophy
lacrimal groove
lacrimal lake
lacrimal nerve
lacrimal papilla
lacrimal punctum
lacrimal sac
La Crosse encephalitis
La Crosse virus
La Crosse virus titer
lactase enzyme
lactate dehydrogenase (LDH)
lactated Ringer's solution
lactational mastitis
lactation hormone
lacteal
lactic acid
  bacillus
  blood
  cerebrospinal fluid
  plasma
  synovial fluid
lactic acid bacillus
lactic acid dehydrogenase (LDH)
lactic acid test
lactic acidosis
lactic dehydrogenase (LDH)
lactiferi, ampullae of tubuli
lactiferous gland
Lactobacillus
Lactobacillus acidophilus
Lactobacillus bifidus
Lactobacillus bulgaricus
lactogen, human placental
lactogenic hormone
lactophenol cotton blue
lactose test
lacuna (pl. lacunae)
  blood
  bone
  cartilage
  intervillous
  osseous
  penis
  resorption
lacunar abscess
lacunar cell
lacunar ligament
LAD (left anterior descending) coronary artery
Ladd band
Ladendorff test for blood
Laënnec cirrhosis
Laënnec pearl
Lafora body
LAK (lymphokine activated killer) cell
LAK cell phenomenon
lake
  bile
  capillary
  mucous
  venous
laked sheep blood
Laki-Lorand factor
lambdoid suture
lamella (pl. lamellae)
  articular
  circumferential
  concentric
  elastic
  enamel
  glandulopreputial

lamella of bone, articular
lamellar body density (LBD) count
lamellar body number density test
lamellar bone
lamellated (layered) pattern
lamellated blood clot
lamellated bone
lamellated thrombus
lamina
lamina cribrosa
lamina propria
laminated clot
laminated keratotic debris
laminated thrombus
laminate induration
lamina terminalis cistern
Lancefield classification of hemolytic streptocci into groups
Lancefield precipitation test
Lancereaux nephritis
lancet, sterile
landmark
  anatomic
  bony
Landouzy-Dejerine atrophy
Landouzy-Dejerine muscular dystrophy
Lane band
Langer line
Langerhans cell
Langerhans, islets of
Langeron iodine solution
Lange test for acetone in urine (*not* Lang)
Langhans cell
Langhans giant cell
Lang test for taurine (*not* Lange)
Lannelongue ligaments
Lansing virus
lanugo
Lanz point
LAP (leucine aminopeptidase)
LAP (leukocyte adhesion protein)
LAP (leukocyte alkaline phosphatase)
laparoscopy, diagnostic
laparotomy
  exploratory
  second-look
Laquer stain
large bowel
large cell carcinoma
large cell, immunoblastic lymphoma
large cell lymphoma
large cleaved cell
large cleaved cell lymphoma
large granule cell
large gut
large intestine
large intestine gland
large noncleaved cell
large noncleaved cell lymphoma
large red kidney
large sweat gland
large trunk muscle
larva migrans
  cutaneous
  visceral
larvae in mucosa of stomach
laryngeal artery
laryngeal atrophy
laryngeal edema
laryngeal gland
laryngeal granuloma
laryngeal nerve
laryngeal nodule
laryngeal part of pharynx
laryngeal polyp
laryngotracheobronchitis
larynx
  appendix of ventricle of
  infraglottic
  ventricle of
  vestibule of
LASA (lipid-associated sialic acid)
laser nephelometry

laser, pumped-dye
lash follicles
Lassa fever
Lassa virus
lata (pl. latae)
 fascia (pl. fasciae latae)
 tensor fascia (pl. latae, tensor fasciae)
Latarget nerve
latent diabetes
latent infection
latent pleurisy
latent virus
lateral alveolar abscess
lateral antebrachial cutaneous nerve
lateral aperture
lateral arcuate ligament
lateral atlantoaxial joint
lateral calcaneal artery
lateral canal
lateral circumflex artery of thigh
lateral collateral ligament of ankle
lateral costal artery
lateral costotransverse ligament
lateral crus (pl. crura)
lateral crus of superficial inguinal ring
lateral cuneiform bone
lateral cutaneous branch of intercostal nerve
lateral eminence
lateral epicondyle
lateral femoral circumflex artery
lateral fornix of vagina
lateral gutter
lateral horn
lateral ligament of malleus
lateral ligament of bladder
lateral lobe of prostate
lateral lumbocostal arch
lateral lumbosacral ligament
lateral malleolar ligament
lateral nasal artery
lateral oblique fascia
lateral palpebral artery
lateral palpebral ligament
lateral periodontal abscess
lateral plantar artery
lateral puboprostatic ligament
lateral recess
lateral reflection of colon
lateral sacrococcygeal ligament
lateral semicircular canal
lateral striate artery
lateral sulcus
lateral talocalcaneal ligament
lateral tarsal artery
lateral temporomandibular ligament
lateral third of inguinal ligament
lateral thoracic artery
lateral umbilical fold
lateral umbilical ligament
lateral vaginal wall smear
lateral ventricle of cerebrum
lateral wall of nasal cavity
late secretory endometrium
latex agglutination (LA)
latex agglutination test for antibody
latex beads, agglutination of
latex fixation test
latex particles coated with antigen
latissimus dorsi muscle
lattice cell
laudable pus
Lauth canal
Lauth ligament
lavage
 bronchoalveolar
 gastric
 tracheobronchial
layer
 basal
 basal cell
 blastodermic
 choriocapillary
 choroid

layer *(continued)*
  circular
  columnar
  conjunctival
  corneal
  cornified
  elastic
  enamel
  ependymal
  epithelial
  epithelial choroid
  epitrichial
  fibrous
  fusiform
  ganglionic
  germ
  germinative
  malpighian
  membranous deep
  papillary
  parietal
  prickle cell
  reticular
  subcutaneous
  subserosal
  superficial fatty
  visceral
layered
L cell
LCIS (lobular carcinoma in situ)
LCM (lymphocytic choriomeningitis)
  virus
LCT (long chain triglycerides)
LDH (lactate dehydrogenase)
LDH1 (LDH_1) isoenzyme
LDH2 (LDH_2) isoenzyme
LDL (low density lipoprotein)
LDL cholesterol (LDLC)
LE (leukocyte esterase)
LE (lupus erythematosus)
LE cell
LE cell prep (preparation)
lead (Pb)
  blood
  urinary
lead citrate
lead hydroxide stain
lead level in blood
lead level in urine
lead poisoning
lead stomatitis
leaflet, valve
leakage
leaking from vessel
leaking of red blood cells
leaky mitral valve
lean body mass
leaping atrophy
leather bottle stomach
leaves of diaphragm
leaves of mesentery
Leber optic atrophy
Lechini test for blood in urine
lecithin/sphingomyelin (L/S) ratio
Lecythophora hoffmannii
Lecythophora mutabilis
Leder stain
ledge, enamel
Lee cutting biopsy needle
Lee test for rennin
Lee tissue biopsy needle
Leeuwenhoek canal
Lee-White clotting method
Lee-White clotting time
Lee-White coagulation time
LE factor
left anterior descending (LAD)
  coronary artery
left atrium
left auricle
left border of heart
left colic artery
left colic flexure
left colon

left colonic flexure
left crus (pl. crura)
left gastric artery
left gastroepiploic artery
left gutter
left heart
left hemisphere
left hepatic vein (LHV)
left lobe of liver
left lower quadrant (LLQ)
left main bronchus
left shift on WBC count
left superior vena cava ligament
left triangular ligament
left upper outer quadrant
left upper quadrant (LUQ)
left vena cava ligament
left ventricle of heart
left ventricular hypertrophy (LVH)
Legal test for acetone
Legg-Calvé-Perthes disease
Legionella anisa
Legionella bozemanii
Legionella dumoffii
Legionella feeleii
Legionella gormanii
Legionella jordanis
Legionella longbeachae
Legionella micdadei
Legionella oakridgensis
Legionella pneumophila
Legionella sainthelensis
Legionella wadsworthii
legionellosis
legionnaire's bacillus
legionnaire's disease
Leifson flagella stain
Leiner dermatitis
leiomyoma (pl. leiomyomata)
  benign
  cytologically bland
  epithelioid
leiomyoma *(continued)*
  submucous
  subserosal
  uterine
leiomyoma uteri
leiomyosarcoma
Leishman-Donovan body
Leishmania brasiliensis (or *braziliensis*)
Leishmania donovani
Leishmania tropica
leishmaniasis
  cutaneous
  mucocutaneous
  visceral
leishmanin test
Leishman chrome cell
Leishman stain
Lendrum phloxine–tartrazine stain
length
  crown-heel
  crown-rump
lengthwise
Lennert lymphoma
lenticular ansa
lenticular artery
lenticular bone
lenticular carcinoma
lenticular glands of stomach
lenticular glands of tongue
lenticular loop
lenticulostriate artery
lentiform bone
lentiginous
lentigo
  malignant
  nevoid
  senile
  solar
lentigo maligna
lentigo maligna melanoma
Lentivirinae
Lentivirus, lentivirus

- Leon virus
- leopard retina
- Leo test for free hydrochloric acid
- LE panniculitis
- Lepehne-Pickworth stain
- *Leporipoxvirus*
- lepra bacillus
- lepra cell
- lepromatous leprosy
- lepromin test
- leprosy (Hansen disease)
    - borderline
    - indeterminate
    - intermediate
    - Lucio
    - tuberculoid
    - water-buffalo
- leprosy bacillus
- leptomeningeal fibrosis
- leptomeninges
- *Leptospira biflexa*
- *Leptospira icterohemorrhagiae*
- *Leptospira interrogans*
- leptospirosis
- *Leptotrichia*
- *Leptotrichia buccalis*
- LES (lower esophageal sphincter)
- Lesgaft space
- Lesgaft triangle
- lesion
    - angiocentric immunoproliferative
    - Armanni-Ebstein
    - Baehr-Lohlein
    - Bankart
    - benign lymphoepithelial
    - bird's nest
    - blastic
    - Blumenthal
    - Bracht-Wachter
    - bull's-eye
    - cardiac valvular
    - caviar

- lesion *(continued)*
    - central
    - coin (of lungs)
    - Councilman
    - depigmented
    - Dieulafoy
    - Duret
    - Ebstein
    - erythematous
    - flat
    - freckle-like
    - Ghon primary
    - gross
    - Hill-Sachs
    - histologic
    - impaction
    - indiscriminate
    - infiltrating
    - irritative
    - Janeway
    - lichenoid
    - linear cutaneous
    - local
    - Löhlein-Baehr
    - lower motor neuron
    - lytic
    - Mallory-Weiss
    - molecular
    - mongolian spot-like
    - napkin-ring
    - necrotic
    - onion scale
    - onionskin
    - organic
    - papillary
    - papular
    - papulonecrotic
    - partial
    - peripheral
    - pigmented (melanotic)
    - precancerous
    - primary

lesion *(continued)*
- punctate keratotic
- purulent
- radial sclerosing
- ring-wall
- satellite
- skin
- solitary
- squamous intraepithelial
- structural
- supranuclear
- systemic
- target
- total
- trophic
- tuberculoid
- upper motor neuron
- vulvar
- wire-loop

lesser curvature of stomach
lesser multangular bone
lesser omentum
lesser palatine artery
lesser palatine foramina
lesser palatine nerve
lesser pancreas
lesser peritoneal sac
lesser sac of peritoneal cavity
Lesser test
lesser trochanter of femur
lesser tubercle
LET (leukocyte esterase test)
lethal disease
lethal gene
lethal factor
Letterer-Siwe disease
leucine aminopeptidase (LAP)
leucine test
leukemia
- acute
- acute granulocytic
- acute lymphoblastic (ALL)
- acute lymphocytic
- acute megakaryoblastic
- acute monocytic
- acute myeloblastic
- acute myelogenous (AML)
- acute myelomonocytic
- acute promyelocytic
- acute undifferentiated (AUL)
- adult T-cell/lymphoma (ATL)
- aleukemic
- basophilic
- B-cell type
- Burkitt-like
- chronic
- chronic lymphocytic (CLL)
- chronic myelomonocytic
- common type
- eosinophilic
- granulocytic
- hairy cell
- lymphatic
- lymphoblastic
- lymphocytic
- mast cell
- micromyeloblastic
- monocytic
- myeloblastic
- myelocytic
- myelogenous
- Naegeli monocytic
- nonlymphocytic
- null cell type
- plasma cell
- plasmacytic
- pre-B-cell type
- promyelocytic
- Rieder cell
- T-cell type
- undifferentiated

leukemia classification
leukemia cutis

leukemic
leukemid
leukemogen
leukemogenesis
leukemogenic
leukemoid reaction
leukencephalitis
leukexosis
leukin
leukoagglutinin
leukoblast
leukoblastosis
leukocidin
  Neisser-Wechsberg
  Panton-Valentine (P-V)
leukocrit
leukocyte
  acidophil
  acidophilic
  agranular
  basophilic
  beta
  circulating
  endothelial
  eosinophil
  eosinophilic
  fecal
  granular
  heterophilic
  lymphoid
  mast
  migration of
  motile
  neutrophilic
  nongranular
  nonmotile
  peripheral
  polymorphonuclear
  polymorphonuclear karyorrhectic
  Türk irritation
leukocyte acid phosphatase,
  tartrate resistant
leukocyte adherence assay
leukocyte adhesion protein (LAP)
leukocyte alkaline phosphatase (LAP)
leukocyte ascorbic acid (LAA)
leukocyte bactericidal assay
leukocyte differential count
  basophils
  eosinophils
  lymphocytes
  monocytes
  myelocytes
  neutrophils
    bands
    segs
leukocyte/erythrocyte ratio
leukocyte esterase (LE) in urine
leukocyte esterase test (LET)
leukocyte-poor red blood cells
leukocyte surface receptors
leukocythemia
leukocytic infiltration of submucosa
leukocytic sarcoma
leukocytic trapping of bacteria
leukocytoblast
leukocytogenesis
leukocytoid
leukocytolysin
leukocytolysis
leukocytolytic
leukocytoma
leukocytopenia
leukocytopoiesis
leukocytosis
  absolute
  agonal
  basophilic
  mononuclear
  neutrophilic
  pathologic
  physiologic
  pure
  relative

leukocytosis *(continued)*
  terminal
  toxic
leukocytosis-promoting factor
leukocytotactic
leukocytotaxis
leukocytotherapy
leukocytotoxicity
leukocytotropic
leukocyturia
leukoderma
  occupational
  postinflammatory
  syphilitic
leukodermatous
leukodystrophy
  globoid cell
  hereditary adult-onset
  hereditary cerebral
  Krabbe
  metachromatic
  spongiform
  sudanophilic
leukoedema
leukoencephalitis
leukoencephalopathy
  necrotizing
  progressive multifocal (PML)
  subacute sclerosing
leukoerythroblastosis
leukogram
leukokeratosis
leukokinesis
leukokinetic
leukokinetics
leukopedesis
leukopenia
leukopenic factor
leukopenic index
leukophagocytosis
leukoplakia
leukopoiesis
leukopoietic
leukopoietin
leukoprecipitin
leukorrhagia
leukorrhea
leukosarcoma
leukoscope
leukosis
leukotactic
leukotaxis
leukothrombin
leukotoxic
leukotoxicity
leukotoxin
Levaditi stain
levator muscle
level
  blood alcohol
  panic
  peak and trough
  PIVKA-II
  plasma lipoprotein
  red blood cell cholinesterase
  therapeutic
  toxic
  trough
level of umbilicus
Leventhal-Stein syndrome
Levine alkaline Congo red method
Levinson test for tuberculous meningitis
Lewis blood group
Lewis hydrophagocytosis phenomenon
Lewy body
Lewy inclusion body
Leyden neuritis
Leyden-Charcot crystal
Leydig cell
LFT, LFTs (liver function test)(s)
LH (luteinizing hormone)
LHV (left hepatic vein)
Liacopoulos phenomenon
Libman-Sacks verrucous endocarditis

lice and nits on body hair
lice and nits on pubic hair
lice and nits on scalp hair
lichen planus
lichenification
lichenoid dermatitis
lichenoid lesion
lichenoid papules
lichenoid pityriasis
Lichtheim disease
Lichtheim syndrome
Lieben-Ralfe test for acetone
Lieben test for acetone in urine
Lieberkühn crypt
Lieberkühn gland
Liebermann-Burchard test for cholesterol
Liebermann test for proteins
Liebermeister groove
Liebig test for cystine
lienal artery
lienophrenic ligament
lienorenal ligament
lienteric diarrhea
lienteric stool
Liesegang phenomenon
Lieutaud trigone
lifeless eye
lifelong obesity
lifesaving drugs
life span, shortening
lifestyle (noun)
life support (noun)
life-support system
life-threatening condition
life-threatening disease
Li-Fraumeni syndrome (LFS)
ligament
  accessory
  accessory plantar
  accessory volar
  alar

ligament *(continued)*
  alveolodental
  anatomy
  annular
  anococcygeal
  anterior calcaneoastragaloid
  anterior costotransverse
  anterior costovertebral
  anterior costoxiphoid
  anterior cruciate
  anterior inferior tibiofibular
  anterior longitudinal
  anterior radioulnar
  anterior talotibial
  anterior tibiotalar
  apical
  apical ligament of dens
  Arantius
  arcuate popliteal
  arcuate pubic
  arterial
  auricular
  axis
  Bardinet
  Barkow
  Bellini
  Berry
  Bertin
  Bichat
  bifurcate
  bifurcated
  Bigelow
  Botallo
  Bourgery
  broad l. of uterus
  Brodie
  Burns
  calcaneocuboid
  calcaneofibular
  calcaneonavicular
  calcaneotibial
  Caldani

ligament *(continued)*
Campbell
Camper
capsular
Carcassonne
cardinal
caroticoclinoid
carpometacarpal
casserian
Casser
caudal
ceratocricoid
cervical
check
cholecystoduodenal
chondroxiphoid
ciliary
Civinini
Clado
Cloquet
collateral
Colles
conjugate
conoid
Cooper
coracoacromial
coracoclavicular
coracohumeral
corniculopharyngeal
coronary
costoclavicular
costocolic
costotransverse
costoxiphoid
cotyloid
Cowper
cricopharyngeal
cricosantorinian
cricothyroid
cricotracheal
crucial
cruciate

ligament *(continued)*
cruciform
Cruveilhier
cuboideonavicular
cuneocuboid
cuneonavicular
cystoduodenal
deep dorsal sacrococcygeal
deep posterior sacrococcygeal
deep transverse metacarpal
deep transverse metatarsal
deltoid
Denonvilliers
dentate
denticulate
Denucé
diaphragmatic
dorsal calcaneocuboid
dorsal carpal
dorsal carpometacarpal
dorsal cuboideonavicular
dorsal cuneocuboid
dorsal cuneonavicular
dorsal metacarpal
dorsal metatarsal
dorsal radiocarpal
dorsal sacroiliac
dorsal talonavicular
Douglas
duodenal
duodenorenal
epihyal
external
external collateral (of wrist)
extracapsular
falciform
fallopian
femoral
Ferrein
fibular collateral
Flood
fundiform

igament *(continued)*
gastrocolic
gastrodiaphragmatic
gastrohepatic
gastrolienal
gastropancreatic
gastrophrenic
gastrosplenic
genital
genitoinguinal
Gerdy
Gillette suspensory
Gimbernat
gingivodental
glenohumeral
glenoid
glossoepiglottic
Günz (Guenz)
Günzberg (Guenzberg)
hammock
Helmholtz axis
Hensing
hepatic
hepatocolic
hepatocystocolic
hepatoduodenal
hepatoesophageal
hepatogastric
hepatogastroduodenal
hepatophrenic
hepatorenal
hepatoumbilical
Hesselbach
Hey
Holl
Hueck
Humphry
Hunter
Huschke
hyalocapsular
hyoepiglottic
hypsiloid

ligament *(continued)*
iliofemoral
iliolumbar
iliopectineal
iliotibial l. of Maissiat
iliotrochanteric
inferior calcaneonavicular
inferior pubic
inferior transverse scapular
infundibulo-ovarian
infundibulopelvic
inguinal
intercapital
intercarpal
interclavicular
interclinoid
intercornual
intercostal
intercuneiform
interfoveolar
internal collateral
interosseous
interosseous cuneocuboid
interosseous cuneometatarsal
interosseous lunotriquetral
interosseous metacarpal
interosseous metatarsal
interosseous sacroiliac
interosseous talocalcaneal
interosseous tibiofibular
interspinous
intertransverse
intra-articular
intra-articular sternocostal
intrascapular
ischiocapsular
ischiofemoral
Jarjavay
jugal
Krause
laciniate
lacunar

ligament *(continued)*
- Lannelongue
- lateral arcuate
- lateral costotransverse
- lateral lumbosacral
- lateral malleolar
- lateral palpebral
- lateral puboprostatic
- lateral sacrococcygeal
- lateral talocalcaneal
- lateral temporomandibular
- lateral umbilical
- Lauth
- left superior vena cava
- left triangular
- left vena cava
- lienophrenic
- lienorenal
- Lisfranc
- Lockwood
- long plantar
- longitudinal
- lumbocostal
- lunotriquetral
- Luschka
- Mackenrodt
- Maissiat
- Mauchart
- Meckel
- medial
- medial arcuate
- medial collateral
- medial palpebral
- medial puboprostatic
- medial talocalcaneal
- medial umbilical
- median arcuate
- meniscofemoral
- middle costotransverse
- middle umbilical
- mucosal suspensory
- nuchal

ligament *(continued)*
- oblique
- oblique popliteal
- occipitoaxial
- odontoid
- orbicular
- ovarian
- palmar
- palmar carpal
- palmar carpometacarpal
- palmar metacarpal
- palmar radiocarpal
- palmar ulnocarpal
- patellar
- pectinate
- pectineal
- peridental
- periodontal
- peritoneal
- Petit
- Pétrequin
- phrenicocolic
- phrenicolienal
- phrenicosplenic
- phrenoesophageal
- phrenogastric
- phrenosplenic
- pisohamate
- pisometacarpal
- pisounciform
- pisouncinate
- plantar
- plantar calcaneocuboid
- plantar calcaneonavicular
- plantar cuboideonavicular
- plantar cuneocuboid
- plantar cuneonavicular
- plantar metatarsal
- posterior
- posterior costotransverse
- posterior costotransverse ligament
- posterior cricoarytenoid

ligament *(continued)*
posterior cruciate
posterior longitudinal
posterior meniscofemoral
posterior occipitoaxial
posterior sacroiliac
posterior sacrosciatic
posterior sternoclavicular
posterior talofibular
posterior talotibial
posterior tibiofibular
posterior tibiotalar
Poupart
pterygomandibular
pterygospinal
pterygospinous
pubocapsular
pubocervical
pubofemoral
puboprostatic
pubovesical
pulmonary
quadrate
radial collateral
radiate
radiate sternocostal
radiocarpal
radiolunotriquetral
radioscaphocapitate
radioscapholunate
reflected inguinal
reflecting edge of
reflex
reflex inguinal
Retzius
rhomboid
right triangular
ring
Robert
round
sacrodural
sacrospinous

ligament *(continued)*
sacrotuberous
Santorini
Sappey
scapholunate
Schlemm
serous
sheath
Simonart
Soemmerring
sphenomandibular
spinoglenoid
spiral
splenocolic
splenorenal
spring
Stanley cervical
stellate
sternoclavicular
sternopericardial
stylohyoid
stylomandibular
stylomaxillary
superficial dorsal sacrococcygeal
superficial posterior sacrococcygeal
superficial transverse metacarpal
superficial transverse metartarsal
superior
superior costotransverse
superior pubic
superior transverse scapular
suprascapular
supraspinous
suspensory
sutural
synovial
talocalcaneal
talonavicular
tarsal
tarsometatarsal
temporomandibular
Teutleben

ligament *(continued)*
  Thompson
  thyroepiglottic
  thyrohyoid
  tibial collateral
  tibiocalcaneal
  tibiofibular
  tibionavicular
  transverse
  transverse atlantal
  transverse carpal
  transverse crural
  transverse genicular
  transverse humeral
  transverse metacarpal
  transverse metatarsal
  transverse perineal
  transverse tibiofibular
  trapezoid
  triangular
  Tuffier inferior
  ulnar collateral
  ulnocarpal
  ulnolunate
  ulnotriquetral
  umbilical
  urachal
  uterine
    broad
    cardinal
    round
  uterosacral
  uterovesical
  venous
  ventral sacrococcygeal
  ventral sacroiliac
  ventricular
  vertebropelvic
  vesicoumbilical
  vesicouterine
  vestibular
  vocal

ligament *(continued)*
  volar
  volar carpal
  Walther oblique
  Weitbrecht
  Winslow
  Wrisberg
  xiphicostal
  xiphoid
  Y-shaped
  Zaglas
  Zinn
ligament of Scarpa
ligament of Struthers
ligament of Testut
ligament of Treitz
ligament shelving edge, Poupart
ligand
ligation, tubal
ligature, elastic
ligature needle
light
  black
  infrared
  polarized
  reflected
  refracted
  Tyndall
  ultraviolet
  white
  Wood
light cell
light cells of thyroid
light-chain proteinuria
light gray stool
light microscope
light microscopy
light scatter gate
ligneous
lilac rash
Lillie allochrome connective tissue
  stain

Lillie azure–eosin stain
Lillie ferrous iron stain
Lillie sulfuric acid Nile blue stain
limb
  afferent
  ampullary
  efferent
  jejunal
  lower
  phantom
  Roux-en-Y jejunal
  sagittal
  upper
limb lead
limb muscle
limb stump
limbus fossae ovalis
limit of resection
limiting membrane
limits, within normal (WNL)
limnemia (chronic malaria)
limp
Limulus amebocyte lysate assay
limulus lysate test
Limulus polyphemus
limulus test
Lindemann test for acetoacetic acid in urine
line (pl. lines)
  absorption
  accretion
  alveolonasal
  anocutaneous
  anorectal
  arcuate
  axillary
  azygos venous
  basinasal
  Beau
  Brödel white
  Brücke
  calcification
line *(continued)*
  cell
  cement
  cervical
  Chaussier
  Clapton
  cleavage
  contour
  copper
  Corrigan
  costoclavicular
  costophrenic septal
  dentate
  developmental
  Eberth
  epiphysial
  established cell
  Frommann
  Hunter
  iliopectineal
  incremental
  Langer
  midaxillary
  midclavicular
  midscapular
  milk
  pectinate
  period
  polypropylene
  pubic hair
  pubococcygeal
  Retzius
  Rex-Cantli-Serege
  semilunar
  skin
  suture
  white l. of Toldt
  Z
  Zahn
linea alba
linea nigra
lineae (pl. of linea)

linear cutaneous lesion
linear defect
linear epidermal nevus
linear fraction
linear fracture
linear IgA bullous disease
linear morphea
line of arrested growth
line of Ebner
line of ilium, arcuate
line of Kaes
line of resection
line of Retzius
line of Toldt
line of Zahn
line test for rickets
lingua (tongue)
lingua apex
lingua nigra (black tongue)
lingual aponeurosis
lingual artery, deep
lingual atrophy
lingual bone
lingual frenulum
lingual goiter
lingual muscle
lingual papilla
lingual root
lingual septum
lingual tonsil
lingual vein
lingula (pl. lingulae)
lining cell
lining, ependymal
linitis plastica
lip
  articular
  cleft
  hypoplastic
  lower
  rhombic
  upper
lipase
  pancreatic
  serum
lipase enzyme
lipase test for liver function
lipedematous alopecia
lipemic
lipid-associated sialic acid (LASA)
lipid compound
lipid island
lipid-laden macrophages
lipid material, macrophages stuffed with
lipid metabolism, disorders of
lipid-mobilizing hormone
lipidosis
lipid pigment
lipid profile
lipid test on venous blood
liplike projections of cartilage
lipoatrophic diabetes
lipoatrophy
lipoblast
lipocyte
lipodystrophy, familial
lipofuscin
lipogenous diabetes
lipoid, anisotropic
lipoid granuloma
lipoid nephrosis
lipoid pneumonia
lipoid pneumonitis
lipoid proteinosis
lipoid substance
lipoidal degeneration
lipolytic enzyme
lipoma
lipomatosis
lipomatous-like tissue
lipomatous nevus
lipomatous polyp
lipophage

lipophagic granuloma
lipopolysaccharide (LPS)
lipoprotein (LP)
  alpha$_1$–
  beta
  high density (HDL)
  low density (LDL)
  very low density (VLDL)
lipoprotein electrophoresis (LPE)
lipoproteinemia
lipoprotein metabolism, disorder of
liposarcoma
lipotropic factor
lipotropic hormone
lipping of vertebrae
lips of hilum
Lipschütz body
Lipschütz cell
lipuria
liquefaction degeneration
liquefaction, gas
liquefaction necrosis
liquefaction of debris
liquefying
liquid chromatography
liquid material
liquid nitrogen
liquor folliculi
liquid stool
Lisfranc joint
Lisfranc ligament
Lison-Dunn stain
Listeria monocytogenes
listeriosis
Lister tubercle
liter (L)
lithium-carmine stain
litmus milk test for pancreatic lipase
littoral cell
Littré gland
livedoid dermatitis
livedo, postmortem

liver
  albuminoid
  bare area of
  biliary cirrhotic
  black
  blue
  brimstone
  bronze
  capsule of
  caudate lobe of
  centrilobular region of
  cirrhosis of
  degenerative
  degraded
  diaphragmatic surface of
  dome of
  duodenal impression on
  fatty
  floating
  foamy
  frosted
  green
  hobnail
  icing
  infantile
  iron
  lardaceous
  left lobe of
  metastasis to
  nutmeg
  pigmented
  polycystic
  quadrate lobe of
  renal impression on
  right lobe of
  sago
  stasis
  sugar-icing
  undersurface of
  visceral surface of
  wandering
  waxy

liver adenocarcinoma
liver bed, surface of
liver bile
liver cell
liver cell plate
liver cirrhosis
liver death
liver edge
liver enzyme (glucuronosyltransferase)
liver fluke
liver function test
liver impression
liver iron store
liverlike lung
liver lobule, central vein of
liver panel
liver parenchyma
liver profile
liver segment
liver transplant
liver tumor
livid
lividity
  dependent
  postmortem
livedo reticularis–digital infarct
livedo vasculitis
Livingston triangle
livor mortis
LKS (liver, kidneys, and spleen)
L-L factor (XIII)
LLQ (left lower quadrant)
Loa loa
lobar artery
lobar atrophy
lobar bronchi
lobar consolidation
lobar pneumonia
lobe
  azygos
  caudate (liver)
  cuneiform
lobe *(continued)*
  falciform
  fetal
  flocculonodular
  frontal
  inferior
  left
  occipital
  polyalveolar
  pulmonary
  Riedel
  right
  superior
lobe bronchus
lobectomy
lobed nuclei
Loboa loboi
lobster-claw deformity
lobular architecture
lobular panniculitis
lobular parenchyma
lobular pattern
lobular pneumonia
lobulated
lobulation
lobule
  ansiform
  biventral
  central
  crescentic
  hepatic
  portal
  respiratory
  semilunar
lobule of epididymis
local death
local hormone
localized myeloma
localized nodular synovitis
localized osteitis fibrosa
localized pemphigoid of Brunsting-Perry

localized thickenings of Bruch membrane
local lesion
locally invasive tumor
local metastasis
locked-in syndrome
locked knee
Lockwood ligament
loculated fluid
Locffler (Löffler)
Loeffler caustic stain
Loeffler coagulated serum medium
Loeffler methylene blue stain
Loeffler serum
Loeffler stain
Loevit cell
Loewe test for urine glucose
Löffler (Loeffler)
Löhlein-Baehr lesion
loiasis (Calabar swelling)
loin
long-acting thyroid stimulating (LATS) hormone test
long axis of spleen
long bone
long chain fatty acid–CoA ligase
long chain triglycerides (LCT)
long ciliary artery
long plantar ligament
long spinous process
long thoracic artery
longitudinal anastomosis
longitudinal arc of skull
longitudinal axis
longitudinal band
longitudinal canals of modiolus
longitudinal cerebral fissure
longitudinal ligament, anterior
longitudinal muscle coat
longitudinal oval pelvis
longitudinal raphe
longitudinal section
loop
- afferent
- bowel
- capillary
- cervical
- closed
- colonic
- duodenal
- efferent
- gamma
- Gerdy interatrial
- Henle
- Hyrtl
- intestinal
- jejunal
- lenticular
- Meyer
- Meyer-Archambault
- open
- peduncular
- pressure-volume
- puborectalis
- sentinel
- sigmoid
- Storck
- subclavian
- transverse colon
- ventricular
- Vieussens

loose connective tissue
looseness
loose stool
lordosis
lordotic proteinuria
Lorrain Smith stain
loss of striations
louse (pl. lice)
- body
- hair
- pubic

louse-borne typhus
low birth weight

low density lipoprotein (LDL)
low density lipoprotein receptors
Löwenberg canal
Lowenthal test for glucose not in urine
lower esophageal sphincter (LES)
lower extremity arteries
lower extremity articulation
lower extremity joint
lower limb
lower lip
lower motor neuron lesion
lower nephron nephrosis
lower respiratory tract smear
lowest splanchnic nerve
low frequency blood group
low-grade dysplasia
low-grade malignancy
low normal test result
low-power field (lpf)
low-viscosity fluid
LP (lumbar puncture)
lpf (low-power field)
LPS (lipopolysaccharide)
LPS-receptor system
L/S (lecithin/sphingomyelin)
L/S ratio in amniotic fluid
lubricant-secreting membrane
lucidum, stratum
Lucio leprosy
Lucio phenomenon
Lucké carcinoma
Lücke test for hippuric acid
Lucké virus
Ludwig angina
Ludwig labyrinth
lues (syphilis) myocarditis
luetic abscess
Luft potassium permanganate fixative
Lugol solution
Lukes-Butler classification of non-Hodgkin lymphoma
Lukes-Collins classification of non-Hodgkin lymphoma
lumbar aponeurosis
lumbar artery
lumbar lymph node
lumborum muscle, quadratus
lumbar nerve
lumbar puncture (LP)
lumbar region
lumbar rib
lumbar vein, ascending
lumbar vertebrae (L1 through L5)
lumberman's itch
lumbocostal aponeurosis
lumbocostal arch
lumbocostal ligament
lumbocostoabdominal triangle
lumbosacral arch
lumbosacral articulation
lumbosacral joint
lumbosacral ligament
lumbosacral trunk
lumen (pl. lumens, lumina)
lumiaggregometry
lumina (pl. of lumen)
luminal
lumpectomy
lumpy skin disease
Luna-Ishak stain
Luna modification of Bodian stain
lunate bone
lunate facet
Lundh test for pancreatic function
lung
  airless
  atelectatic
  bird-breeder's
  black
  book
  cardiac
  cheese handler's
  coal-miner's

lung *(continued)*
- drowned
- dull purple
- emphysematous
- farmer's
- fibrinoid
- fissures of
- grain handler's
- hemorrhagic consolidation of
- hilum of
- honeycomb
- humidifier
- hyperlucent
- hypoplastic
- malt worker's
- mason's
- meat wrapper's
- miller's
- miner's
- normal gas exchange in
- pigeon-breeder's
- rudimentary
- shock
- shrunken
- silo-filler's
- silver finisher's
- smoker's
- thresher's
- vanishing
- welder's
- wet
- white

lung abscess
lung adenocarcinoma
lung apex
lung base
lung capacity
lung flukes
lung mass
lung parenchyma
lung plague
lung root
lung tumor
lunotriquetral joint
lunotriquetral ligament
lunula ossicle
lunule
lupoid hepatitis
lupus anticoagulant
lupus band test
lupus erythematosus (LE)
- chilblain
- cutaneous
- discoid (DLE)
- disseminated
- drug-induced
- hypertrophic
- systemic (SLE)

lupus erythematosus cell (LE cell)
lupus erythematosus cell preparation test (LE prep)
lupus erythematosus profundus (lupus panniculitis)
lupus erythematosus tumidus
lupus hypertrophicus
lupus nephritis
lupus nephrosis
lupus pernio
lupus tumidus
lupus vulgaris
LUQ (left upper quadrant)
Luschka crypt
Luschka gland
Luschka joint
Luschka ligament
Luschka tissue
Lust peroneal nerve phenomenon
luteal cell
luteal phase
luteal phase defect
lutein cell
lutein cyst
luteinization
luteinizing hormone (LH)

luteinizing hormone/follicle-stimulating hormone-releasing factor (LH/FSH-RF)
luteinizing hormone-releasing hormone (LH-RH, LRH)
luteinizing theca cell
Lutembacher syndrome
luteotropic hormone
luteum, corpus
Lutheran blood group
Lutkens sphincter
Luttke test for free hydrochloric acid in gastric juice
Luxol fast blue
LVH (left ventricular hypertrophy)
Lyle and Curtman test for blood
Lyme disease
lymph
  aplastic
  chyle
  corpuscular
  croupous
  dental
  euplastic
  inflammatory
  intercellular
  intravascular
"lymphs" (slang for lymphocytes)
lymphadenitis
  caseous
  mesenteric
  necrotizing granulomatous
  nonbacterial regional
  tuberculoid
  tuberculous
lymphadenoid goiter
lymphadenoma cells
lymphadenopathy
lymphadenopathy-associated virus (LAV)
lymphangioendothelioma
lymphangioma, cutaneous
lymphangitis
  ascending
  descending
lymphatic abscess
lymphatic, afferent
lymphatic cortex
lymphatic duct
lymphatic edema
lymphatic fluid
lymphatic gland
lymphatic leukemia
lymphatic medulla
lymphatic metastasis
lymphatic network
lymphatic nodules, aggregated
lymphatic obstruction
lymphatic sarcoma
lymphatics of scrotum
lymphatic system
lymphatic tissue
lymphaticum, angioma
lymphatic vessel
lymphatic vessels thickened
lymph capillary
lymph cell
lymph duct
lymphedema
lymph gland
lymph node
  abdominal
  accessory
  anorectal
  aortic
  apical
  appendicular
  auricular
  axillary
  bifurcation
  Bouchard
  brachial
  bronchopulmonary
  buccal

lymph node *(continued)*
buccinator
caval
celiac
central
cervical paratracheal
Cloquet inguinal
common iliac
companion
cubital
cystic
Delphian
deltopectoral
diaphragmatic
epicolic
epigastric
external iliac
facial
fibular
gastric
gastroduodenal
gastroepiploic
gastro-omental
gluteal
hemolymph
hepatic
hilar
ileocolic
iliac
iliac circumflex
infrahyoid
inguinal
intercostal
interiliac
internal iliac
interpectoral
jugular
jugulodigastric
jugulo-omohyoid
lumbar
malar
mandibular

lymph node *(continued)*
mastoid
mediastinal
nasolabial
obturator
occipital
palpable regional
pancreatic
pancreaticoduodenal
pancreaticolienal
pancreaticosplenic
paracardial
paracolic
paramammary
pararectal
parasternal
paratracheal
parauterine
paravaginal
paravesicular
paratracheal
parietal
parotid
pectoral
pelvic
pericardial
phrenic
popliteal
postaortic
postcaval
postvesicular
preaortic
precaval
prececal
prepericardial
pretracheal
prevertebral
prevesicular
pulmonary
pyloric
rectal
regional

lymph node *(continued)*
- retroaortic
- retroauricular
- retrocecal
- retropharyngeal
- retrorectal
- sacral
- sentinel
- sigmoid
- solitary
- splenic
- submandibular
- submental
- subscapular
- superficial inguinal
- supraclavicular
- supratrochlear
- thyroid
- tracheal
- tracheobronchial
- vesicular
- visceral

lymph node aspiration
lymph node metastasis
lymph node permeability factor
lymph node sinus
lymphoblast
lymphoblastic leukemia
lymphoblastic lymphoma
Lymphocryptovirus
lymphocyte
- atypical
- B
- CD4+
- circulating
- mature
- sinusoidal
- T
- T4
- thymus-dependent
- thymus-independent

lymphocyte-associated virus
lymphocyte-like cell
lymphocyte proliferation test
lymphocyte subset assay
lymphocyte transformation test
lymphocytic choriomeningitis
lymphocytic infiltrate
lymphocytic infiltration of dermis
lymphocytic infiltration of skin
lymphocytic interstitial pneumonitis
lymphocytic leukemia
lymphocytic lymphoma
- plasmacytoid
- poorly differentiated
- well differentiated

lymphocytic myocarditis
lymphocytic thyroiditis
lymphocytopheresis
lymphocytosis, relative
lymphocytotoxic antibody
lymphogenous embolism
lymphogenous metastasis
lymphoglandular body
lymphogranuloma venereum
lymphohistiocytic infiltrate
lymphoid cell
lymphoid follicle
lymphoid hyperplasia
lymphoid interstitial pneumonia
lymphoid leukocyte
lymphoid microabscess
lymphoid polyp
lymphoid tissue, aggregations of
lymphoid tumor
lymphokine-activated killer (LAK) cell
lymphoma
- adult T-cell
- African
- B-cell
- B-cell monocytoid
- Burkitt
- centrocytic
- cleaved cell

lymphoma *(continued)*
- diffuse
- diffuse large cell
- diffuse mixed small and large cell
- diffuse small cleaved cell
- follicular
- follicular center cell
- follicular mixed small cleaved
- follicular predominantly large cell
- follicular predominantly small cell
- giant follicle
- granulomatous
- histiocytic
- Hodgkin
- intermediate lymphocytic
- large cell, immunoblastic
- large cleaved cell
- large noncleaved cell
- Lennert
- lymphoblastic
- lymphocytic plasmacytoid
- lymphocytic poorly differentiated
- lymphocytic well differentiated
- malignant
- mantle zone
- Mediterranean
- mixed lymphocytic-histiocytic
- nodular
- non-Hodgkin
- pleomorphic
- primary of central nervous system
- small B-cell
- small cleaved cell
- small lymphocytic
- small noncleaved cell
- T-cell
  - convoluted
  - cutaneous
  - small lymphocytic
- U-cell
- undefined
- undifferentiated

lymphoma cutis
lymphomatoid papulosis
lymphomatosis
lymphomatous
lymphomyxoma
lymphonodulus (pl. lymphonoduli)
lymphopathy, ataxic
lymphopenia
lymphoplasia
lymphoplasmapheresis
lymphopoiesis
lymphoproliferative
lymphoreticular cell
lymphoreticular tissue
lymphoreticulosis
lymphorrhage
lymphorrhagia
lymphorrhea
lymphorrhoid
lymphosarcoma
lymphostasis
lymphotaxis
lymphotrophy
lymphotropic
lymph plexus
lymph tissue
lymph trunk, bronchomediastinal
lymphvascular
lymph vessel
lysate of blood cells
lyse, lysed
lysing
lysis, euglobulin clot
lysis of cells
lysosomal protease
lysosome
lysozyme
lyssa inclusion body
Lyssavirus
"lytes" (slang for electrolytes)
lytic lesion
lytic virus

M, m

Macalister muscle
Macchiavello stain
MacConkey agar
Macdonald test for liver function
MAC EIA (IgM antibody capture enzyme immunoassay)
macerate
macerated fetus
maceration
Machado-Guerreiro test for Chagas disease
Machado test for Chagas disease
Mach band
Mackenrodt ligament
Mackenzie point
Maclagan thymol turbidity test
MacLean–de Wesselow urea concentration test
MacLean test for lactic acid in gastric juice
MacMunn test for indican
MacNeal tetrachrome blood stain
macrocytic anemia
macrocytosis
macroglia cell
macroglobulin
macroglobulinemia, Waldenström
macroglossia
macrognathia
macrolobular cirrhosis
macrometastasis
macrophage
    alveolar
    armed
    fixed
    free
    hemosiderin-laden
    inflammatory
    lipid-laden
    pulmonary
macrophage-activating factor
macrophage colony-stimulating factor
macrophage inflammatory protein
macrophage migration inhibition test
macrophages stuffed with lipid material
macroscopic diagnosis
macroscopic hematuria
macroscopic report
macrosomia
MACS immunomagnetic cell sorter
macula (pl. maculae)
macula, false
macular artery
macular atrophy

macular degeneration
macule
maculopapular exanthem
maculopapular rash
MacWilliam test for albumin
Madayag biopsy needle
Madelung deformity
Madelung neck
Madurella mycetomatis
maduromycosis
Magendie space
magna, lacuna
magnesionitric test for albumin in urine
magnesium (Mg)
Magpie test
mahogany-colored stool
Maier sinus
main artery
main pancreatic duct (MPD)
main stem bronchus
maintenance protein
Maissiat band
Maissiat ligament
Maissiat tract
Majocchi disease
Majocchi granuloma
major branch
major calyx
major duodenal papilla
major, pelvis
major salivary gland
major vessel
majus (pl. majora)
  labium (pl. labia)
  omentum
malabsorption
  congenital lactose
  glucose-galactose
  sucrose-isomaltose, congenital
malabsorption of fats
malabsorption of vitamin B_{12}
malabsorption state
malabsorption syndrome
Malacarne space
malachite green
malar bone
malaria
  acute
  algid
  autochthonous
  avian
  benign tertian
  bilious remittent
  cerebral
  congenital
  double tertian
  dysenteric algid
  falciparum
  gastric algid
  hemolytic
  hemorrhagic
  induced
  intermittent
  malignant tertian
  nonan
  ovale
  pernicious
  quartan
  quotidian
  relapsing
  remittent
  tertian
  therapeutic
  transfusion
  vivax
malarial cachexia
malarial cirrhosis
malarial granuloma
malaria-like illness
malarial knobs
malarial pigment
malarial pneumonitis
malaria smear
malariotherapy

malar rash
malar skin
Malassezia furfur
Malassezia pachydermatis
Malbin-Sternheimer stain
Maldonado–San Jose stain
male pattern alopecia
male pattern baldness
male pelvis
male reproductive system
male sex cell
malformation
  Arnold-Chiari
  cystic adenomatoid
  dancer foot
  Dieulafoy vascular
malignancy
  aggressive
  borderline
  grading of
  hematologic
  hematopoietic
  high-grade
  intraocular
  low-grade
  metastatic
  primary
  prostatic
  staging of
malignant atrophic papulosis
malignant cell
malignant change
malignant degeneration
malignant edema
malignant fibrous histiocytoma
malignant glioma tumor
malignant hyperphenylalaninemia
malignant hypertension
malignant lentigo
malignant lymphoma
malignant melanoma
malignant melanoma in situ
malignant melanoma metastatic to heart
malignant mesothelioma
malignant mole
malignant neoplasm
malignant nephrosclerosis
malignant pheochromocytoma
malignant teratoma of heart
malignant tertian malaria
malleolar artery
malleus bone
malleus, ligaments of
Mallory aniline blue stain
Mallory-Azan stain
Mallory body
Mallory collagen stain
Mallory hemofuchsin stain
Mallory hyalin body
Mallory iodine stain
Mallory iron stain
Mallory phloxine stain
Mallory phosphotungstic acid-hematoxylin stain
Mallory trichrome stain
Mallory triple stain
Mallory-Weiss lesion
Mallory-Weiss syndrome
Mallory-Weiss tear
malnutrition
malodorous stool
Malot test
malpighian body
malpighian cell
malpighian corpuscle
malpighian follicle
malpighian gland
malpighian layer
malrotation of intestine
Malta fever
maltose test
malunion of fracture fragments
mamillary body

mammary abscess
mammary adenoma
mammary adenosis
mammary artery
mammary atrophy
mammary cyst
mammary duct obstruction
mammary dysplasia
mammary gland
mammotropic factor
mammotropic hormone
Manchurian fever
Mancini iodine technique
mandible
  alveolar border of
  angle of
mandible bone
mandible joint
mandibular arch
mandibular artery
mandibular canal
mandibular disk
mandibular gland
mandibular incisor angle, Frankfort
mandibulofacial dysostosis
manganese (Mn)
manganese pneumonitis
mango dermatitis
Mann methyl blue-eosin stain
Mann-Whitney test
Mann-Whitney-Wilcoxon test
Manson pyosis
mantle, brain
mantle zone lymphoma
Mantoux intracutaneous tuberculin test
Mantoux skin test
manubriosternal articulation
manubriosternal joint
manubrium, inferior border of
manubrium of sternum
many-sided
maple syrup odor in urine
maple syrup urine disease
maprotiline
marantic clot
marasmus
marble bone disease
marble bones
Marburg disease
Marburg virus
Marchand adrenal gland
Marchand wandering cell
Marchi fixative
Marchi method of staining
Maréchal test for bile pigments in urine
Marfan syndrome
margin
margin of pupil
margin of resection
marginal artery
marginal artery of colon
marginal artery of Drummond
marginal osteophyte
marginal sinus
marginatum erythema
Marie-Strümpell (Struempell) disease
marine dermatitis
mark, Unna
marked focal hyperkeratosis
marker (see *tumor marker*)
markings, haustral
maroon-colored stool
Marquis test for morphine
marrow
  bone
  depressed
  erythroid hyperplasia of
  fat
  gelatinized
  hyperplasia of
  red
  spinal
  yellow
marrow aspiration

- marrow canal
- marrow cell
- marrow harvesting, stem cell
- Martinotti cell
- masculine pelvis
- mask, ecchymotic
- masked virus
- mass
  - appendiceal
  - apperceptive
  - body cell
  - brittle
  - concentrically laminated
  - conical
  - cystic
  - elongated
  - encapsulated
  - firm
  - fleecy
  - friable
  - fungating
  - glistening
  - injection
  - inner cell
  - irregular
  - lean body
  - lung
  - molar
  - molecular
  - multilocular
  - nodular
  - pearly white
  - relative molecular
  - sex chromatin
  - shiny
  - slowly enlarging
  - stonelike
  - tigroid
- mass effect
- masseteric artery
- Masset test for bile pigments in urine
- mass infection
- massive coagulation
- massive deposits of glycogen in muscle
- massive embolism
- massive hepatic necrosis
- massive pneumonia
- massive pulmonary hemorrhagic edema
- mass of congealed blood
- Masson argentaffin stain
- Masson-Fontana ammoniacal silver stain
- Masson trichrome stain
- mass spectrometry
- mast cell
- mast cell leukemia
- master gland
- mast leukocyte
- masticate
- mastitis
  - acute
  - chronic
  - cystic
  - gargantuan
  - glandular
  - interstitial
  - lactational
  - parenchymatous
  - periductal
  - phlegmonous
  - plasma cell
  - puerperal
  - retromammary
  - stagnation
  - submammary
  - suppurative
- mastocytosis, diffuse cutaneous
- mastoid abscess
- mastoid air cells, epithelium-lined
- mastoid antrum
- mastoid artery
- mastoid bone
- mastoid cell

mastoid fontanelle
mastoid process
mastoiditis
mater (note: one *t*)
  dura
  pia
material
  amorphous
  base
  breadlike
  calcareous
  coffee-grounds
  colloid
  cross-reacting (CRM)
  cytoplasmic
  dried out
  eosinophilic
  extracellular (ECM)
  fluid
  foamy
  foreign
  functional
  gelatinous
  gel-like
  genetic
  globoid
  gritty
  grumous
  hemorrhagic
  homogeneous
  inspissated
  jelly-like
  liquid
  lumpy
  mucoid
  myxoid
  noncellular
  nonfibrous
  purulent
  refractile
  sandy
  sarcoplasmic
material *(continued)*
  semisolid
  thickened
  tissue equivalent
maternal diabetes
maternal phenylketonuria
Mathews test for lactose and glucose
matrix
  amphophilic
  bone
  cartilage
  cytoplasmic
  extracellular (ECM)
  interterritorial
  mitochondrial
  nail
  sarcoplasmic
  solid
  territorial
matrix band
matrix cell
matrix granule
matrix hyaline
matrix of collagenic fibers
matt or matte
matter
  gray
  white
matting
maturation
maturation index
mature lymphocyte
maturity-onset diabetes
maturity-onset diabetes of youth (MODY)
Mauchart ligament
Maumené test for glucose
Maurer dots
Mauthner cell
maxilla (pl. maxillae)
maxillary antrum
maxillary artery

- maxillary articulation
- maxillary bone
- maxillary canal
- maxillary nerve
- maxilloturbinal bone
- Maximow fixative
- Maximow solution
- Maximow stain
- maximum breathing capacity
- maximus, gluteus
- Mayaro virus
- Mayer hematoxylin
- Mayer hematoxylin counterstain
- Mayer mucicarmine
- Mayer stain
- Mayerhofer test
- Mayer test for alkaloids
- May-Grünwald-Giemsa stain
- mazoplasia
- Mazzotti test for onchocerciasis
- M band
- MB band
- MBC (minimum bactericidal concentration)
- MB fraction
- MB isoenzyme
- MBP (myelin basic protein)
- MCB Tissue Freeze
- McBurney point
- McCort sign
- McCoy cell
- mcg (microgram)
- MCH (mean corpuscular hemoglobin)
- MCHC (mean corpuscular hemoglobin concentration)
- McKrae strain of herpesvirus
- McLeod blood phenotype
- MCV (mean corpuscular volume)
- MD (muscular dystrophy)
- MDM2 expression
- meadow dermatitis
- meadow grass dermatitis
- meal
  - barium
  - fatty
  - opaque
  - retention
  - test
- mealy
- mean corpuscular hemoglobin (MCH)
- mean corpuscular hemoglobin concentration (MCHC)
- mean corpuscular volume (MCV)
- mean platelet volume (MPV)
- measles (rubeola)
- measles encephalitis
- measles-like viruses
- measles virus
- measurement
  - axial extinction
  - slit-scan
- meatus
  - acoustic
  - external auditory
- meaty appearance
- meaty texture
- mechanical vector
- mechanism
  - deglutition
  - Frank-Starling
  - humeral
  - immune
  - sphincteric
  - swallowing
- Meckel band
- Meckel diverticulitis
- Meckel diverticulum
- Meckel ligament
- Meckel space
- meconium plug
- meconium-stained amniotic fluid
- meconium-stained membrane
- medial antebrachial cutaneous nerve
- medial arcuate ligament

medial atlantoaxial joint
medial circumflex artery of thigh
medial collateral ligament of elbow
medial crus (pl. crura)
medial crus of superficial inguinal ring
medial cuneiform bone
medial cutaneous nerve
medial cutaneous nerve of arm
medial cystic necrosis
medial eminence
medial epicondyle
medial frontobasal artery
medial ligament of knee
medial ligament of talocrural joint
medial lumbocostal arch
medial necrosis of large arteries
medial palpebral artery
medial palpebral ligament
medial puboprostatic ligament
medial striate artery
medial surface of lung
medial surface, vertebral part of
medial talocalcaneal ligament
medial tarsal artery
medial umbilical fold
medial umbilical ligament
medial wall of nasal cavity
median antebranchial vein
median aperture
median arcuate ligament
median eminence
median groove
median lobe of prostate
median plane
median raphe
median sacral artery
median umbilical fold
media, otitis
mediastinal artery
mediastinal fibrosis
mediastinal lymph node
mediastinal pleura
mediastinal pleurisy
mediastinitis
  fibrous
  indurative
mediastinodiaphragmatic pleural reflection
mediastinum
mediate transfusion
media tunica
medical mycology
medical surveillance
medical technologist
medicolegal autopsy
Mediterranean anemia
Mediterranean lymphoma
medium (pl. media)
  agar
  AimV serum-free
  alkaline
  Apathy mounting
  artificial
  balsam mounting
  Bruns glucose
  Clarite mounting
  clear (or clearing)
  contrast
  culture
  embedding
  HAT (hypoxanthine, aminopterin, thymidine)
  homogeneous
  infiltration
  jelly-like
  Loeffler
  mounting
  nutrient
  Permount mounting
  refractile
  Sabouraud culture
  Spurr
  Stuart
  Thayer-Martin

medium *(continued)*
- transparent
- transport

medium chain fatty acid (MCFA)
medium chain triglycerides (MCT)
medius, scalenus
medulla (pl. medullas, medullae)
- adrenal
- dusky
- lymphatic
- ovarian
- renal
- spinal

medulla oblongata
medulla of bone
medulla of kidney
medulla of lymph node
medulla of thymus
medullary artery
medullary bone
medullary canal
medullary carcinoma
medullary cavity
medullary cord
medullary ray
medullary sarcoma
medullary sinus
medullary sponge kidney
medullary substance
medullary zone
medulloblastoma
medusae, caput
megacolon, congenital
megakaryocyte
megakaryocyte progenitor cell
megakaryopoiesis
megaloblastic anemia
megaloblastic bone marrow
megaspore mother cell
meibomian cyst
meibomian froth
meibomian gland
Meigs syndrome
Meigs test for fat in milk
meiosis
Meirowsky phenomenon
Meissner corpuscle
Meissner plexus in submucosa
melanin-containing cell
melanin deposition
melanin incontinence
melanin synthesis, defect in
melanin test
melanoblasts
melanocyte
melanocyte-stimulating hormone
melanocytic nevus
melanocytoma, dermal
melanocytosis
melanoma
- acral-lentiginous
- amelanotic
- benign juvenile
- benign uveal
- desmoplastic malignant
- halo
- intraocular
- juvenile
- lentigo maligna
- malignant
- malignant lentigo
- minimal deviation
- mucosal
- nodular
- ocular
- staging of malignant
- subungual
- superficial spreading
- uveal

melanomatosis
melanophage
melanosis
melanosis coli
melanosome

melanotic freckle, Hutchinson
melanotic pigment
melanotic prurigo
melanotropic
melanotropin release-inhibiting hormone (MIH)
melanotropin-releasing factor
melanotropin-releasing hormone (MRH)
melasma
melatonin
melenic stool
mellitus, diabetes
membrane
  allantoid
  alveolodental
  anal
  arachnoid
  arachnoidal
  areolar
  atlanto-occipital
  basement
  basilar
  boundary
  Bowman
  Bruch
  bucconasal
  buccopharyngeal
  cell
  chorioallantoic
  cloacal
  closing
  cricothyroid
  cricotracheal
  cricovocal
  croupous
  deciduous
  Descemet
  diphtheritic
  drum
  dysmenorrheal
  egg

membrane *(continued)*
  elastic
  embryonic
  enamel
  epipapillary
  exocelomic
  external intercostal
  false
  fenestrated
  fertilization
  fetal
  fibrous
  flaccid
  gelatinous otoli sthic
  germ
  germinal
  glomerular capillary
  hyaline
  inner
  innermost intercostal
  intact
  internal elastic
  internal intercostal
  interosseous
  limiting
  localized thickenings of Bruch
  Millipore
  mucous
  nitrocellulose
  nuclear
  obturator
  otolithic
  outer
  perforated tympanic
  perineal
  phrenoesophageal
  placental
  plasma
  pleuroperitoneal
  polyvinylidene difluoride
  serous
  suprapleural

membrane *(continued)*
  synovial
  tympanic
membrane permeability
membranoproliferative glomerulonephritis
membranous deep layer
membranous glomerulonephritis
membranous labyrinth
membranous pneumonocyte
membranous pregnancy
membranous stomatitis
membranous urethra
memory cell
MEN (multiple endocrine neoplasia)
  type I (Wermer syndrome)
  type II (Sipple syndrome)
  type III (mucosal neuroma syndrome)
Mendel test
Menghini needle
meningeal adhesion
meningeal artery
meningeal carcinoma
meningeal petechiae
meningeal plague
meningeal tuberculosis
meninges (pl. of meninx)
meningioma
  angioblastic
  cerebellopontine angle
  clival
  convexity
  cystic
  falcine
  falx
  fibroblastic
  fibrous
  malignant
  meningotheliomatous
  parasagittal
  posterior fossa

meningioma *(continued)*
  psammomatous
  suprasellar
  syncytial
  tentorial
  transitional
meningioma of olfactory groove
meningioma of sphenoid ridge
meningitis
  aseptic
  bacterial
  basilar
  benign lymphocytic
  cerebral
  cerebrospinal
  chronic
  coccidioidal
  cryptococcal
  eosinophilic
  epidemic cerebrospinal
  gummatous
  Haemophilus influenzae
  meningococcal
  Mollaret
  mumps
  neoplastic
  occlusive
  otitic
  plague
  pneumococcal
  purulent
  pyogenic
  Quincke
  serous
  spinal
  sterile
  syphilitic
  tuberculous
  viral
meningitis necrotoxica reactiva
meningitis ossificans
meningoarteritis

meningocele
  anterior
  cranial
  sacral
  spinal
  spurious
  traumatic
meningocephalitis (also, meningoencephalitis)
meningocerebritis
meningococcal meningitis
meningococcal myocarditis
meningococcal septicemia
meningococcus
meningoencephalitis
meningoencephalomyelitis
meningomyelocele
meningothelial cell
meningotheliomatous meningioma
meningothelium
meningotyphoid fever
meninx (pl. meninges)
meniscal horn
menisci (pl. of meniscus)
meniscofemoral ligament
meniscus (pl. menisci)
  articular
  diverging
meniscus homologue
menstrual endometrium
menstrual stage
menstruation
mental artery
mental canal
mental deterioration
mental impairment
mental retardation
mental spine of maxilla
mentolabial sulcus
mEq (milliequivalent)
mEq/L (milliequivalents per liter)
M/E (myeloid/erythroid) ratio
mercurial stomatitis
mercuric chloride
mercuric salts
mercury poisoning
mercury test
Merkel-Ranvier cell
Merkel tactile cell
Merkel tactile disk
mermaid deformity
merocrine gland
Mery gland
Merzbacher-Pelizaeus disease
mesangial cell
mesangial cell fibronectin
mesangial cell proliferation
mesangium
mesarteritis, Mönckeberg
mesatipellic pelvis
mesencephalic artery
mesencephalon
mesenchyma
mesenchymal cell
mesenchymal model
mesenchymal tissue
mesenchymoma
  benign
  malignant
mesenteric artery
mesenteric gland
mesenteric plexus
mesenteric pregnancy
mesenteric soft tissue
mesenteric triangle
mesenteric vein
mesentery
  fan-shaped
  leaves of
  root of
  ventral
mesentery of appendix
mesentery of ileum
mesentery of jejunum

- meshwork of connective tissue
- meshwork of glial fibrils as repair material
- mesoappendix
- mesocardium, arterial
- mesocolic band
- mesocolic gland
- mesocolon
- mesocolonic fat tissue
- mesoderm
  - extraembryonic
  - gastral
- mesodermal factor
- mesogastrium, dorsal
- mesoglial cell
- mesorectum
- mesosalpinx
- mesosigmoid colon
- mesothelial cell
- mesothelial cyst
- mesothelioma of pleura
- mesothelium
- mesothial cell
- mesovarium
- Mester test for rheumatic disease
- metabisulfite test for sickle cell hemoglobin
- metabolic acidosis
- metabolic alkalosis
- metabolic cirrhosis
- metabolic coma
- metabolic disorder
- metabolic disturbance of acid-base balance
- metabolic encephalopathy
- metabolic insult
- metabolism
  - abnormal glucose
  - basal
  - carbohydrate
  - carbon dioxide
  - electrolyte
- metabolism *(continued)*
  - energy
  - glucose
  - inborn error of
  - intermediary
  - mucopolysaccharide
  - primary
  - protein
  - respiratory
  - secondary
- metacarpal artery
- metacarpal bone
- metacarpophalangeal articulation
- metacarpophalangeal joint
- metacarpus (pl. metacarpi)
- metachromatic leukodystrophy
- metachromatic stain
- metahypophysial diabetes
- metamorphosis
  - fatty
  - platelet
  - retrograde
  - tissue
  - viscous
- metamyelocyte
- metanephric diverticulum
- metanephrines in urine
- metaphyseal artery
- metaphyseal dysplasia
- metaphysis (pl. metaphyses)
  - agnogenic myeloid
  - apocrine
  - apocrine (of breast)
  - autoparenchymatous
  - celomic
  - columnar
  - fundic
  - intestinal
  - myeloid
  - primary myeloid
  - secondary myeloid
  - squamous

metaplastic squamous cell epithelium
metapneumonic pleurisy
metastasis (pl. metastases)
  calcareous
  drop
  hematogenous
  local
  lymphatic
  lymph node
  pulsating
  satellite
  widespread
metastasis staging
metastasis to bone
metastasis to brain
metastasis to liver
metastasis to lung
metastatic abscess
metastatic calcification
metastatic carcinoma
metastatic disease
metastatic inflammation
metastatic malignancy
metastatic orchitis
metastatic pneumonia
metastatic polyp
metastatic tuberculous abscess
metastatic tumor
metatarsal artery
metatarsal bone
metatarsal plantar artery
metatarsophalangeal articulation
metatarsophalangeal joint
metatarsus (pl. metatarsi)
metazoal myocarditis
methanol (methyl alcohol)
methanol-based polychrome stain
methanol fixative
metHb (methemoglobin)
methemalbumin
methemalbuminemia
methemoglobin (metHb)
methemoglobinemia
  acquired
  congenital
  enterogenous
  hereditary
  primary
  secondary
methemoglobinuria
methicillin-resistant *Staphylococcus aureus* (MRSA)
methionine test
method (staining) (see *solution, stain*)
  ABC peroxidase
  Abell-Kendall
  absorption
  Altmann-Gersh
  AMEX (of processing and embedding)
  Ashby
  Bielschowsky
  Billheimer assay
  capillary gap
  cell separation
  cooled-knife
  copper sulfate
  disk sensitivity
  Filley
  Gallyas
  immunofluorescence
  Jenner
  Klumpp & Bieth
  Kokoskin modified Weber
  Lee-White
  Marshall
  Millipore
  Nuclepore
  PAP
  Parham
  peroxidase/antiperoxidase protein labeling
  phenol/chloroform
  RNAzolB (of RNA extraction)

method *(continued)*
- Sainte-Marie (of alcoholic fixation and paraffin embedding)
- strong trichrome staining
- thermodilution
- Torrance and Bothwell
- Towbin (of immunoblotting)
- Warthin-Starry tissue staining
- Weber staining
- Westergren
- Wijsman (of end-labeling)
- Wu
- Ziehl-Neelsen

methyl alcohol
methylene blue stain
- Kühne
- Loeffler
- polychrome

methyl green–pyronin stain
methylphenylhydrazine test for fructose
methyl red test
methylumbelliferylglucuronide (MUG)
methyl violet stain
metopic suture
metrotrophic test
Mett test for estimating pepsin
metyrapone test
Mexican hat cell
Mexican spotted fever
Meyenburg complex
Meyer-Archambault loop
Meyer loop
Meynert cell
mg/dl (milligrams per deciliter)
Mg (magnesium)
MHA-TP (microhemagglutinin-*Treponema pallidum*) test
MIC (minimum inhibitory concentration)
mice, joint
Michaelis stain
Michailow test for proteins
Michel transport fixative
microabscess
- dermal
- lymphoid
- Munro
- Pautrier

microabscess of lung
microabscess of skin
microaerophilic
microaneurysm of retina, capillary
microangiopathy, diabetic
microbe
microbial
microbiology
microchemotaxis chamber
Micrococcus
microcytosis
microcytotoxicity assay
microfilaria
microfilariae in blood
microfilariae in subcutaneous tissue, skin, eye
microfocus
microglandular
microglia
microglial cell
micrognathia
microgram (mcg)
microhemagglutination test for *Treponema pallidum* (MHA-TP)
microhematocrit
microinfarcts of spleen
microinvasion
microinvasive carcinoma
microinvasive carcinoma classification
microkatal
microliter (μL)
microlobular cirrhosis
micrometastasis
micrometer (μm)
micromolar

micromole (μmol)
micromyeloblastic leukemia
micronodular cirrhosis of liver
micronodular fibrotic pattern
microorganism, pathogenic (see *pathogen*)
microprecipitation test
microscope
  BHS-RFC A3 fluorescence
  cervical
  confocal epifluorescence
  darkfield
  electron
  fluorescence
  JEOL 100 CX electron
  light
  Olympus B-Max
  phase-contrast
  Phillips 300 transmission electron
  polarizing
  Sarastro-2000 confocal scanning
  transmission electron
  Vanox fluorescence
  Vanox-T
  Zeiss Axiolab light
microscopic clefts
microscopic diagnosis
microscopic hematuria
microscopy
  confocal laser scanning
  darkfield
  electron
  fluorescent
  intravital
  light
microsomal antibodies, thyroid
microsomal TRC antibody titer
microsomes
microsomia
Microsporum
Microsporum amazonicum
Microsporum audouinii
Microsporum boullardii
Microsporum canis
Microsporum cookei
Microsporum equinum
Microsporum faeni
Microsporum ferrugineum
Microsporum floccosum
Microsporum fulvum
Microsporum gallinae
Microsporum gypseum
Microsporum nanum
Microsporum persicolor
Microsporum praecox
Microsporum racemosum
Microsporum ripariae
Microsporum vanbreuseghemii
Microtainer (B-D Microtainer)
microtome
  freezing
  rocking
  rotary
  sliding
microtubule-associated protein (MAP)
microvesicular fat
microvesiculation
microvillus (pl. microvilli)
midabdominal wall
midaxillary line
midbody
midbrain
midcarpal joint
midcarpal portal
midclavicular line
midcolon
midcycle cervical mucus
middle capsular artery
middle cardiac vein
middle cell
middle cerebral artery
middle collateral artery
middle costotransverse ligament
middle cuneiform bone

middle ear
middle ethmoidal air cell
middle extrahepatic bile duct
middle genicular artery
middle hemorrhoidal artery
middle lobe bronchus
middle meatus
middle mediastinum
middle meningeal artery
middle nasal concha
middle radioulnar joint
middle rectal artery
middle rectal vein
middle sacral artery
middle suprarenal artery
middle temporal artery
middle turbinated bone
middle umbilical ligament
middle vesical artery
midepigastric area
midepigastrium
midesophagus
midface
midfoot
midfrontal
midget bipolar cell
midgut
midgut artery
midinguinal point
midlateral
midline abdominal crease
midline granuloma
midpoint of clavicle
midportion
mid-pretibial
midrectal area
midscapular line
midsection
midsigmoid colon
midstream urine specimen
midtarsal
midtarsal joint
midthigh
midzonal hepatic necrosis
Mielke bleeding time
Mignon eosinophilic granuloma
migrating abscess
migrating neuritis
migration inhibition test
migration inhibitory factor (MIF)
migration inhibitory factor (MIF) test
migration of leukocytes
migration, transepithelial
migratory cell
migratory pneumonia
migratory polyarthritis
Mikulicz cell
Mikulicz syndrome
miliaria
miliary abscess
miliary aneurysm
miliary embolism
miliary fever
miliary granuloma
miliary pattern
miliary tubercles
miliary tuberculosis
milker node virus
milk fever
milk-filled cyst
milk line
milk protein antibody
milk teeth
Millard test for albumin
Miller-Galante knee
Miller-Kurzrok test
milliequivalent (mEq)
milliequivalents per liter (mEq/L)
Milligan trichrome stain
milliliter (mL, ml)
millimeter (mm)
millimole (mmol)
millimoles per liter (mmol/L)
milliosmole (mOsm)

Millipore filter
Millipore membrane
Millipore method
Millonig phosphate-buffered formalin
Millon-Nasse test for protein
Millon test for proteins and
  nitrogenous compounds
Mima polymorpha (now *Acinetobacter*
  calcoaceticus, var. *lwoffi*)
mineralocorticoid
minilaparotomy
minimal deviation melanoma
minimum bactericidal concentration
  (MBC) culture
minimum inhibitory concentration
  (MIC)
minimum lethal concentration (MLC)
minor (pl. minora)
  labia
  pelvis
minor calyx
minor duodenal papilla
mirror image breast biopsy
mirror-image cell
mismatched blood transfusion
missed abortion
mites in cutaneous burrows
mites in skin scrapings
mitochondria
mitochondrial antibody
mitochondrial gene
mitochondrial matrix
mitogen
mitosis (pl. mitoses), multipolar
mitotic activity
mitotic division
mitotic figures, bizarre
mitotic index
mitotic rate
mitral arcade
mitral cell
mitral orifice
mitral stenosis
mitral valve
mitral valvular leaflet
Mitscherlich test for phosphorus
  in stomach
Mittendorf dot
mIU (milli-international unit)
mixed agglutination test
mixed cell sarcoma
mixed flora
mixed gland
mixed infection
mixed leukocyte culture (MLC)
mixed lymphocyte culture (MLC) test
mixed lymphocytic-histiocytic
  lymphoma
mixed phase endometrium
mixed proteinuria
mL, ml (milliliter)
MLC (minimum lethal concentration)
mm (millimeter)
MM band
MM isoenzyme
MM virus
mm^3 (cubic millimeter)
mmol (millimole)
mmol/L (millimoles per liter)
Mn (manganese)
MNS blood group
mobile gallbladder
moderator band
Modic disk abnormality classification
modicum
modifier gene
MODY (maturity-onset diabetes
  of youth)
Mohrenheim space
Mohr test for hydrochloric acid
  in stomach contents
Mohs surgery
moist scaling
Mokola virus

mol (mole)
molar gland
molar mass
molar pregnancy
molar tissue
mold
mold fungus
mole (mol) (measurement)
  blood
  Breus
  cystic
  false
  fleshy
  hairy
  hydatidiform
  invasive
  malignant
  pigmented
  stone
  true
  tubal
  vesicular
molecular death
molecular lesion
molecular mass
molecular weight
Molisch test for urine glucose
Mollaret meningitis
Moll gland
Molluscipoxvirus
molluscum body
molluscum contagiosum
molluscum contagiosum virus
Moloney test
molybdenum
Mönckeberg arteriosclerosis
Mönckeberg calcification
Mönckeberg degeneration
Mönckeberg sclerosis
Mondor disease
mongolian spot-like lesion
mongolism
Monilia (former name of *Candida*)
Monilia sitophila
moniliaceous
moniliasis
monkeypox virus
"mono" (slang for infectious mononucleosis)
"monos" (slang for monocytes)
monoamino-monocarboxylic acids, impaired transport of
monoblast
monoclonal antibody (see *antibody*)
monoclonal gammopathy
monoclonal immunoglobulin
monoclonal immunoglobulin light chains in serum
monoclonal light chains
monoclonal peak
monocyte
monocyte chemoattractant protein-1 (MCP-1)
monocyte derived neutrophil chemotactic (MDNCF)
monocytic leukemia
monocytoid cell
monocytopenia
monocytosis
Mono-Diff test
monolayer
monoleptic fever
monomorphous oval cell
mononeuritis
mononuclear and neutrophilic exudate
mononuclear cell infiltrate
mononuclear cells in circulating blood
mononuclear infiltrate
mononucleosis
monoptychic gland
monosaccharide
Monoscreen test
monosexual
monosome

monosomic
monosomy
Monospot test (also, MonoSpot)
Monosticon Dri-Dot test
Monsel solution
mons pubis
monstrocellular nuclei
Montenegro test
Montgomery gland
moon face (facies)
Moore test for carbohydrate
Mooser cell
Morax-Axenfeld bacillus
Moraxella atlantae
Moraxella catarrhalis
Moraxella lacunata
Moraxella nonliquefaciens
Moraxella osloensis
Moraxella phenylpyruvica
Moraxella urethralis
morbid obesity
morbilliform
Morbillivirus, morbillivirus
mordant (see *stain*)
mordant solution
Morel ear
Morelli test (exudate v. transudate) (*not* Moretti)
Moretti test for typhoid fever
morgagnian cyst
Morgagni appendix
Morgagni crypt
Morgagni gland
Morgagni hydatid
Morgagni nodule
Morgagni ventricle
Morgan bacillus
Morganella
Morganella morganii
morgue
moribund
Morison pouch
Moritz test
Mörner test for tyrosine
morphea (localized scleroderma)
  generalized
  guttate
  linear
morphogenic field
morphologic change
morphologic classification
morphology
Morquio disease
mortar kidney
mortem (see *antemortem* and *postmortem*)
Mortierella wolfii
mortis
  algor
  livor
  rigor
mortise
mortise joint
morula (pl. morulae)
mosaic fungus
mosaic pattern
mosaic wart
Mosenthal test
Mosler diabetes
mOsm (milliosmole)
mosquito
  Culex
  Wyeomyia melanocephala
mosquito-borne febrile exanthem
mosquito-borne virus
mossy cell
moth-eaten alopecia of secondary syphilis
mother cell
motile
motile bacillus
motile leukocyte
motile sperm
motility, sperm

motility test
motor cell
motor cortex
motor end plates
motor fiber
motor neuron, cell body of
motor root
motor supply
motor unit
Mott cell
mottled appearance
Motulsky dye reduction test
mound, infraumbilical
mount, KOH (potassium hydroxide)
mounted
mounting medium
mounting of tissue section
mouth, foot, and hand disease
mouth of processus vaginalis
movable articulation
movable joint
movable kidney
movement, ameboid
movers, prime
Mowry colloidal iron stain
moyamoya
Mozart ear
MPD (main pancreatic duct)
MP, MCP (metacarpophalangeal) joint
MP, MTP (metatarsophalangeal) joint
M protein
MPV (mean platelet volume)
MRSA (methicillin-resistant *Staphylococcus aureus*)
MSB trichrome stain
MSTS (Musculoskeletal Tumor Society) staging system
M-25 virus
μL (microliter)
μmol (micromole)
Much bacillus
Much granule
mucicarmine
mucilaginous gum
mucin clot formation
mucin clot test
mucin, gastric
mucinoid degeneration
mucinosis
  follicular
  papular
mucinous adenocarcinoma
mucinous carcinoma
mucinous cystadenocarcinoma
mucinous degeneration
mucinous nest
mucin-secreting columnar cell
mucin stain
mucoalbuminous cell
mucocutaneous lymph node syndrome
mucocutaneous pigmentation
mucoid degeneration
mucoid impaction of bronchus
mucoid material
mucoid stool
mucoperichondrium
mucopolysaccharide metabolism
mucopolysaccharides, excessive production of
mucopolysaccharides in intima of arteries
mucoprotein
mucopurulent exudate in alveoli
mucopus (mucus and pus)
Mucor
Mucor ramosissimus
Mucor rouxianus
mucormycosis
mucorrhea
mucosa (mucous membrane)
  alimentary
  alveolar
  antral
  auditory

mucosa *(continued)*
  bronchial
  buccal
  bulging of
  cardiac m. of stomach
  colorectal
  endocervical
  foveolar gastric
  foveolosulciolar gastric
  gallbladder
  gingival
  intestinal
  oxyntic
  pyloric
  rectal
  sulciolar gastric
  urinary
  vaginal
mucosal bridge
mucosal disease virus
mucosal folds
mucosal hyperemia
mucosal hyperplasia
mucosal injection
mucosal island (on x-ray)
mucosal junction, squamocolumnar
mucosal melanoma
mucosal necrosis
mucosal patch
mucosal pattern
mucosal ring, esophageal
mucosal suspensory ligament
mucosal ulcer
mucosal zone
mucoserous cell
mucous cell
mucous cyst
mucous degeneration
mucous diarrhea
mucous gland
mucous glands of auditory tube
mucous glands of duodenum
mucous glands of eustachian tube
mucous lake of stomach
mucous membrane
mucous neck cell
mucous plug
mucous polyp
mucous salivary gland
mucous shred
mucous stool
mucous strand
mucous surface
mucoviscidosis
mucus (noun)
  cervical
  midcycle cervical
  ovulatory
mucus-secreting cell
mucus-secreting epithelium
mucus-secreting gland
mud, biliary
MUG (methylumbelliferylglucuronide)
mulberry cell
mulberry ovary
mulberry-shaped intracytoplasmic
  inclusion
Mulder test for glucose
Müller (Mueller)
Müller canal
müllerian cyst
müllerian duct
Müller radial cell
Müller solution
Müller trigone
multangular bone
multiaxial articulation
multiaxial joint
multicellular gland
multicellular organism
multicentric osteosarcoma
multi-colony-stimulating factor
  (multi-CSF)
multifaceted

multifocal area
multifocal encephalomalacia
multifocal osteitis fibrosa
multilobular cirrhosis
multilocular cyst
multiloculated cyst
multiloculated pustule
multinodular goiter
multinucleate cell
multinucleate giant cell
multinucleate giant cells with cytoplasmic inclusions
multinucleate globoid cell
multinucleated giant cell
multiparity
multipennate muscle
multiple embolism
multiple endocrine neoplasia (MEN)
  type I (Wermer syndrome)
  type II (Sipple syndrome)
  type III (mucosal neuroma syndrome)
multiple familial polyposis
multiple idiopathic hemorrhagic sarcoma
multiple intestinal polyposis
multiple myeloma
multiple myositis
multiple neuritis
multiple organ failure
multiple osteochondromatosis
multiple pregnancy
multiple-puncture intracutaneous tuberculin test
multiple sclerosis
multiple stain
multiple system atrophy
multiple trauma
multipolar cell
multipolar mitosis
multiseptate, brown distorted hyphae
multiseptate gallbladder
multiseptate hyphae
Multistix
multisystem failure
mummification
mumps
mumps encephalitis
mumps meningitis
mumps meningoencephalitis
mumps sensitivity test
mumps virus
Munro abscess
Munro microabscess
Munro point
mural aneurysm
mural cell
mural kidney
mural pregnancy
mural thrombus
muramidase
Murayama test
murine leukemia virus
murine typhus
murmur grades
Murray Valley encephalitis virus
muscle (see Table of Muscles for anatomical names)
  abdominal
  accessory
  Aeby
  agonistic
  Albinus
  anterior
  antigravity
  auricular
  axillary
  Bell
  bipennate
  Bochdalek
  Bovero ("sucking")
  Bowman
  Braune
  Brücke

muscle *(continued)*
bulbocavernosus
canine
cardiac
Casser
casserian
cervical
Crampton
Chassaignac
chin
Coiter
deep
detrusor
digastric
dorsal
Dupré
Duverney
emergency
external
fast (white)
fixation
fixator
Folius
Gantzer
Gavard
greater
Guthrie
Hilton
Horner
Houston
iliococcygeal
iliocostal
inferior
internal
interosseous
interspinal
intertransverse
intra-auricular
involuntary
ischiocavernosus
Jung
Klein

muscle *(continued)*
lateral
lesser
levator
longitudinal
major
Macalister
Marcacci
medial
Merkel
middle
minor
Müller (Mueller)
multipennate
nonstriated
oblique
Ochsner
Oddi
Oehl
opposing
organic
Phillips
posterior
Pozzi
pubococcygeal
quadrate
red (slow)
Reisseisen
ribbon
rider
Riolan
Rouget
round
Ruysch
Santorini
sartorius
scalp
Sebileau
semimembranous
semispinal
semitendinous
short

muscle *(continued)*
  Sibson
  skeletal
  slow (red)
  smaller
  smooth
  Soemmerring
  somatic
  spindle-shaped
  strap
  striated
  "sucking" (Bovero)
  superficial
  synergic
  synergistic
  tailor's
  Theile
  Tod
  Toynbee
  transverse
  Treitz
  triangular
  trigonal
  true back
  two-bellied
  unipennate
  unstriated
  unstriped
  Valsalva
  ventral
  vertical
  visceral
  vocal
  voluntary
  white (fast)
  Wilson
  wrinkler
  yoked
muscle cell
muscle coat
  circular
  longitudinal
muscle contusion
muscle cramp
muscle enzyme
muscle fiber
  cardiac
  skeletal
  sling
muscle rigidity
muscle shortening
muscle tearing
muscle tissue
muscle twitching
muscle wasting
muscular artery
muscular atrophy
muscular degeneration
muscular dystrophy
  Dejerine-Landouzy
  Duchenne
  Erb
  Landouzy-Dejerine
muscular ring, esophageal
muscular spasticity and rigidity
muscular tube
muscular twig
musculature
musculi (pl. of musculus)
musculophrenic artery
musculophrenic vessel
musculoskeletal
musculotendinous
musculotendinous crura
musculotubal canal
musculus (pl. musculi) (see Table of Muscles)
musculus uvulae
mushroom cap
mushroom caps of mucus-like pseudomembrane
mushroom-like excrescence
mushroom poisoning
mushy stool

mutant gene
mutant protein
mutant tumor suppressor
mutton fat KPs (keratic precipitates)
myalgia
myasthenia gravis
Mycelia sterilia
mycelial fungus
mycelium
MycoAKT latex bead agglutination test
mycobacteria
mycobacterial antibody
Mycobacterium asiaticum
Mycobacterium avium
Mycobacterium avium-intracellulare (MAI) complex
Mycobacterium bovis
Mycobacterium celatum
Mycobacterium chelonei (formerly *Mycobacterium abscessus*)
Mycobacterium cookii
Mycobacterium flavescens
Mycobacterium fortuitum
Mycobacterium gastri
Mycobacterium genavense
Mycobacterium gordonae
Mycobacterium haemophilum
Mycobacterium intracellulare
Mycobacterium kansasii
Mycobacterium leprae
Mycobacterium malmoense
Mycobacterium marinum
Mycobacterium microti
Mycobacterium paratuberculosis
Mycobacterium phlei
Mycobacterium scrofulaceum
Mycobacterium shimoidei
Mycobacterium simiae
Mycobacterium smegmatis
Mycobacterium szulgai
Mycobacterium terrae
Mycobacterium triviale
Mycobacterium tuberculosis
Mycobacterium ulcerans
Mycobacterium xenopi
Mycocentrospora acerina
mycologic test for sugar in urine
mycoplasma (pl. mycoplasmata)
Mycoplasma buccale
Mycoplasma faucium
Mycoplasma fermentans
Mycoplasma genitalium
Mycoplasma hominis
mycoplasmal pneumonia
Mycoplasma orale
Mycoplasma pharyngis
Mycoplasma pneumoniae
Mycoplasma salivarium
mycosis (pl. mycoses)
mycosis cell
mycosis cutis chronica
mycosis fungoides
mycosis intestinalis
mycotic aneurysm
mycotic keratitis
mycotic stomatitis
mycotoxicosis
mydriasis
myelination, incomplete (of nerve fibers in brain and spinal cord)
myelin basic protein (MBP)
myelin degeneration of peripheral nerves
myelinic degeneration
myelin kidney
myelinogenic field
myelin oligodendrocyte glycoprotein
myelin sheath
myelitic
myelitis
  acute
  ascending
  bulbar
  cavitary

- myelitis *(continued)*
  - central
  - chronic
  - compression
  - concussion
  - cornual
  - diffuse
  - disseminated
  - hemorrhagic
  - neuro-optic
  - periependymal
  - postinfectious
  - postvaccinal
  - subacute
  - subacute necrotic
  - syphilitic
  - transverse
  - viral
- myeloblast
- myeloblastic leukemia
- myeloblastic protein
- myelocele
- myelocytic leukemia
- myelofibrosis
- myelogenic osteopathy
- myelogenic sarcoma
- myelogenous leukemia
- myeloid cell
- myeloid leukocyte
- myeloid metaplasia
- myeloid sarcoma
- myeloid tissue
- myeloma
  - giant cell
  - indolent
  - localized
  - multiple
  - plasma cell
  - sclerosing
  - solitary
- myeloma cell
- myeloma kidney
- myeloma protein
- myelomonocytic leukemia
- myelopathic muscular atrophy
- myeloperoxidase
- myeloproliferative disease
- Myers and Fine test for amylolytic activity
- Mylius test for bile acids
- mylohyoid artery
- myoblast
- myoblastoma
- myocardial depressant
- myocardial fiber
- myocardial hypertrophy
- myocardial infarction
- myocardial ischemia
- myocardial necrosis
- myocardial scarring
- myocarditis (MC)
  - acute bacterial
  - acute interstitial
  - acute isolated
  - acute rheumatic
  - aseptic (of newborn)
  - bacterial
  - chronic
  - chronic hypertrophic
  - chronic interstitial
  - chronic pernicious
  - coxsackievirus
  - diphtheritic
  - eosinophilic
  - fibroid
  - fibrous
  - Fiedler
  - fragmentation
  - fungal
  - giant cell
  - granulomatous
  - *Histoplasma*
  - hypersensitivity
  - idiopathic

myocarditis *(continued)*
- infectious
- infective
- inflammatory
- influenzal
- interstitial
- isolated diffuse
- Löffler (Loeffler)
- lues
- lymphocytic
- meningococcal
- metazoal
- neutrophilic
- nonspecific granulomatous
- parenchymatous
- peripartum
- pernicious
- pneumococcal
- protozoal
- rheumatic
- rickettsial
- senile
- septic
- spirochetal
- staphylococcal
- subepicardial
- syphilitic
- toxic
- toxoplasmotic
- *Trichinella*
- tuberculoid
- tuberculous
- viral

myocardium
- senile
- stunned

myocellular area
myoclonic encephalopathy
myocyte
myocyte necrosis
myocytic lysosome
myocytolysis, focal
myoendocarditis
- acute
- subacute

myoepithelial cell
myofiber
myofibrillar area
myofilament protein
myoglobin in urine
myoid cell
myoma (pl. myomata)
myomastoid artery
myomatous polyp
myometrial gland
myometrium, uterine
myopathic atrophy
myopericarditis
myosarcoma
myosin
myosin heavy chain
myosin light chain
myositis
- acute disseminated
- acute progressive
- inclusion body
- infectious
- interstitial
- multiple
- parenchymatous
- primary multiple
- progressive ossifying
- proliferative
- rheumatoid
- spontaneous bacterial
- trichinous

myositis fibrosa
myositis ossificans
myositis serosa
myotome
myotubular myopathy
myxedema
myxedema heart
myxoid cyst

myxoid degeneration
myxoid fibroma
myxolipoma
myxoliposarcoma
myxoma (pl. myxomas, myxomata)
myxoma syndrome with facial freckling
myxomatous degeneration
myxomatous tumor
myxopapilloma
myxosarcoma
myxovirus

N, n

Naboth gland
nabothian cyst
nabothian follicle
nabothian gland
NADH diaphorase
NADH methemoglobin reductase
nadir
Naegeli monocytic leukemia
Nägele pelvis
Nageotte cells
nail bed
nail fungal infection
nail matrix
Nairovirus
Najjar-Crigler syndrome
Nakanishi stain
Nakayama test for bile pigments
naked virus
Nakiwogo virus
nalidixic acid
nanogram (ng)
nanoliter (nL)
nanometer (nm)
nanomole (nmol)
NAP (neutrophil activating protein)
nape nevus
naphthalene poisoning
naphthol-ASD chloroacetate esterase
naphthol green B stain
naphthol yellow S stain
napkin (diaper) dermatitis
napkin-ring lesion
narcotic abuse
narcotism, intravenous
naris (pl. nares)
narrow-angle glaucoma
nasal ala
nasal aperture
nasal arch
nasal artery
nasal bone
nasal canal
nasal cavity
nasal concha
nasal fossa
nasal gland
nasal part of pharynx
nasal polyp
nasal secretions
nasal septum
nasal smear
nasion
nasobregmatic arc
nasolabial sulcus

nasolacrimal canal
nasolacrimal duct
naso-occipital arc
nasopalatine artery
nasopalatine canal
nasopalatine nerve
nasopharyngeal carcinoma
nasopharyngeal culture
nasopharyngeal flora
nasopharyngeal secretions
nasopharynx
native albumin
native protein
natural body fluid
natural death
natural killer (NK) cell
natural killer cell stimulating factor (NKSF)
nausea
Nauta stain
navicular bone of hand
navicular fossa
N-b band
NBT (nitroblue tetrazolium)
NCL-Arp monoclonal antibody
NCL-Cdm
NCL-ER-LHZ monoclonal antibody
NCL-PGR monoclonal antibody
NCL-pS2
Necator americanus
neck
- dental
- femoral
- Madelung
- bladder
- gallbladder
- pancreas
- rib
- surgical
- transverse artery of
- webbed
- wry

necklike
neck of femur
neck of gallbladder
neck of humerus, anatomical
necrobacillosis
necrobiosis
necrobiotic core
necrocytosis
necrocytotoxin
necrogenic
necrolysis
necrophilia
necrophilic
necropneumonia
necropsy
necrosis
- acute tubular
- arteriolar
- aseptic
- avascular
- bacillary
- Balser fatty
- bilateral cortical
- bloodless zone of
- bridging
- caseous
- central
- centrilobular
- cheesy
- coagulation
- colliquative
- contraction band
- cystic medial
- diffuse
- dry
- epiphyseal ischemic
- Erdheim cystic medial
- exanthematous
- fat
- fibrinoid
- focal
- focal hepatic

necrosis *(continued)*
focal hepatocellular n. with hemorrhagic cysts
frank
gangrenous
gangrenous pulp
hemorrhagic
hepatic
hyaline
indurative
infectious pancreatic
ischemic
liquefaction
localized
massive hepatic
medial cystic
midzonal
mucosal
myocardial
Paget quiet
papillary
peripheral
peripheral hepatic
phosphorus
piecemeal
postpartum pituitary
pressure
progressive emphysematous
radiation
renal tubular
septic
stromal
subacute hepatic
subcutaneous fat
submassive hepatic
superficial
syphilitic
total
tracheobronchial mucosal
Zenker
zonal
necrosis of bladder epithelium
necrosis of bladder mucosa
necrosis of ductal epithelium
necrosis of hepatocytes
necrosis of muscle
necrosis of muscle cells
necrosis of small bowel mucosa
necrosis of tissue
necrotic "anchovy paste" material in hepatic abscess
necrotic bone
necrotic debris
necrotic inflammation
necrotic lesion in retina
necrotic tissue
necrotizing and suppurative osteomyelitis of maxilla and mandible
necrotizing arteriolitis in kidney
necrotizing arteritis
necrotizing fasciitis
necrotizing gastritis
necrotizing gingivitis
necrotizing glomerulonephritis
necrotizing granulomatous lymphadenitis
necrotizing nephrosis
necrotizing papillitis
necrotizing pneumonia
needle
Abrams
aneurysm
aspirating
Brockenbrough
cataract
Chiba aspiration biopsy
Cook aspiration biopsy
Cope
cutting biopsy
Deschamps
discission
double-pointed
fine

needle *(continued)*
  Franseen
  Greene biopsy
  Hagedorn
  hollow
  hypodermic
  Jamshidi biopsy
  Lee cutting biopsy
  ligature
  Madayag biopsy
  Menghini
  Reverdin
  Rotex cutting biopsy
  Seldinger
  Silverman
  Skinny
  swaged
  transseptal
  Trucut cutting biopsy
  Turner biopsy
  Vim-Silverman
  Westcott cutting biopsy
needle aspiration, fine-
needle biopsy, fine-
needle core biopsy
needle puncture
needle puncture wound
Neer shoulder fractures I, II, III classification
negative
  false
  Rh
negative charge
negative control
negative stain
negative strand virus
Negri bodies in neurons
Negri inclusion body
Neisseria
Neisseria catarrhalis
Neisseria cinerea
Neisseria elongata
Neisseria flavescens
Neisseria gonorrhoeae
Neisseria lactamica
Neisseria meningitidis
Neisseria mucosa
Neisseria sicca
Neisseria subflava
Neisser stain
Neisser-Wechsberg leukocidin
Neisser-Wechsberg phenomenon
Nélaton fold
Nélaton sphincter
Nencki test for indole
neonatal diagnosis
neonatal hepatitis
neonatal jaundice
neonatal lupus
neoplasia
  cervical intraepithelial (CIN)
  lobular
  gestational trophoblastic (GTN)
  multiple endocrine (MEN)
    type I (Wermer syndrome)
    type II (Sipple syndrome)
    type III (mucosal neuroma syndrome)
  vaginal intraepithelial (VIN)
neoplasm
  benign
  encapsulated
  firm
  functioning
  gonadal
  grading
  hormone-dependent
  lethal
  malignant
  ovarian
  premalignant
  spherical
  staging
  well-circumscribed

neoplastic cell
neoplastic cyst
neoplastic meningitis
neoplastic tissue
Neoprobe cancer detector device
neorectum
Neotestudina rosatii
neovascularization
nephelometry
nephritic factor
nephritis
  acute
  arteriosclerotic
  azotemic
  bacterial
  Balkan
  capsular
  caseous
  cheesy
  chloro-azotemic
  chronic
  congenital
  croupous
  degenerative
  exudative
  fibrolipomatous
  glomerular
  glomerulocapsular
  hemorrhagic
  interstitial
  Lancereaux
  lupus
  parenchymatous
  pneumococcus
  potassium-losing
  productive
  salt-losing
  saturnine
  scarlatinal
  subacute
  suppurative
  syphilitic
nephritis *(continued)*
  transfusion
  tubal
  tuberculous
  vascular
nephritis dolorosa
nephritis gravidarum
nephritogenic strains of betahemolytic streptococci
nephroblastoma
nephrocalcinosis
nephrogenic zone
nephrogenous proteinuria
nephropathy, diabetic
nephrosclerosis
  arterial
  arteriolar
  benign
  hyperplastic arteriolar
  malignant
  senile
nephrosis
  acute
  amyloid
  cholemic
  Epstein
  glycogen
  hydropic
  hypokalemic
  infectious avian
  lower nephron
  lupus
  necrotizing
  osmotic
  toxic
  vacuolar
nephrotic syndrome
nerve (see Table of Nerves)
nerve cell
nerve cell degeneration
nerve degeneration
nerve fasciculus

nerve fiber
nerve fibril
nerve growth factor (NGF)
nerve plexus
nerve root
nerve sheath cell
nerve supply, parasympathetic
nerve tissue damage
nerve tissue degeneration
nerve tissue inflammation
nerve tracts, disruption of
nerve trunk
nervous pregnancy
nervous system
  autonomic
  central
nest
  Brunn
  cell
  epithelial
  isogenous
  mucinous
nests and clumps
nests of radially disposed cells
net knot
network
  articular
  cell
  lymphatic
  venous
Neubauer artery
Neufeld capsular swelling
Neukomm test for bile acids
Neumann cell
neural arc
neural factor
neural (neuroid) nevus
neural arch
neural atrophy
neural canal
neuralgic amyotrophy
neural groove
neural tube
neural tube defect
neurenteric canal
neurilemma
neurilemma cell
neurilemmitis
neurilemoma
  acoustic
  Antoni type A
  Antoni type B
neurinoma, acoustic
neuritic muscular atrophy
neuritic pain
neuritic plaque
neuritis (pl. neuritides)
  adventitial
  ascending
  brachial
  descending
  dietetic
  Eichhorst
  fallopian
  Gombault
  hereditary optic
  interstitial hypertrophic
  intraocular
  Leyden
  migrating
  multiple
  optic
  orbital optic
  parenchymatous
  periaxial
  peripheral
  postfebrile
  postocular optic
  radiation
  radicular
  retrobulbar optic
  sciatic
  segmental
  serum

neuritis *(continued)*
- shoulder-girdle
- syphilitic
- toxic
- traumatic
- vestibular

neuritis migrans
neuroastrocytoma
neuroblastoma
neurocentral joint
neurocentral junction
neurodegenerative disease
neuroendocrine cell
neuroendocrine transducer cell
neuroepithelial cell
neurofibril
neurofibrillary tangle
neurofibroma
neurofibromatosis
neurofibrosarcoma
neurofilament
neurofilament triplet protein
neurogenic bladder
neurogenic diabetes
neurogenic sarcoma
neuroglia
neuroglial cell
neurohypophyseal tract of hypothalamus
neurohypophysis
neuroma, acoustic
neuromuscular cell
neuromuscular excitability
neuromuscular junction
neuromyelitis, optic
neuron
- autonomic motor
- commissural
- degenerating
- gamma motor
- motor
- spinal

neuronal degeneration
neuronitis
neuronophagia of anterior horn cells of spinal cord
neuron-specific enolase
neuro-optic myelitis
neuropathic atrophy
neuropathic joint
neuropathy
- diabetic
- peripheral
- segmental (demyelination)

neuropore, caudal
neurosecretory cell
neurosyphilis
neurotonic congestion
neurotrophic atrophy
neurotropic hormone
neurotropic virus
neurovascular bundle
Neusser granule
neutral (buffered) formalin
neutralization test
neutral red stain
neutral zone
neutropenia
neutrophil
- band
- filamented
- giant
- immature
- juvenile
- nonfilamented
- rod
- segmented
- stab
- unsegmented

neutrophil activating protein (NAP)
neutrophil alkaline phosphatase
neutrophil chemotactant factor
neutrophilia
neutrophilic exudate

neutrophilic infiltrate
neutrophilic leukocyte
neutrophilic myocarditis
nevocyte
nevocytic nevus
nevoid lentigo
nevolipoma
nevus (pl. nevi)
  achromic
  acquired
  amelanotic
  anemic
  balloon cell
  basal cell
  bathing trunk
  Becker
  benign pigmented
  blue
  blue rubber-bleb
  capillary
  cellular blue
  choroidal
  comedo
  compound
  congenital
  connective tissue
  dermal
  dysplastic
  fatty
  flame
  giant hairy
  giant pigmented
  hairy
  halo
  intradermal
  Ito
  Jadassohn
  Jadassohn-Tièche
  junction
  juvenile
  linear epidermal
  melanocytic

nevus *(continued)*
  nape
  neural (neuroid)
  nevocytic
  oral epithelial
  organoid
  Ota
  pigmented
  pigmented hairy
  pigmented hairy epidermal
  port-wine
  sebaceous
  spider
  spindle and epithelioid cell
  spindle cell
  Spitz
  stellar
  strawberry
  Sutton
  systematized
  Unna
  uveal
  vascular
  verrucous
  white sponge
  woolly-hair
nevus cell
  A-type
  B-type
  C-type
nevus-type giant cell
new bone formation
newborn
  gonococcal ophthalmia of the
  hemolytic disease of the
newborn pneumonitis virus
Newcastle disease virus
Newcastle-Manchester bacillus
newly woven bone
NF (neurofibromatosis)
NF1 tumor suppressor gene
NF2 tumor suppressor gene

ng (nanogram)
niacin (nicotinic acid)
niacin test for *Mycobacterium tuberculosis*
niche, Barclay
niche en plateau
nickel dermatitis
nickel grid
Nickerson-Kveim test
nicking
Nicolle stain
nidus
nidus of inflamed tissue
nidus of necrotic tissue
nidus of stone formation
Niemann-Pick cell
Niemann-Pick disease
nigra
- linea
- substantia
- tinea

Nikolsky sign
Nile blue fat stain
ninhydrin reagent
ninhydrin-Schiff stain
ninhydrin test
Nippe test for blood
nipple
- accessory
- supernumerary

nipple-areola complex
nipple inversion
nipplelike projections
Nissl body
Nissl degeneration
Nissl granule
Nissl method of staining
Nissl stain
Nissl substance
nitrate reduction test
Nitrazine positive test
Nitrazine test
nitric acid
nitric acid–magnesium sulfate test
nitric acid test for albumin
nitrites test in saliva
nitroblue tetrazolium (NBT) test
nitrocellulose membrane
nitrogen
- alpha amino
- blood urea (BUN)
- liquid
- total

nitrogen gas
nitrogenous compounds test
nitrogenous waste
nitrogen oxide poisoning
nitrogen waste
nitropropiol test for urine glucose
nitroprusside reaction
nitroprusside test for cysteine
nitroso-indole-nitrate test
NK (natural killer) cell
nL (nanoliter)
nm (nanometer)
nmol (nanomole)
N-Multistix
N-myc oncogene
Nobel agar
Nobel stain
Nobel test for acetoacetic acid and acetone
Nocardia
Nocardia asteroides
Nocardia brasiliensis
Nocardia caviae
nocardiosis
nodal artery
nodal fever
nodal tissue
node (see also *lymph node*)
- abdominal lymph
- accessory lymph
- anorectal lymph

node *(continued)*
- aortic lymph
- apical lymph
- appendicular lymph
- Aschoff AV (atrioventricular)
- atrioventricular
- auricular lymph
- AV (atrioventricular)
- axillary lymph
- bifurcation lymph
- Bouchard
- brachial lymph
- bronchopulmonary lymph
- buccal lymph
- buccinator lymph
- caval lymph
- celiac lymph
- central lymph
- cervical paratracheal lymph
- Cloquet inguinal lymph
- common iliac lymph
- companion lymph
- coronary
- cubital lymph
- cystic lymph
- Delphian lymph
- deltopectoral lymph
- diaphragmatic lymph
- Dürck
- epicolic lymph
- epigastric lymph
- epitrochlear
- Ewald
- external iliac lymph
- facial lymph
- fibular lymph
- Flack
- foraminal
- gastric lymph
- gastroduodenal lymph
- gastroepiploic lymph
- gastro-omental lymph

node *(continued)*
- gluteal lymph
- gouty
- Haygarth
- Heberden
- hemal
- hemolymph
- Hensen
- hepatic lymph
- hilar lymph
- ileocolic lymph
- iliac circumflex lymph
- iliac lymph
- infraclavicular
- infrahyoid lymph
- inguinal lymph
- intercostal lymph
- interiliac lymph
- interpectoral lymph
- jugular lymph
- jugulodigastric lymph
- jugulo-omohyoid lymph
- juxtaintestinal
- Keith
- Keith-Flack
- lacunar
- lumbar lymph
- lymph
- malar lymph
- mandibular lymph
- mastoid lymph
- Meynet
- nasolabial lymph
- obturator lymph
- occipital lymph
- Osler
- pancreatic lymph
- pancreaticoduodenal lymph
- pancreaticolienal lymph
- paracardial lymph
- paracolic lymph
- paramammary lymph

node *(continued)*
- pararectal lymph
- parasternal lymph
- paratracheal lymph
- parauterine lymph
- paravaginal lymph
- paravesicular lymph
- parietal lymph
- parotid lymph
- Parrot
- pectoral lymph
- pelvic lymph
- pericardial lymph
- peroneal
- phrenic lymph
- popliteal lymph
- postaortic lymph
- postcaval lymph
- postvesicular lymph
- preaortic lymph
- precaval lymph
- prececal lymph
- prelaryngeal
- prepericardial lymph
- pretracheal
- pretracheal lymph
- prevertebral lymph
- prevesicular lymph
- pulmonary juxtaesophageal lymph
- pulmonary lymph
- pyloric lymph
- Ranvier
- rectal lymph
- retroaortic lymph
- retroauricular lymph
- retrocecal lymph
- retropharyngeal lymph
- retropyloric
- retrorectal lymph node
- Rosenmüller
- Rotter
- SA (sinoatrial)

node *(continued)*
- sacral lymph
- Schmorl
- sentinel
- sigmoid lymph
- signal
- singer
- sinoatrial
- sinus
- splenic lymph
- subcarinal
- submandibular lymph
- submental lymph
- subpyloric
- subscapular lymph
- supraclavicular lymph
- suprapyloric
- supratrochlear lymph
- syphilitic
- teacher
- thyroid lymph
- tibial
- tracheal lymph
- tracheobronchial lymph
- Troisier
- vesicular lymph
- Virchow
- visceral lymph

node of epiploic foramen
node of His, atrioventricular
node of neck of gallbladder
node of Tawara
nodosum (pl. nodosa)
- erythema
- periarteritis
- polyarteritis (PAN)

nodular aneurysm
nodular deposit in cartilage
nodular embryo
nodular excrescence
nodular fibrotic reaction
nodular goiter

nodularity
nodular lymphoma
nodular melanoma
nodular nonsuppurative panniculitis
nodular proliferation
nodular subepidermal fibrosis
nodular texture
nodular thickening of alveolar septa
nodule
  aggregated lymphatic
  Arantius
  cold
  cortical
  cutaneous
  Dalen-Fuchs
  discrete
  easily compressible
  erectile
  fibrous
  Fraenkel typhus
  Gandy-Gamma
  hard
  hemangiomatous
  Hoboken
  hot
  indiscrete
  Koeppe
  laryngeal
  lymphatic
  Morgagni
  myometrial
  nondiscrete
  Picker
  red
  respiratory
  rheumatoid
  rubbery
  Schmorl
  singer's
  Sister Joseph
  soapy
  solitary

nodule *(continued)*
  surfer's
  teacher's
  thin-walled hemangiomatous
  tobacco
  tuberculous
  typhoid
  typhus
  warm
  waxy
Noguchi test for globulin
nomogram
non-A, non-B hepatitis
non-A, non-B hepatitis virus
non-alpha, non-beta pancreatic islet cell
nonan malaria
nonbacterial pneumonia
non-beta cell
nonbloody stool
noncaseating
noncellular material
nonclonogenic cell
noncondylomatous
noncoronary cusp
nondeciduate placenta
nondiscrete nodule
nonenveloped virus
nonfibrous material
nonfilamented neutrophil
nonfunctioning tissue
nongerminal tissue
nonglandular cell
nongonococcal urethritis
nongranular leukocyte
non-heme iron protein
non-Hodgkin's lymphoma
non-hormone-producing neoplasms of pituitary
Nonidet P40
noninfectious conjunctivitis
noninfectivity

noninvasive
nonisolated proteinuria
nonkeratinizing epithelium
nonlamellar bone
nonlamellated bone
nonlipid histiocytosis
nonlymphocytic leukemia
nonmalignant cell
nonmeconium-stained membrane
nonmotile leukocyte
nonmyelinated axons of nerve cells
non-necrotizing granuloma
non-necrotizing granulomatous
  inflammation
non-neoplastic cyst
non-nerve cell
non-nodular
nonobese population
nonoccluded virus
non-oncogenic virus
nonpathogenic organisms
nonpenetrating wound
nonrachitic bowleg
non-small cell lung carcinoma
  (NSCLC)
nonspecialized cell
nonspecific antigen
nonspecific granulomatous myocarditis
nonspecific protein
nonspecific stomatitis
nonspecific vaginitis
nonstriated muscle
nonthrombocytopenic purpura
nontoxic goiter
nontreponemal antigen test
nonunion of bone fragments
nonunion of fracture
nonvenereal skin disease
nonviable fetus
nonviable tissue
noradrenaline
no-reflow phenomenon
norepinephrine
normal
  borderline
  high
  low
normal calcification
normal flora
normal gas exchange in lungs
normal human plasma
normal range
normal solution
normal test result
normetanephrine, total
normoblast, polychromatophilic
normoblastic
normoblastosis
normocalcemia
normocapnia
normocephalic
normocholesterolemia
normochromasia
normochromia
normochromic anemia
normocrinic
normocyte
normocytic anemia
normocytosis
normoerythrocyte
normoglycemia
normokalemia
normolipidemic
normoorthocytosis
normoskeocytosis
normospermic
normosthenuria
normotest
normotrophic
normouricemia
normouricuria
normovolemia
Norris corpuscle
North American blastomycosis

Northern blot (NB)
Northern blot analysis
Northern blot procedure
Northern blot test
Northern blotting
Northern hybridization
Norwalk disease
Norwalk gastroenteritis
Norwalk virus
nose, alar cartilages of
nosebleed
nosocomial infection
nosocomial pneumonia
nosomycosis
nosoparasite
nosopoietic
nosotoxic
nosotoxicity
nosotoxicosis
notch
  acetabular
  angular
  antegonial
  aortic
  auricular
  cardiac
  cerebellar
  clavicular
  costal
  cotyloid
  craniofacial
  dicrotic
  digastric
  ethmoidal
  fibular
  frontal
  radial sigmoid
  sciatic
  sigmoid
notched incisor teeth
notching of rib
notch of spleen
notochordal canal
novobiocin resistance
NSCLC (non-small cell lung carcinoma)
N-terminus
nuchal ligament
nuchal line
nuchal rigidity
Nuck, canal of
nuclear/cytoplasmic ratio
nuclear disintegration
nuclear dust
nuclear fast red
nuclear membrane
nuclear morphometry
nuclear outline
nuclear polarity
nuclear rim fluorescence
nuclear:cytoplasmic ratio
nucleated cell
nucleated erythrocyte
nucleated red blood cell (RBC)
nucleocytoplasmic
nucleolar fluorescence
nucleolus (pl. nucleoli)
nucleoplasmic index
nucleoprotein
Nuclepore filter
Nuclepore method
Nuclepore prep
nucleus (pl. nuclei)
  abducens
  accessory cuneate
  accessory olivary
  almond
  amygdaloid
  arcuate
  atypical
  auditory
  band-shaped
  benzene
  bizarre

nucleus *(continued)*
- branchimotor
- caudate
- centrally located
- centromedian
- chromatin
- cochlear
- cuneate
- dentate
- descending
- diploid
- dorsomedial
- dorsomedial hypothalamic
- droplet
- eccentrically located
- emboliform
- germ
- horseshoe-shaped
- hyperchromatic
- monstrocellular
- oval
- pleomorphic
- plump
- prominent
- pseudostratified
- pulposus
- pyknotic
- vesicular

nucleus of Perlia
Nuel space
Nuhn gland
null cell
null cell lymphoblastic leukemia
null type non-Hodgkin lymphoma
number, accession
numeric atrophy
nummular eczematous dermatitis
nurse cell
nutmeg appearance
nutmeg liver
nutmeg pattern
nutrient artery
nutrient broth
nutrient canal
nutrient medium
nutritional cirrhosis
nutritional deficiency
nutritional deficiency syndrome
nutritional disorders
NYHA (New York Heart Association) classification of congestive heart failure
Nyiri test

O, o

O (oxygen)
oat cell
oat cell carcinoma
O-banding
O'Beirne sphincter
Obermayer test for indican in urine
Obermueller test for cholesterol
obesity
- adult-onset
- alimentary
- endogenous
- exogenous
- hyperinsulinar
- hyperinterrenal
- hyperplasmic
- hyperplastic-hypertrophic
- hypertrophic
- hypogonad
- hypoplasmic
- hypothyroid
- lifelong
- morbid
- simple

obesity-associated diabetes
oblique abdominis muscle
oblique fasciculus of pons
oblique fissure of lung
oblique ligament of elbow joint
oblique muscle
oblique pericardial sinus
oblique popliteal ligament
oblique vein
obliterans, thromboangiitis
obliterated hypogastric artery
obliterated umbilical artery
obliterating pericarditis
obliteration, fibrous
obliteration of blood vessels
obliteration of cavity
obliteration of passage
obliteration of structure
obliterative bronchiolitis
obliterative endarteritis
obliterative inflammation
obliterative vasculitis
obstetric canal
obstruction
- arterial
- biliary
- cardiac
- closed-loop
- false colonic
- gastric
- hepatic

obstruction *(continued)*
- intestinal
- lymphatic
- mammary duct
- mechanical
- otic
- pancreatic duct
- renal
- respiratory
- urinary
- venous

obstructive jaundice
obstructive pneumonia
obstructive uropathy
obturating embolism
obturator artery
obturator canal
obturator fascia
obturator foramen
obturator membrane
obturator nerve
occipital artery
occipital belly
occipital bone
occipital eminence
occipital fontantelle
occipital lobe
occipital myotome
occipital node
occipital pole
occipital sinus
occipitoatloid
occipitoaxial ligament
occipitofrontal
occiput
occluding spring embolism
occlusal surface
occlusal zone
occlusion, buccal
occlusive meningitis
occult blood in stool
occult blood in urine
occult blood, positive test for
occupational dermatitis
occupational leukoderma
ochronosis
Ochsner muscle
Ochsner ring
O.C.T. compound
OCT (oxytocin challenge) test
ocular hypertension
ocular melanoma
ocular pemphigoid
ocular sclera
Oddi, sphincter of
odontoid bone
odontoid ligament
odontoma
- ameloblastic
- composite
- fibrous
- radicular

odorant binding protein
odoriferous glands of prepuce
odorless gas
OI (osteogenesis imperfecta)
oil-aspiration pneumonia
oil embolism
oil gland
oil red O
oily stool
Oken, canal of
OKT (Ortho-Kung T)
OKT antibody
OKT cell
OKT4 monoclonal antibody
OKT8 monoclonal antibody
olecranon bursa
olecranon bursitis
olecranon fossa
oleic acid–^{131}I absorption test
Olerud and Molander fracture classification
olfactory area of nose

olfactory bulb
olfactory canal
olfactory cell
olfactory nerve
olfactory receptor cell
olfactory sulcus
olfactory tract
oligakisuria
oligemia
oligochromemia
oligoclonal band
oligocystic
oligodendrocyte
oligodendroglia cell
oligodendroglioma
oligodynamic
oligohydruria
oligohypermenorrhea
oligohypomenorrhea
oligomeganephronia
oligomenorrhea
oligomeric plasmid
oligonucleotide probe
oligophosphaturia
oligotrophia
oliguria
olivary nuclei, accessory
olive (also, oliva)
Oliver test for albumin
Olympus B-Max microscope
omega-3 fatty acid
Omenn syndrome
omental artery
omental band
omental bursa
omental tuberosity
omentum
- colic
- gastric
- gastrocolic
- gastrohepatic
- gastrosplenic

omentum *(continued)*
- greater (omentum majus)
- lesser (omentum minus)
- pancreaticosplenic
- splenogastric

omphalomesenteric artery
Omsk hemorrhagic fever
Omsk hemorrhagic fever virus
Onchocerca volvulus
onchocerciasis
oncocyte
oncocytoma
oncofetal antigen, pancreatic (POA)
oncogene (gene)
- bcl-2
- N-myc
- nm23-H1
- p53
- Philadelphia chromosome
- ras

oncogene code
oncogenesis
oncogenic virus
oncogenous osteomalacia
oncotropic
oncovirus
one-stage prothrombin time
onion mite dermatitis
onion scale lesion
onionskin appearance of new bone formation
onionskin lesion
Onodi cell
onychomycosis
O'nyong-nyong virus
oocyte
oophorocystosis
oozing from vessel
oozing of fluid
opacification
opacified
opacify

opacifying
opacities
  cloudy "snowflake"
  diffuse
  lenticular
opacity of lens
opalescent
Opalski cell
opaque cornea
OPD4 monoclonal antibody
open-angle glaucoma
open biopsy
open comedo
opening
  aortic
  cardiac
opening cell block
  esophageal
  external urethral
  femoral
  internal urethral
  saphenous
  ureteral
  vaginal
opening of His, atrioventricular
opening of superior vena cava
open loop
open wound
operative diagnosis
operator gene
ophthalmia neonatorum
ophthalmia of the newborn, gonococcal
ophthalmia, sympathetic
ophthalmic artery
Opisthorchis sinensis
opportunistic infection
opportunistic infection in immuno-deficiency
opportunistic microorganism
opsonic index
opsonizing antibody
optic atrophy
optic canal
optic chiasm
optic chiasma
optic cup
optic degeneration
optic disk (or disc)
optic fundus
optic nerve
optic neuritis
optic neuromyelitis
optic radiation
optic tract
optic vesicle
Optilyse one-step staining system
optochin disk
optochin sensitivity test
ora serrata retinae
oral administration of medication
oral cavity
oral cavity proper
oral enanthem
oral epithelial nevus
oral fissure
Oral Fluid Vironostika HIV-1 Microelisa System
oral lactose tolerance test
oral mucosa
oral orifice
oral papilloma
oral part of pharynx
oral smear
oral ulcers
oral vestibule
"oramine"—see *auramine*
orange G
orange, gentian
orange stick
OraSure HIV-1 oral specimen collection device
orbicular bone
orbicular ligament
orbit

orbital artery
orbital canal
orbital fissure
orbital gyri
orbital optic neuritis
orbital plate
orbitosphenoidal bone
Orbivirus, orbivirus
orcein
orchitis
  metastatic
  spermatogenic granulomatous
  traumatic
orchitis variolosa
orf (contagious pustular dermatitis)
orf virus
organ
  accessory
  annulospiral
  cell
  circumventricular
  Corti
  critical
  donor
  enamel
  end
  extraperitoneal
  floating
  genital
  poles of
  reticuloendothelial
  retroperitoneal
  vestigial
organ capsule
organelle, cellular
organic acid
organic lesion
organism (see *pathogen* for list)
  acid-fast
  blood-borne
  intracellular
  multicellular
organism *(continued)*
  nonpathogenic
  pathogenic
    bacterium
    fungus
    parasite
    rickettsia
    virus
  pleuropneumonia-like (PPLO)
  pyogenic
  unicellular
  urease-producing
  virulent
organized clot
organized thrombus
organogenesis
organoid array
organoid nevus
organophosphate pesticides
organophosphate poisoning
organosilane-coated glass slide
Oriental sore
orienting reflex
orifice
  anal
  aortic
  atrioventricular
  cardiac
  esophagogastric
  external urethral
  gastroduodenal
  golf-hole ureteral
  ileocecal
  internal urethral
  mitral
  pharyngeal
  pulmonary
  pyloric
  tricuspid
  ureteral or ureteric
  urethral
  vaginal

orofacial fistula
orofacial herpes
"oromine"—see *auramine*
oropharynx
Oropouche virus
orosomucoid test
Oroya fever
orphan virus
Orth fixative
orthochromatic
orthodontic device
orthomyxovirus
orthostatic proteinuria
Orth solution
Orth stain
Orungo virus
os (pl. ossa), cervical
  external
  internal
os coxae (hip bone)
Osgood-Haskins test for albumin
Osgood-Schlatter disease
Osler-Weber-Rendu disease
Osm (osmole)
osmic acid
osmium tetroxide
osmium tetroxide phosphate
osmolality
  serum
  urinary
  urine
osmolality ratio, urine/serum
osmolarity
osmole (Osm)
osmosis
osmotic activity of total solute content
osmotic edema
osmotic fragility test (RBC fragility)
osmotic fragility test for spherocytosis
osmotic nephrosis
osmotic pressure
os pubis, ascending ramus of
ossa (pl. of os)
osseocartilaginous thoracic cage
osseous cell
osseous labyrinth
osseous polyp
osseous portion of auditory tube
ossicle
  auditory
  epactal
  lunula
ossicles of ear
ossificans, myositis
ossification
  abnormal
  enchondral
  intracartilaginous
  intramembranous
  irregular enchondral
  primary center of
  secondary center of
ossification center
osteitis
  acute
  alveolar
  chronic
  condensing
  cortical
  hematogenous
  sclerosing
  vascular
osteitis deformans
osteitis fibrosa cystica
osteitis pubis
osteitis tuberculosa multiplex cystica
osteoaneurysm
osteoarthritis
osteoarthritis grading
osteoarthropathy
  hypertrophic pulmonary
  idiopathic hypertrophic
osteoblast
osteoblastic osteosarcoma

osteoblastoma
osteocachexia
osteocalcin
osteocampsia
osteocele
osteochondral
osteochondritis dissecans
osteochondritis
  juvenile deforming metatarso-
    phalangeal
  syphilitic
osteochondritis necroticans
osteochondrodysplasia
osteochondrodystrophia deformans
osteochondrodystrophy
osteochondrofibroma
osteochondrogenic cell
osteochondrolysis
osteochondroma, fibrosing
osteochondromatosis
  multiple
  synovial
osteochondromyxoma
osteochondrosarcoma
osteochondrosis deformans tibiae
osteoclast
osteoclast activating factor
osteoclastoma
osteocystoma
osteocyte
osteodermia
osteodysplasty
osteodystrophy, renal
osteogenesis imperfecta (OI)
osteogenic cell
osteogenic sarcoma
osteohemachromatosis
osteoid osteoma
osteoid tissue
osteoid trabeculae
osteolipochondroma
osteolysis, focal
osteolytic
osteoma
  cavalryman's
  compact
  giant osteoid
  ivory
  osteoid
  spongy
osteoma cutis
osteomalacia
  antacid-induced
  anticonvulsant
  familial hypophosphatemic
  hepatic
  oncogenous
  puerperal
  renal tubular
  senile
osteomalacic pelvis
osteomyelitis
  chronic diffuse sclerosing
  chronic focal sclerosing
  conchiolin
  focal sclerosing
  Garré
  hematogenous
  salmonella
  sclerosing nonsuppurative
  typhoid
osteomyelitis variolosa
osteomyelodysplasia
osteomyxochondroma
osteon
osteonecrosis
osteopathia striata
osteopathy
  disseminated condensing
  hunger
  myelogenic
osteopenia
osteoperiostitis
osteopetrosis

osteophlebitis
osteophyma
osteophyte, marginal
osteophytosis
osteoporosis
  disuse
  juvenile
  postmenopausal
  post-traumatic
  senile
osteoporosis of bone
osteoporotic bone
osteoprogenitor cell
osteopulmonary arthropathy
osteoradionecrosis
osteorrhagia
osteosarcoma
  chondroblastic
  classical
  extraosseous
  fibroblastic
  high-grade surface
  intracortical
  intraosseous low-grade
  jaw
  juxtacortical
  multicentric
  osteoblastic
  parosteal
  periosteal
  small cell
  synchronous multicentric
  telangiectatic
osteosarcomatosis
osteosclerosis
osteosclerotic anemia
osteosis cutis
osteosis, parathyroid
osteosynovitis
osteothrombophlebitis
osteothrombosis
Osterberg test
ostium (pl. ostia)
  abdominal
  aortic
  auditory tube of pharyngeal
  uterine
Ota nevus
otic abscess
otic atrophy
otic degeneration
otic dystrophy
otic ganglion
otic labyrinth
otic obstruction
otitic meningitis
otitis externa
otitis interna
otitis media, purulent
otitis, serous
otocyst
otogenous abscess
otolithic membrane
otomycosis
otorrhea, cerebrospinal fluid
otosclerosis
ototoxic
Ouchterlony double diffusion method
Ouchterlony test
outer lipoprotein bilayer
outer membrane
outer pigment cell layer
outflow, sacral parasympathetic
outlet
  pelvic
  pyloric
  thoracic
outpouching of joint capsule
outpouching of tendon sheath
outpouring of fluid
output, cardiac
ova and parasites (O&P) test
oval cell
ovale malaria

oval foramen
oval-form colonic groove
ovalis
  annulus
  fossa (saphenous opening)
  limbus fossae
oval nucleus
ovalocyte
ovalocytosis
oval shape
oval-shaped
oval window
ovarian abscess
ovarian adenocarcinoma
ovarian artery
ovarian cortex
ovarian cyst
ovarian fibroma
ovarian fimbria
ovarian follicle
ovarian follicle atresia
ovarian fossa
ovarian hormone
ovarian ligament
ovarian medulla
ovarian nerve
ovarian plexus of nerves
ovarian pregnancy
ovarian tumor
ovario-abdominal pregnancy
ovariocentesis
ovary (pl. ovaries)
  atrophied
  atrophy of
  cyst of
  embryonic
  ligament of
  mulberry
  polycystic
  suspensory ligament of
ovary teratocarcinoma
ovary teratoma
overdevelopment, genetically induced
overdevelopment of bone tissue
overflow proteinuria
overgrowth of poorly mineralized osteoid
overhydration
overnutrition
overriding aorta
overt diabetes
oviduct
oviductal pregnancy
ovoid articulation
ovotestis
ovulatory mucus
ovum (pl. ova)
  blighted
  fertilized
OvuQUICK test
oxalate plasma
oxalic acid
ox cell hemolysin test
oxidase test
oxide nitrogen
oxygen (O)
  arterial
  partial pressure of (PO_2)
oxygenated blood
oxygenated hemoglobin
oxygen capacity
oxygen-carrying capacity of blood
oxygen-carrying material of red blood cells
oxygen deficiency
oxygen saturation
oxygen tension (hypoxemia)
oxyhemoglobin
oxyntic cell
oxyntic gland
oxyntic mucosa
oxyphil cell
oxyphilic
oxytocin challenge test (OCT)

P, p

P (phosphorus)
Pab 1801 immunostain
pacemaker cell
pacemaker region, gastric
pachyderma of vocal cord
pachymeninges
packed cells, volume of
packed human blood cells
packed red blood cells
pad
  abdominal
  antimesenteric fat
  electrode
  fat
  fibrocartilaginous
pad of fat, ischiorectal
Padykula-Herman stain
Paecilomyces javanicus
Paecilomyces lilacinus
Paecilomyces variotii
Paecilomyces viridis
Paget cell
Paget disease, extramammary
Paget disease of bone
Paget disease of breast
Paget-Eccleston stain
Paget quiet necrosis
pagetoid cell
pagetoid fashion
PAI (plasminogen activator inhibitor)
pain fiber
painful hematuria
painless hematuria
painless indurated ulcer
paired parietal branches
paired visceral branches
palatal abscess
palatal arch
palate
  bony
  Byzantine arch
  cleft
  hard
  smoker's
  soft
palatine aponeurosis
palatine artery
palatine bone
palatine canal
palatine foramen
palatine gland
palatine nerve
palatine process
palatine raphe

palatine root
palatine shelf
palatine tonsil
palatoglossal arch
palatoglossus muscle
palatomaxillary canal
palatopharyngeal arch
palatopharyngeal fold
palatopharyngeus muscle
palatovaginal canal
pale cytoplasm
pale myocardium
pale stool
palisade cell
palisade formation
palisades of proliferating cells
palisading, peripheral
palmar aponeurosis
palmar arch artery
palmar carpal ligament
palmar carpometacarpal ligament
palmar crease
palmar interosseous artery
palmar ligament
palmar metacarpal ligament
palmar radiocarpal ligament
palmar ulnocarpal ligament
Palmer acid test for peptic ulcer
palmin test for pancreatic efficiency
palpable
palpate
palpatory proteinuria
palpebra (pl. palpebrae)
palpebral arch
palpebral artery
palpebral conjunctiva
palpebral fascia
palpebral fissure
palpebral gland
palpebral raphe
pampiniform
pampiniform plexus
PAN (polyarteritis nodosa)
pancake kidney
pancervical smear
pancreas
  aberrant
  accessory
  annular
  anterior surface of
  Aselli
  beta-cells of the
  biopsy of
  degeneration of
  dorsal
  head of
  heterotopic
  inferior surface of
  lesser
  neck of
  posterior surface of
  tail of
  uncinate process of
  ventral
  Willis
  Winslow
pancreas divisum
pancreas transplant
pancreatic abscess
pancreatic acini atrophy
pancreatic bud
pancreatic calculus
pancreatic carcinoma
pancreatic cyst
pancreatic diabetes
pancreatic duct
  accessory
  duodenal end of dorsal
  duodenal end of main
  main
  obstruction of
  proximal part of dorsal
pancreatic duct sphincter
pancreatic enzyme

pancreatic function test
pancreatic hormone
pancreatic islet
pancreatic islet cell
pancreatic juice
pancreatic lipase
pancreaticobiliary common channel
pancreaticobiliary ductal junction
pancreaticobiliary sphincter
pancreaticobiliary tract
pancreatic obstruction
pancreaticoduodenal artery
pancreaticolienal lymph nodes
pancreatic oncofetal antigen (POA)
pancreaticosplenic gland
pancreaticosplenic lymph nodes
pancreaticosplenic omentum
pancreatic phlegmon
pancreatic polypeptide (PP)
pancreatic pseudocyst
pancreatic tumor
pancreatic vein
pancreatin
pancreatitis
  acute
  acute hemorrhagic
  acute interstitial
  calcareous
  centrilobar
  chronic
  chronic relapsing
  interstitial
  necrotizing
  perilobar
  purulent
pancreatoblastoma
pancrelipase
pancreozymin-secretin test
panculture
pancystitis
pancytopenia
panduriform placenta
panel
  arthritis
  chemistry
  electrolyte
  enzyme
  fasting chemistry
  febrile agglutinin
  liver
  rheumatoid (rheumatology)
  rheumatology
  test
  thyroid
panel cell
panel coagulation
panencephalitis
  Pette-Döring
  subacute sclerosing (SSPE)
Paneth granular cell
panhypopituitarism
panic level
panlobular emphysema
Panner disease
panniculitis
  LE (lupus erythematosus)
  lobular
  nodular nonsuppurative
  relapsing febrile nodular
    nonsuppurative
  septal
  subacute nodular migratory
  Weber-Christian
panniculus
panniculus adiposus
panniculus carnosus
pannus formation
pannus of eye
pannus of joint
pannus subcutaneous
panophthalmitis
panoptic stain
panosteitis
pantaloon embolism

Panton-Valentine leukocidin
PAP (Papanicolaou)
PAP smear
PAP stain (or test)
PAP (peroxidase-antiperoxidase) technique for detecting antigen or antibody in tissue sections
PAP (prostatic acid phosphatase)
paper chromatography
paper electrophoresis
papilla (pl. papillae)
  acoustic
  bile
  circumvallate
  clavate
  conical
  dentinal
  dermal
  filiform
  foliate
  fungiform
  lingual
  major duodenal
  minor duodenal
  renal
  urethral
papilla of Vater
papillary adenocarcinoma
papillary carcinoma
papillary cluster of cells
papillary cystadenocarcinoma
papillary cystic adenoma
papillary dermis
papillary hyperplasia of follicles
papillary hypertrophy of conjunctiva
papillary layer of dermis
papillary lesion
papillary muscle
papillary necrosis
papillary proliferation
papillary tumor
papillated surface
papillation
papillitis
  necrotizing
  necrotizing renal
papilloadenocystoma
papillocarcinoma
papilloma
  basal cell
  benign squamous
  choroid plexus
  cockscomb (also coxcomb)
  cutaneous
  duct
  fibroepithelial
  friable
  Hopmann
  intracanalicular
  intracystic
  intraductal
  inverted
  inverted ductal
  oral
  soft
  squamous
  transitional cell
  villous
  warty
papilloma of bladder
papilloma of vocal cord
papillomatosis, confluent reticulated
papillomatosis/epitheliosis, intraductal
papillomatous benign tumor
papilloma virus (also, papillomavirus)
Papnet test
papovavirus
pappataci fever virus
Pappenheimer body
Pappenheim stain
papular dermatitis of pregnancy
papular eruption
papular erythema and scaling
papular fever

papular lesion
papule
  fluid-filled
  lichenoid
  minute
  pedunculated
  pruritic urticarial (of pregnancy)
  rust-colored
  sessile
  transitory
papulonecrotic lesion
papulosis
  bowenoid
  lymphomatoid
  malignant atrophic
papulosquamous
papulovesicular dermatitis
papulovesicular eruption
para 1 (primipara)
para 2 (secundipara)
para-aortic region
paracarmine stain
paracecal appendix
paracentesis
paracentric inversion
parachute deformity
Paracoccidioides brasiliensis
paracoccidioidomycosis
paracolic gutter
paracolic lymph nodes
paracolon bacilli
paracystic
paracystic pouch
paracytic
paradidymis
paradoxical embolism
paraduodenal fold
paraduodenal recess
paradysentery bacillus
parafascicular (PF) nucleus
paraffin
paraffin block
paraffin section
paraffin tumor
paraffin wax
paraffinoma
parafollicular cell
paraformaldehyde
parafrenal abscess
parafrenal gland
paraganglioma
paraganglion (pl. paraganglia)
paraganglionic cell
Paragon stain
paragonimiasis
Paragonimus westermani
parainfluenza 2 virus
parainfluenza 3 virus
parainfluenza 4 virus
parainfluenza virus (PIV)
parakeratosis
parallel pelvic plane
paraluteal cell
paralutein cell
paralysis
paralysis agitans
paramedial
paramedian
paramesonephric duct
parameter
parametrial abscess
parametric abscess
parametrium
Paramyxovirus, paramyxovirus
paranasal sinus
paraneoplasia
paraneoplastic pemphigus
paraneoplastic syndrome
paranephric abscess
paraneural infiltration
paraphimosis
Paraplast embedding medium
Parapoxvirus
paraproctitis

paraproteinemia
parapsoriasis en plaque
pararectal fossa
pararectal lymph node
pararectal pouch
parasagittal meningioma
parasite (see *pathogen* for list)
parasite, bloodsucking intestinal
parasite cyst
parasites in crypts of Lieberkühn
parasitic infiltration
parasitic worms
parasitism, intestinal
parasitize
parasitology
parasternal lymph node
parasympathetic cardiac nerve
parasympathetic ganglion
parasympathetic nerve supply
parasympathetic secretomotor fiber
parasympathetic system
parathormone hormone
parathyroid adenoma
parathyroid gland
parathyroid hormone (PTH, parathormone)
parathyroid hormonelike protein
parathyroid hyperplasia of
parathyroid-like polypeptide
parathyroid osteosis
parathyroid tumor
paratubal cyst
paratyphoid bacillus
paratyphoid fever
paraumbilical region
paraumbilical vein
paraurethral canal
paraurethral duct
paraurethral gland
paravaccinia virus
paravertebral body
paravertebral ganglion
paravertebral groove
paravertebral nerve plexus
paravesical fossa
paravesical pouch
parchment induration
parenchyma
parenchymal cell
parenchymal hemorrhage
parenchymal tissue
parenchymatous degeneration
parenchymatous goiter
parenchymatous inflammation
parenchymatous mastitis
parenchymatous myocarditis
parenchymatous nephritis
parenchymatous neuritis
parenchymatous pneumonia
parent cell
parenteric fever
paresthesia
Parham method of Fab fragment preparation
parietal bone
parietal branches
    paired
    unpaired
parietal cell
parietal cell antibody
parietal convolution, ascending
parietal eye
parietal layer
parietal parenchyma
parietal pelvic fascia
parietal pericardium
parietal peritoneum
parietal pleura
parietal pregnancy
parietal tuber
parieto-occipital artery
parieto-occipital sulcus
parieto-temporal artery
Park aneurysm

Parkinson disease
parkinsonism
Park-Williams bacillus
Park-Williams fixative
Parlodion embedding medium
Parona space
parosteal osteosarcoma
parotid abscess
parotid bed
parotid gland
parotid lymph node
parotidoscirrhus
parotid sheath
parotitis
  acute suppurative
  epidemic
parovarian cyst
paroxysmal cold hemoglobinuria
paroxysmal cough
paroxysmal hemoglobinuria
paroxysmal nocturnal hemoglobinuria
paroxysmal proteinuria
parrot fever
part (portion) (see *pars* in reference books for anatomical structures)
partial lesion
partial pressure of carbon dioxide (PCO_2)
partial pressure of oxygen in arterial blood (PO_2)
partial protein
partial-thickness tear
partial thromboplastin time (PTT) test
particle
  beta
  chromatin
  Dane
  elementary
  ribonucleoprotein
particulate matter
partition, gastric
parturient canal
parturition
Parvovirus
parvovirus B19, human
parvum
PAS (periodic acid-Schiff) stain
PAS III flow cytometer
passage, biliary
passive clot
passive congestion
passive cutaneous anaphylaxis
passive hyperemia
passive pneumonia
passive protection test
Pasteur pipette
Pasteurella haemolytica
Pasteurella multocida
Pasteurella pestis
Pasteurella pneumotropica
Pasteurella pseudotuberculosis
Pasteurella ureae
pasteurellosis
patch (pl. patches)
  cotton-wool
  fibrotic
  Peyer
  transdermal (for glucose monitoring)
  yellow crusted
patches of vascularization
patch test
patchy intercellular edema
patella
  bipartite
  floating
patellar bone
patellar ligament
patellofemoral articulation
patent
patent ductus arteriosus
patent foramen ovale
paternity test
path, condyle

pathogen (including bacteria, fungi, parasites, and viruses)
Abel bacillus
Abelson murine leukemia virus
abortus bacillus
Absidia corymbifera
Acanthamoeba
Achromobacter xylosoxidans
acid-fast bacillus (AFB)
Acinetobacter calcoaceticus var. *anitratus* (formerly *Herellea vaginicola)*
Acinetobacter calcoaceticus var. *lwoffi* (formerly *Mima polymorpha)*
Acremonium
Acremonium falciforme
Acremonium kiliense
Acremonium recifei
Acremonium restrictum
Acrodermatitis enteropathica
Actinobacillus actinomycetem comitans
Actinobacillus equuli
Actinobacillus hominis
Actinobacillus lignieresii
Actinobacillus suis
Actinomadura
Actinomyces
Actinomyces gonidiaformis
Actinomyces israelii
Actinomyces meyeri
Actinomyces naeslundii
Actinomyces odontolyticus
Actinomyces viscosus
adenovirus
Aerobacter (old name for *Enterobacter)*
Aerobacter aerogenes
Aerobacter cloacae
Aerobacter liquefaciens
Aerococcus

pathogen *(continued)*
Aeromonas caviae
Aeromonas hydrophila
Aeromonas salmonicida
Aeromonas shigelloides (see *Plesiomonas shigelloides)*
Aeromonas sobria
Afipia felis
Agaricus
Agrimonia eupatoria
Ajellomyces capsulatus
Ajellomyces dermatitidis
Alcaligenes denitrificans
Alcaligenes faecalis
Alcaligenes odorans
Alphavirus
Alternaria
Alternaria alternata
Alteromonas putrefaciens
Amanita
Amanita bisporigera
Amanita muscaria
Amanita ocreata
Amanita phalloides
Amanita verna
Amanita virosa
Amoeba
Anaerobiospirillum succiniciproducens
Ancylostoma
Ancylostoma americanum
Ancylostoma brasiliense
Ancylostoma braziliense
Ancylostoma caninum
Ancylostoma dermatitis
Ancylostoma duodenale
Anisakis marina
Arachnia
Arachnia propionica
arbovirus
arenavirus
Argentine hemorrhagic fever virus

pathogen *(continued)*
Arizona hinshawii
anthrax bacillus
arterivirus
Arthrinium
Arthroderma
Arthropoda
arthropod-borne virus
Ascaris lumbricoides
Aspergillus
Aspergillus flavus
Aspergillus fumigatus
Aspergillus glaucus
Aspergillus niger
Aspergillus terreus
Aureobasidium pullulans
avian leukosis virus
Avipoxvirus
Babesia
Babesia bigemina
Babesia microti
Bacillus anthracis
Bacillus cereus
Bacillus megaterium
Bacillus subtilis
Bacteroides
Bacteroides asaccharolyticus
Bacteroides bivius
Bacteroides buccae
Bacteroides corporis
Bacteroides corrodens (Bacteroides ureolyticus)
Bacteroides denticola
Bacteroides disiens
Bacteroides distasonis
Bacteroides eggerthii
Bacteroides fragilis
Bacteroides gingivalis
Bacteroides intermedius
Bacteroides loescheii
Bacteroides melaninogenicus
Bacteroides oralis

pathogen *(continued)*
Bacteroides oris
Bacteroides ovatus
Bacteroides ruminicola
Bacteroides thetaiotaomicron
Bacteroides uniformis
Bacteroides ureolyticus
Bacteroides vulgatus
Balantidium coli
Bang bacillus
Barr-Epstein virus
Bartonella bacilliformis
Basidiobolus ranarum
Battey bacillus
beta-hemolytic streptococci
Bifidobacterium
Bipolaris australiensis
Bipolaris hawaiiensis
Bipolaris spicifera
BK DNA virus
Blastomyces dermatitidis
Blastoschizomyces pseudotrichosporon
blue pus bacillus
bluetongue virus
Boas-Oppler bacillus
Bolivian hemorrhagic fever virus
Bordet-Gengou bacillus
Bordetella bronchiseptica
Bordetella parapertussis
Bordetella pertussis
Bornholm disease
Borrelia burgdorferi
Borrelia hermsii
Borrelia kochii
Borrelia mazzottii
Borrelia parkeri
Borrelia recurrentis
Borrelia turicatae
Botryodiplodia theobromae
Branhamella catarrhalis (formerly *Neisseria catarrhalis*)

pathogen *(continued)*

Brucella abortus
Brucella canis
Brucella melitensis
Brucella suis
Bunyavirus, bunyavirus
butter bacillus
Calicivirus, calicivirus
California encephalitis virus
Calmette-Guérin bacillus
Calymmatobacterium granulomatis (formerly *Donovania granulomatis)*
Campylobacter cinaedi
Campylobacter coli
Campylobacter fennelliae
Campylobacter fetus (formerly *Vibrio fetus*)
Campylobacter jejuni
Campylobacter laridis
Campylobacter parahaemolyticus
Campylobacter vulnificus
Candida
Candida albicans
Candida guilliermondii
Candida krusei
Candida lusitaniae
Candida parapsilosis
Candida pseudotropicalis
Candida pulcherrima
Candida ravautii
Candida rugosa
Candida stellatoidea
Candida tropicalis
Candida viswanathii
Capnocytophaga canimorsus
Capnocytophaga ochracea
Capripoxvirus
Cardiobacterium hominis
Cedecea
Cedecea davisae
Cedecea lapagei

pathogen *(continued)*

Cedecea neteri
Chaetoconidium
chikungunya virus
Chlamydia pneumoniae
Chlamydia psittaci
Chlamydia trachomatis
Chromobacterium violaceum
Chrysosporium
Chrysosporium parvum
Citrobacter
Citrobacter amalonaticus
Citrobacter diversus
Citrobacter freundii
Cladosporium
Cladosporium bantianum
Cladosporium carrionii
Cladosporium cladosporioides
Cladosporium trichoides
Cladosporium werneckii
Clonorchis sinensis
Clostridium
Clostridium bifermentans
Clostridium botulinum
Clostridium butyricum
Clostridium cadaveris
Clostridium difficile
Clostridium histolyticum
Clostridium innocuum
Clostridium novyi
Clostridium paraputrificum
Clostridium perfringens
Clostridium putrificum
Clostridium ramosum
Clostridium septicum
Clostridium sordellii
Clostridium sphenoides
Clostridium subterminale
Clostridium tertium
Clostridium tetani
Clostridium welchii
club-shaped bacillus

pathogen *(continued)*
Coccidioides immitis
coliform bacillus
Colorado tick fever virus
Comamonas terrigena
common cold virus
Conidiobolus coronatus
Conidiobolus incongruus
Coprinus cinereus
corkscrew-shaped bacteria
Coronavirus, coronavirus
Corynebacterium acnes
Corynebacterium bovis
Corynebacterium diphtheriae
Corynebacterium equi
Corynebacterium haemolyticum
Corynebacterium minutissimum
Corynebacterium pseudodiphtheriticum
Corynebacterium pseudotuberculosis
Corynebacterium ulcerans
Corynebacterium xerosis
Coxiella burnetii
Coxsackie virus
Crimean-Congo hemorrhagic fever virus
Crithidia luciliae
croup-associated virus (CA v.)
Cryptococcus
Cryptococcus albidus
Cryptococcus laurentii
Cryptococcus luteolus
Cryptococcus neoformans
Cryptosporidium
Curvularia geniculata
Curvularia lunata
Curvularia pallescens
Curvularia senegalensis
Curvularia verruculosa
cytomegalovirus
Dactylaria

pathogen *(continued)*
dengue virus
Dermatophilus
Dermatophilus congolensis
dermatophytic fungi
dermotropic virus
DF-2 bacillus
Dibothriocephalus latus
Dientamoeba fragilis
diphtheria bacillus
Diplococcus pneumoniae
DNA virus
DNA tumor virus
Döderlein bacillus
Donovania granulomatis
Dracunculus medinensis
Ducrey bacillus
dysentery bacillus
Eaton agent
Eberth bacillus
Ebola virus
Echinococcus granulosus
ECHO (enterocytopathogenic human orphan) virus
Edwardsiella
Edwardsiella tarda
Ehrlichia canis
Ehrlichia chaffeensis
Ehrlichia sennetsu
Eikenella corrodens
Eikenella corrodens (formerly *Bacteroides corrodens*, HB-1)
encephalomyocarditis virus
Entamoeba histolytica
enteric bacillus
enteric orphan viruses
Enterobacter (formerly *Aerobacter*)
Enterobacter aerogenes
Enterobacter agglomerans
Enterobacter cloacae
Enterobacter gergoviae

pathogen *(continued)*
- *Enterobacter hafniae*
- *Enterobacter liquefaciens*
- *Enterobacter sakazakii*
- *Enterobacteriaceae*
- *Enterobius vermicularis*
- *Enterococcus* (pl. *Enterococci*)
- *Enterococcus avium*
- *Enterococcus faecalis*
- *Enterococcus faecium*
- enterocytopathogenic human orphan (ECHO) virus
- *Enterovirus*, enterovirus
- epidemic keratoconjunctivitis virus
- *Epidermophyton*
- *Epidermophyton floccosum*
- *Epidermophyton stockdaleae*
- Epstein-Barr virus (EBV)
- *Erysipelothrix rhusiopathiae*
- Escherich bacillus
- *Escherichia coli (E. coli)*
- *Escherichia fergusonii*
- *Escherichia hermannii*
- *Escherichia vulneris*
- *Eubacterium alactolyticum*
- *Eubacterium lentum*
- *Eubacterium limosum*
- *Ewingella*
- *Exophiala dermatitidis*
- *Exophiala heteromorpha*
- *Exophiala jeanselmei*
- *Exophiala spinifera*
- *Exserohilum rostratum*
- *Fasciola gigantica*
- *Fasciola hepatica*
- *Fasciolopsis buski*
- fibrillary bacteria
- *Filobasidiella neoformans*
- filament-forming bacillus
- *Filovirus*
- *Fissuricella filamenta*

pathogen *(continued)*
- flavivirus
- *Flavobacterium meningosepticum*
- Flexner bacillus
- *Fonsecaea compacta*
- *Fonsecaea dermatitidis*
- *Fonsecaea pedrosoi*
- *Francisella tularensis* (formerly *Pasteurella tularensis*)
- Friedländer bacillus
- Frisch bacillus
- funguslike bacteria
- *Fusarium moniliforme*
- *Fusarium oxysporum*
- *Fusarium solani*
- fusiform bacillus
- *Fusobacterium*
- *Fusobacterium mortiferum*
- *Fusobacterium necrophorum*
- *Fusobacterium nucleatum*
- *Fusobacterium russii*
- *Fusobacterium varium*
- *Gardnerella* vaginitis (formerly *Haemophilus vaginalis* or *Corynebacterium vaginale)*
- Gärtner bacillus
- *Gemella morbillorum*
- *Geotrichum capitatum*
- *Geotrichum fermentans*
- *Geotrichum penicillatum*
- Ghon-Sachs bacillus
- *Giardia lamblia*
- *Gibberella fujikuroi*
- glanders bacillus
- *gram-negative diplococci*
- gram-negative bacillus
- gram-positive bacillus
- grass bacillus
- Guama virus
- Guaroa virus
- *Haemophilus*
- *Haemophilus aegyptius*

pathogen *(continued)*
Haemophilus aphrophilus
Haemophilus ducreyi
Haemophilus haemolyticus
Haemophilus influenzae
Haemophilus parahaemolyticus
Haemophilus parainfluenzae
Haemophilus paraphrophilus
Haemophilus segnis
Haemophilus vaginalis
Hafnia
Hafnia alvei (formerly *Enterobacter hafniae*)
Hansen bacillus
Hantavirus
helical bacteria
Helicobacter pylori
hepatitis A virus (HAV)
hepatitis B virus (HBV)
hepatitis C virus
hepatitis D (delta) virus
hepatitis E virus
Herellea vaginicola (now *Acinetobacter calcoaceticus)*
herpes simplex virus (HSV)
herpesvirus
herpes type 5 virus (cytomegalovirus)
herpes zoster virus (HZV)
Histoplasma capsulatum
Hofmann bacillus
Hormiscium dermatitidis
Hormodendrum dermatitidis
human herpesvirus 3
human herpesvirus 4
human immunodeficiency virus (HIV)
human T-cell leukemia virus
human T-cell lymphoma virus (HTLV I and II)
human T-cell lymphotropic virus type I (HTLV-I)

pathogen *(continued)*
Hymenolepis nana
intracellular bacteria
Isospora belli
Ixodes dammini
Ixodes pacificus
Jamestown Canyon virus
Japanese encephalitis virus
JC DNA virus
Johne bacillus
Kemerovo virus
Kingella denitrificans
Kingella indologenes
Kingella kingae
Kitasato bacillus
Klebsiella
Klebsiella oxytoca
Klebsiella ozaenae
Klebsiella planticola
Klebsiella pneumoniae
Klebsiella rhinoscleromatis
Klebs-Loeffler bacillus
Kluyvera
Kluyvera ascorbata
Kluyvera cryocrescens
Koch bacillus
Koch-Weeks bacillus
Korean hemorrhagic fever virus
Koserella trabulsii
Kyasanur Forest hemorrhagic fever virus
lactic acid bacillus
La Crosse virus
Lactobacillus
Lecythophora hoffmannii
Lecythophora mutabilis
legionnaire's bacillus
Legionella anisa
Legionella bozemanii
Legionella dumoffii
Legionella feelei
Legionella gormanii

pathogen *(continued)*
Legionella jordanis
Legionella longbeachae
Legionella micdadei
Legionella oakridgensis
Legionella pneumonia
Legionella pneumophila
Legionella sainthelensis
Legionella wadsworthii
Leishmania brasiliensis
Leishmania donovani
Leishmania tropica
leprosy bacillus
Leptospira biflexa
Leptospira icterohemorrhagiae
Leptospira interrogans
Leptotrichia
Listeria monocytogenes
Loa loa
Loboa loboi
Lymphocryptovirus
Lyssavirus
lytic virus
M-25 virus
Madurella mycetomatis
Malassezia furfur
Malassezia pachydermatis
Marburg virus
Mayaro virus
measles virus
Micrococcus
Microsporum
Microsporum amazonicum
Microsporum audouinii
Microsporum boullardii
Microsporum canis
Microsporum cookei
Microsporum equinum
Microsporum faeni
Microsporum ferrugineum
Microsporum floccosum
Microsporum fulvum

pathogen *(continued)*
Microsporum gallinae
Microsporum gypseum
Microsporum nanum
Microsporum persicolor
Microsporum praecox
Microsporum racemosum
Microsporum ripariae
Microsporum vanbreuseghemii
Mima polymorpha (now *Acinetobacter calcoaceticus* var. *lwoffi)*
MM virus
Mokola virus
Molluscipoxvirus
molluscum contagiosum virus
Monilia sitophila
Morax-Axenfeld bacillus
Moraxella atlantae
Moraxella catarrhalis
Moraxella lacunata
Moraxella nonliquefaciens
Moraxella osloensis
Moraxella phenylpyruvica
Moraxella urethralis
Morbillivirus, morbillivirus
Morgan bacillus
Morganella
Morganella morganii
Mortierella wolfii
mosquito-borne virus
Much bacillus
Mucor
Mucor ramosissimus
Mucor rouxianus
mumps virus
murine leukemia virus
Murray Valley encephalitis virus
Mycobacterium asiaticum
Mycobacterium avium
Mycobacterium avium-intracellulare (MAI) complex

pathogen *(continued)*
Mycobacterium bovis
Mycobacterium celatum
Mycobacterium chelonei (formerly *Mycobacterium abscessus)*
Mycobacterium flavescens
Mycobacterium fortuitum
Mycobacterium gastri
Mycobacterium genavense
Mycobacterium gordonae
Mycobacterium haemophilum
Mycobacterium intracellulare
Mycobacterium kansasii
Mycobacterium leprae
Mycobacterium malmoense
Mycobacterium marinum
Mycobacterium microti
Mycobacterium paratuberculosis
Mycobacterium phlei
Mycobacterium scrofulaceum
Mycobacterium shimoidei
Mycobacterium simiae
Mycobacterium smegmatis
Mycobacterium szulgai
Mycobacterium terrae
Mycobacterium triviale
Mycobacterium tuberculosis
Mycobacterium ulcerans
Mycobacterium xenopi
Mycocentrospora acerina
Mycoplasma
Mycoplasma buccale
Mycoplasma fauciuim
Mycoplasma fermentans
Mycoplasma genitalium
Mycoplasma hominis
Mycoplasma orale
Mycoplasma pharyngis
Mycoplasma pneumoniae
Mycoplasma salivarium
myxovirus
Nairovirus

pathogen *(continued)*
Nakiwogo virus
Necator
Necator americanus
Neisseria
Neisseria catarrhalis
Neisseria cinerea
Neisseria elongata
Neisseria flavescens
Neisseria gonorrhoeae
Neisseria lactamica
Neisseria meningitidis
Neisseria mucosa
Neisseria sicca
Neisseria subflava
Neotestudina rosatii
newborn pneumonitis virus
Newcastle disease virus
Newcastle-Manchester bacillus
Nocardia
Nocardia asteroides
Nocardia brasiliensis
Nocardia caviae
Norwalk virus
Omsk hemorrhagic fever virus
Onchocerca volvulus
oncogenic virus
oncovirus
O'nyong nyong virus
Opisthorchis sinensis
Orbivirus, orbivirus
orf virus
Oropouche virus
orphan virus
Orthomyxovirus, orthomyxovirus
Orungo virus
Paecilomyces javanicus
Paecilomyces lilacinus
Paecilomyces variotii
Paecilomyces viridis
papilloma virus (also, papilloma virus)

pathogen *(continued)*
- papovavirus
- pappataci fever virus
- *Paracoccidioides brasiliensis*
- *Paragonimus westermanni*
- parainfluenza 2 virus
- parainfluenza 3 virus
- parainfluenza 4 virus
- *Paramyxovirus*, paramyxovirus
- *Parapoxvirus*
- paravaccinia virus
- Park-Williams bacillus
- *Parvovirus,* parvovirus
- parvovirus B19, human
- *Pasteurella haemolytica*
- *Pasteurella multocida*
- *Pasteurella pestis*
- *Pasteurella pneumotropica*
- *Pasteurella pseudotuberculosis*
- *Pasteurella ureae*
- *Pediculus*
- *Pediculus capitis*
- *Pediculus corporis*
- *Pediculus humanus*
- *Pediculus humanus capitis*
- *Pediculus humanus corporis*
- *Pediculus humanus humanus* (yes)
- *Pediculus pubis*
- *Penicillium chrysogenum*
- *Penicillium citrinum*
- *Penicillium commune*
- *Penicillium expansum*
- *Penicillium lilacinum*
- *Penicillium marneffei*
- *Penicillium spinulosum*
- *Peptococcus*
- *Peptococcus niger*
- *Peptostreptococcus*
- *Peptostreptococcus anaerobius*
- *Peptostreptococcus asaccharolyticus*
- *Peptostreptococcus indolicus*
- *Peptostreptococcus lanceolatus*

pathogen *(continued)*
- *Peptostreptococcus magnus*
- *Peptostreptococcus micros*
- *Peptostreptococcus parvulus*
- *Peptostreptococcus prevotii*
- *Peptostreptococcus productus*
- *Pestivirus*
- Pfeiffer bacillus
- *Phaeoannellomyces*
- *Phaeoannellomyces elegans*
- *Phaeoannellomyces werneckii*
- *Phaeococcomyces*
- pharyngoconjunctival fever virus
- *Phaseolus vulgaris*
- *Phialophora bubakii*
- *Phialophora dermatitidis*
- *Phialophora parasitica*
- *Phialophora pedrosoi*
- *Phialophora repens*
- *Phialophora richardsiae*
- *Phialophora verrucosa*
- *Phlebovirus*
- *Phoma cruris-hominis*
- *Phoma eupyrena*
- *Phoma glomerata*
- *Phoma herbarum*
- *Phoma hibernica*
- *Phoma oculo-hominis*
- *Phthirus pubis*
- *Phycomycetes*
- Pichinde virus
- picornavirus
- *Piedraia hortae*
- Piry virus
- *Pityrosporum*
- *Pityrosporum orbiculare*
- *Plasmodium*
- *Plasmodium falciparum*
- *Plasmodium malariae*
- *Plasmodium ovale*
- *Plasmodium vivax*
- Plaut bacillus

pathogen *(continued)*
- *Plesiomonas shigelloides* (formerly *Aeromonas shigelloides)*
- pleuropneumonia-like organism
- Plotz bacillus
- *Pneumococcus*
- *Pneumocystis carinii* (PCP)
- *Pneumovirus*
- poliomyelitis virus
- poliovirus
- polymorphic fungi
- polyoma virus
- *Polyomavirus*, polyomavirus
- Pongola virus
- *Porphyromonas asaccharolytica*
- Powassan virus
- pox virus (also, poxvirus)
- Preisz-Nocard bacillus
- *Prevotella bivia*
- *Prevotella disiens*
- *Prevotella intermedia*
- *Prevotella loeschii*
- *Prevotella melaninogenica*
- *Prevotella oralis*
- *Prevotella oris*
- *Propionibacterium*
- *Propionibacterium acnes* (formerly *Corynebacterium acnes)*
- *Propionibacterium avidum*
- *Propionibacterium freudenreichii*
- *Propionibacterium granulosum*
- *Propionibacterium jensenii*
- *Proteus*
- *Proteus hydrophilus*
- *Proteus inconstans subgroup B*
- *Proteus mirabilis*
- *Proteus morganii*
- *Proteus penneri*
- *Proteus rettgeri*
- *Proteus vulgaris*
- *Proteus zenkeri*
- *Providencia*

pathogen *(continued)*
- *Providencia alcalifaciens*
- *Providencia rettgeri*
- *Providencia stuartii*
- *Pseudallescheria boydii*
- *Pseudochaetosphaeronema larense*
- *Pseudomonas*
- *Pseudomonas acidovorans* (formerly *Comamonas terrigena)*
- *Pseudomonas aeruginosa*
- *Pseudomonas alcaligenes*
- *Pseudomonas cepacia*
- *Pseudomonas diminuta*
- *Pseudomonas fluorescens*
- *Pseudomonas mallei*
- *Pseudomonas maltophilia*
- *Pseudomonas paucimobilis*
- *Pseudomonas pickettii*
- *Pseudomonas pseudoalcaligenes*
- *Pseudomonas pseudomallei*
- *Pseudomonas putida*
- *Pseudomonas putrefaciens*
- *Pseudomonas stutzeri*
- *Pseudomonas testosteroni*
- Pseudomonas-like bacteria
- pseudorabies virus
- pus-forming bacteria
- Puumala virus
- Quaranfil virus
- rabies virus
- *Ramularia*
- REO (respiratory enteric orphan) virus
- reovirus
- respiratory syncytial virus (RSV)
- respiratory virus
- retrovirus
- rhabdovirus
- *Rhinocladiella aquaspersa*
- rhinoscleroma bacillus
- *Rhinosporidium seeberi*

pathogen *(continued)*
Rhinovirus, rhinovirus
Rhizoctonia
Rhizoctonia solani
Rhizomucor pusillus
Rhizopus
Rhizopus arrhizus
Rhizopus microsporus
Rhizopus nigricans
Rhizopus rhizopodiformis
Rhizopus stolonifer
Rhodotorula
Rhodotorula rubra
ribovirus
Rickettsia
Rickettsia akari
Rickettsia australis
Rickettsia conorii
Rickettsia mooseri
Rickettsia prowazekii
Rickettsia rickettsii
Rickettsia sibirica
Rickettsia tsutsugamushi
Rickettsia typhi
Rift Valley fever virus
RNA tumor virus
RNA virus (ribovirus)
Rochalimaea
Rochalimaea henselae
Rochalimaea quintana
Rocio virus
Roseola infantum
Ross River virus
rotavirus
rotavirus antigen
rotavirus DNA virus
Rous-associated virus (RAV)
Rous sarcoma virus (RSV)
Rous virus
rubella virus
Rubivirus

pathogen *(continued)*
Russian autumn encephalitis virus
Russian spring-summer encephalitis virus
SA virus (simian virus SV5)
Saccharomyces cerevisiae
Sachs bacillus
Saksenaea vasiformis
Salisbury common cold virus
salivary gland virus
Salmonella
Salmonella arizonae
Salmonella choleraesuis
Salmonella enteritidis
Salmonella typhi
sandfly fever–Naples virus
sandfly fever–Sicilian virus
Sarcoptes scabiei
satellite virus
Scedosporium apiospermum
Schistosoma
Schistosoma haematobium
Schistosoma japonicum
Schistosoma mansoni
Schmitz bacillus
Schmorl bacillus
Scopulariopsis brevicaulis
Semliki Forest virus
Semunya virus
Sendai virus
Seoul virus
Serratia
Serratia liquefaciens
Serratia marcescens
Serratia rubidaea
Shiga bacillus
Shigella
Shigella boydii
Shigella dysenteriae
Shigella flexneri
Shigella sonnei

pathogen *(continued)*
- Simbu virus
- simian immunodeficiency virus (SIV)
- simian virus 40 (SV40)
- simian virus SV5
- *Simplexvirus*
- Sindbis virus
- slow virus
- smegma bacillus
- Sonne-Duval bacillus
- spiral-shaped bacteria
- *Spirillum*
- *Spirillum minus*
- Spondweni virus
- *Sporothrix schenckii*
- *Sporotrichum schenckii*
- Stanley bacillus
- *Staphylococcus*
- *Staphylococcus albus*
- *Staphylococcus aureus*
- *Staphylococcus auricularis*
- *Staphylococcus capitis*
- *Staphylococcus cohnii*
- *Staphylococcus epidermidis*
- *Staphylococcus haemolyticus*
- *Staphylococcus hominis*
- *Staphylococcus pyogenes*
- *Staphylococcus saccharolyticus*
- *Staphylococcus saprophyticus*
- *Staphylococcus warneri*
- *Staphylococcus xylosus*
- *Stenella araguata*
- St. Louis encephalitis virus
- *Streptobacillus moniliformis*
- *Streptococcus*
- *Streptococcus acidominimus*
- *Streptococcus aecium*
- *Streptococcus agalactiae*
- *Streptococcus anginosus*
- *Streptococcus avium*
- *Streptococcus bovis*

pathogen *(continued)*
- *Streptococcus constellatus*
- *Streptococcus durans*
- *Streptococcus equi*
- *Streptococcus equinus*
- *Streptococcus equisimilis*
- *Streptococcus faecalis*
- *Streptococcus faecium*
- *Streptococcus intermedius*
- Streptococcus M antigen
- *Streptococcus milleri*
- *Streptococcus mitis*
- *Streptococcus morbillorum*
- *Streptococcus mutans*
- *Streptococcus pneumoniae*
- *Streptococcus pyogenes*
- *Streptococcus salivarius*
- *Streptococcus sanguis*
- *Streptococcus uberis*
- *Streptococcus viridans*
- *Streptococcus zooepidemicus*
- *Streptomyces*
- *Streptomyces paraguayensis*
- *Streptomyces somaliensis*
- Strong bacillus
- *Strongyloides stercoralis*
- *Suipoxvirus* (swinepox virus)
- swine influenza virus
- swinepox virus
- Tacaribe virus
- *Taenia saginata*
- *Taenia solium*
- Tahyna virus
- Tamiami virus
- tanapox virus
- *Tatumella*
- *Tatumella ptyseos*
- Teschen virus
- tetanus bacillus
- Theiler virus
- *Thermoactinomyces sacchari*
- tick-borne virus

pathogen *(continued)*
- timothy bacillus
- togavirus
- *Torulopsis candida*
- *Torulopsis glabrata*
- Toscana virus
- *Toxocara canis*
- *Toxoplasma gondii*
- *Treponema*
- *Treponema buccale*
- *Treponema carateum*
- *Treponema pallidum*
- *Treponema pertenue*
- *Treponema vincentii*
- *Trichinella spiralis*
- *Trichomonas*
- *Trichomonas tenax*
- *Trichomonas vaginalis*
- *Trichophyton*
- *Trichophyton ajelloi*
- *Trichophyton concentricum*
- *Trichophyton equinum*
- *Trichophyton fisheri*
- *Trichophyton flavescens*
- *Trichophyton floccosum*
- *Trichophyton georgiae*
- *Trichophyton gloriae*
- *Trichophyton gourvilii*
- *Trichophyton longifusum*
- *Trichophyton mariatii*
- *Trichophyton megninii*
- *Trichophyton mentagrophytes*
- *Trichophyton phaseoliforme*
- *Trichophyton rubrum*
- *Trichophyton schoenleinii*
- *Trichophyton simii*
- *Trichophyton soudanense*
- *Trichophyton terrestre*
- *Trichophyton tonsurans*
- *Trichophyton vanbreuseghemii*
- *Trichophyton verrucosum*
- *Trichophyton violaceum*

pathogen *(continued)*
- *Trichosporon beigelii*
- *trichosporosis*
- *Trichuris*
- *Trichuris trichiura*
- *Trypanosoma*
- *Trypanosoma cruzi*
- *Trypanosoma gambiense*
- *Trypanosoma rhodesiense*
- tumor virus
- 2060 virus
- typhoid bacillus
- U echovirus
- Uganda S arbovirus
- ultravirus
- Uppsala virus
- *Ureaplasma urealyticum*
- vaccinia virus
- varicella-zoster virus (VZV)
- *Varicellavirus*
- variola virus (now extinct)
- *Veillonella*
- *Veillonella parvula*
- *Vesiculovirus*
- *Vibrio alginolyticus*
- *Vibrio cholerae*
- *Vibrio damsela*
- *Vibrio fetus*
- *Vibrio fluvialis*
- *Vibrio hollisae*
- *Vibrio jejuni*
- *Vibrio metschnikovii*
- *Vibrio mimicus*
- *viridans streptococci*
- vole bacillus
- *Wangiella dermatitidis*
- Weeks bacillus
- Welch bacillus
- Wesselsbron virus
- West Nile virus
- Whitmore bacillus
- *Wolinella*

- pathogen *(continued)*
  - *Wucheraria bancrofti*
  - *Wyeomyia melanocephala* mosquito virus
  - *Wyeomyia* virus
  - *Xanthomonas*
  - *Xylohypha bantiana*
  - yabapox virus
  - Yale SK poliovirus
  - *Yatapoxvirus*
  - yellow fever virus
  - *Yersinia*
  - *Yersinia enterocolitica* (formerly *Pasteurella enterocolitica*)
  - *Yersinia frederiksenii*
  - *Yersinia intermedia*
  - *Yersinia kristensenii*
  - *Yersinia pestis* (formerly *Pasteurella pestis*)
  - *Yersinia pestis comitans*
  - *Yersinia pseudotuberculosis* (formerly *Pasteurella pseudotuberculosis*)
  - Zika virus
  - zygomycetous fungus
- pathogenic microorganism
- pathogenic organism
  - bacterium
  - fungus
  - parasite
  - virus
- pathologic atrophy
- pathologic diagnosis
- pathologic fracture
- pathological
- pathologist
- pathology
  - anatomic
  - clinical
  - forensic
  - general
- pathology report
- pathophysiologic
- pattern
  - abdominal wall venous
  - adenoid
  - airspace-filling
  - airway
  - alveolar
  - ballerina-foot
  - basketweave
  - bowel gas
  - branching
  - butterfly
  - cartwheel
  - chromatin
  - cribriform
  - elongate
  - fibrotic
  - fold
  - frondlike
  - gas
  - ground-glass
  - haustral
  - honeycomb
  - hourglass
  - interstitial
  - juvenile
  - lamellated
  - layered
  - lobular
  - micronodular fibrotic
  - miliary
  - mosaic
  - mucosal
  - nutmeg
  - progestational
  - proliferative
  - rugal
  - sawtooth
  - signet ring
  - speckled
  - starry-sky
  - stellate

pattern *(continued)*
  undifferentiated
  vesicular
  wax
patterned alopecia
Patterson test for uremia
patulous
Paul-Bunnell-Davidsohn test
Paul-Bunnell test
Pautrier abscess
Pautrier microabscess
Pauwels femoral neck fracture classification
Pavy test for urine glucose
Pawlik triangle
Pawlik trigone
Pb (lead)
PBC-associated antibody
PBI (protein-bound iodine) test
P blood group
PBS (phosphate-buffered saline)
P cell
PCI (protein C inhibitor)
PCO_2 (partial pressure of carbon dioxide)
PCP (plasma cell pneumonitis)
PCP (*Pneumocystis carinii*) pneumonia
PCR (polymerase chain reaction)
PCT (porphyria cutanea tarda)
PDW (platelet distribution width)
peak and trough level
peak, monoclonal
pearl
  enamel
  epithelial
  horn
  Laënnec
pearl cyst
pearlescent
pearl formation
pearly umbilicated papule
pear-shaped defect in the iris
pea soup stool
peau d'orange
pectinate ligament of iridocorneal angle
pectinate ligament of iris
pectinate line
pectineal ligament
pectoral artery
pectoral girdle
pectoral gland
pectoral muscle
pectoralis major muscle
pectoris, angina
pectus carinatum (pigeon chest)
pectus excavatum (funnel chest)
pectus recurvatum (funnel chest)
pedal bone
pedes (pl. of pes)
pedicle
pediculosis
pediculosis capitis
pediculosis corporis
pediculosis pubis
Pediculus
Pediculus humanus
Pediculus humanus capitis
Pediculus humanus corporis
Pediculus humanus humanus (yes)
pedis, tinea (athlete's foot)
peduncular ansa
peduncular loop
pedunculated fibroid
pedunculated myxoma
pedunculated papule
PEG (polyethylene glycol)
peg-and-socket articulation
peg-and-socket joint
pegs, rete (rete ridges)
Pelger-Huët anomaly
Pelger-Huët cell
pelgeroid
Pelizaeus-Merzbacher disease
pellagra

pellagra-preventing factor
pelleted stool
pelvic abscess
pelvic aperture
pelvic bone
pelvic brim
pelvic canal
pelvic colon
pelvic diaphragm, twigs to
pelvic fascia
pelvic floor, fibromuscular
pelvic inflammatory disease (PID)
pelvic kidney
pelvic organ
pelvic outlet
pelvic peritoneal cavity
pelvic peritoneum
pelvic sacral foramina
pelvic sidewall
pelvic splanchnic nerve
pelvic viscera
pelvirectal abscess
pelvis (pl. pelves, pelvises)
  android
  anthropoid
  assimilation
  beaked
  bony
  brachypellic
  caoutchouc
  contracted
  cordate
  cordiform
  Deventer
  dolichopellic
  dwarf
  false
  female
  flat
  frozen
  funnel-shaped
  greater

pelvis *(continued)*
  gynecoid
  hardened
  heart-shaped
  inverted
  juvenile
  kyphoscoliotic
  kyphotic
  lesser
  longitudinal oval
  lordotic
  male
  masculine
  mesatipellic
  Nagele
  osteomalacic
  platypelloid
  Prague
  pseudo-osteomalacic
  rachitic
  renal
  reniform
  Rokitansky
  scoliotic
  spider
  spondylolisthetic
  transverse oval
  true
  ureteric
pelvis major
pelvis minor
pemphigoid
  benign mucosal
  bullous
  cicatricial
  ocular
pemphigoid of Brunsting-Perry,
  localized
pemphigus
  benign familial chronic
  paraneoplastic
pemphigus antibodies

pemphigus erythematosus
pemphigus foliaceus
pemphigus gangrenosus
pemphigus leprosus
pemphigus vegetans, Hallopeau type
pemphigus vulgaris
pencil-like
pendulous pouch
penetrating trauma
penetrating ulcer
penetrating wound
penetration
penicillate artery
penicillinase test
Penicillium chrysogenum
Penicillium citrinum
Penicillium commune
Penicillium expansum
Penicillium lilacinum
Penicillium marneffei
Penicillium spinulosum
penile atrophy
penile raphe
penis
  bulb of
  bulbospongiosus muscle of
  clubbed
  concealed
  corpora cavernosa
  corpus spongiosum
  crura of
  deep fascia of
  dorsal artery of
  dorsal nerve of
  dorsum of
  double
  glans
  ischiospongiosus muscle of
  root of
  suspensory ligament of
  webbed
penis artery
penis bone
penis lacuna
pennate muscle
pennatus
pentagastrin
pentoses test
Penzoldt-Fischer test
Penzoldt test for acetone
pepsin
pepsin test
pepsinogen (PG I) test
peptic cell
peptic gland
peptic ulcer
  acute
  chronic
peptic ulcer disease
peptide
  adrenocorticotropic
  regulatory
  vasoactive intestinal (VIP)
peptide test
Peptococcus
Peptococcus niger
peptone test
Peptostreptococcus
Peptostreptococcus anaerobius
Peptostreptococcus asaccharolyticus
Peptostreptococcus indolicus
Peptostreptococcus lanceolatus
Peptostreptococcus magnus
Peptostreptococcus micros
Peptostreptococcus parvulus
Peptostreptococcus prevotii
Peptostreptococcus productus
Percoll separation
percutaneous
percutaneous epididymal sperm aspiration
Perdrau method of staining
perforans (pl. perforantes)
perforate

perforated tympanic membrane
perforating abscess
perforating artery of foot
perforating artery of internal mammary
perforating artery of peroneal
perforating artery of profunda femoris
perforating artery of thigh
perforating branch
perforating wound
perforation, frank
perforation of bowel
perfume dermatitis
perfusion, acid
Peria test
perianal region
perianal skin
periangitis
periaortic lymph node
periaortitis
periapical abscess
periappendiceal abscess
periarteritis nodosa
periarteritis, syphilitic
periarticular abscess
periarticular soft tissues
periarticular tissues
periaxial neuritis
Peria test for tyrosine
peribronchial
peribronchial connective tissue
pericallosal artery
pericapillary cell
pericardiacophrenic artery
pericardial artery
pericardial cavity
pericardial cyst
pericardial effusion
pericardial effusion fluid
pericardial fluid
pericardial sac
pericardial sinus
pericardioperitoneal canal
pericarditis
    acute benign
    acute fibrinous
    adhesive
    bacterial
    carcinomatous
    chronic constrictive
    constrictive
    dry
    fibrinous
    hemorrhagic
    internal adhesive
    obliterating
    postmyocardial infarction
    postpericardiotomy
    posttraumatic
    purulent
    rheumatic
    staphylococcal
    tuberculous
    viral
pericarditis with effusion
pericardium
    bread-and-butter
    calcified
    fibrous
    nerves of
    parietal
    serous
    shaggy
    veins of
    visceral
pericecal lymph node
pericellular
pericentral fibrosis
pericentric inversion
pericentromeric region
perichondral bone
perichondrium
perichondroma
pericolonic fat
pericoronal abscess

pericranium
pericyte
pericytial
pericytoma
peridental ligament
periductal inflammation and fibrosis
periductal mastitis
periductal stroma
periencephalitis
periependymal myelitis
periesophagitis
perifolliculitis capitis abscedens et suffodiens (dissecting cellulitis of scalp)
perifolliculitis, superficial pustular
perihepatitis chronica hyperplastica
perihepatitis, gonococcal
perikaryon
perilobar pancreatitis
perilobular duct
perimenopausal female
perimetrium
perimuscular fibrosis
perimysium
perineal artery
perineal branch of posterior femoral cutaneous nerve
perineal branch of pudendal nerve
perineal fascia
perineal membrane
perineal muscle
perineal nerve
perineal space, superficial
perineal tendon, central
perineovaginal fistula
perinephric abscess
perineum
perineural epithelium
perineurium
periocular dermatitis
periodate-lysing-paraformaldehyde fixative
periodic acid-Schiff (PAS) stain
periodic acid-Schiff test
periodic fever
period line
periodonal abscess
periodontal degeneration
periodontal ligament
periodontal membrane
periodontitis
perioplic band
perioral dermatitis
periorbital edema
periorbital tissues
periosteal artery
periosteal bone
periosteal nerve
periosteal osteosarcoma
periosteal sarcoma
periosteoma
periosteum, alveolar
periosteum of rib
periostitis, proliferative
periotic bone
peripancreatic area
peripartum myocarditis
peripelvic adipose tissue
peripheral aneurysm
peripheral blood
peripheral blood smear
peripheral embolism
peripheral hepatic necrosis
peripheral lesion
peripheral necrosis
peripheral nerve
peripheral neuritis
peripheral neuropathy
peripheral palisading
peripheral protein
peripheral smear
peripheral zone
periphery
peripleuritic abscess

peripolar cell
periportal area
periportal cellular component
periportal cirrhosis
periportal component
periportal fibrosis
perirectal abscess
perirectal fat
perirenal fat
perisigmoid colon
perisinusoidal space
perisplenic soft tissue
peristalsis
peristaltic contraction
peristaltic rushes
peristaltic wave
perithelial cell
perithelioma
peritoneal abscess
peritoneal band
peritoneal cavity
  greater sac of
  lesser sac of
peritoneal effusion fluid
peritoneal fluid
peritoneal fold
peritoneal gutter
peritoneal ligament
peritoneal recess
peritoneal reflection
peritoneal sac
peritoneal scarring
peritoneal seeding
peritoneal space
peritoneum
  double-layered sheets of
  parietal
  pelvic
  visceral
peritonitis
peritonsillar abscess
peritubular contractile cell
periungual desquamation
periureteral abscess
periurethral cellulitis
periurethral phlegmon
perivascular canal
perivascular cuffing
perivascular goiter
perivascular lymphocytic infiltrate
perivascular mononuclear infiltrate
perivascular round-cell infiltrate
perivascular space
perivascularity
periventricular zone
perlèche
Perls Prussian blue stain
Perls test
permanent molar, first
permanent section
permanent teeth
permeable
permissive cell
Permount mounting medium
pernicious anemia
pernicious malaria
pernicious myocarditis
peroneal artery
peroneal atrophy
peroneal bone
peroneal nerve phenomenon
peroxidase-antiperoxidase (PAP) labeling method
peroxidase stain
peroxidase test
perpendicular plate of ethmoid bone
per se
persistent atrioventricular canal
persistent common atrioventricular canal
persistent hematuria
persistent truncus arteriosus
Perspex
Perthes-Legg-Calvé disease

pertussis (whooping cough)
pertussoid eosinophilic pneumonia
per volume units
pessary cell
pesticide, organophosphate
Pestivirus
petechia (pl. petechiae)
petechial angioma
petechial fever
petechial hemorrhage of viscera
Petit canal
Petit ligament
Pétrequin ligament
Petri dish
Petri test for proteins
petrobasilar articulation
petrobasilar joint
petroleum distillates poisoning
petro-occipital joint
petro-occipital suture
petrosal artery, superficial
petrosal bone
petrosal sinus
petrous bone
petrous ridge
Pette-Döring panencephalitis
Pettenkofer test for bile acids in urine
Petzetaki test for typhoid fever
Peyer gland
Peyer patches in ileum
Peyer plaque
Peyronie disease
PF (parafascicular) nucleus
Pfeiffer bacillus
Pfeiffer phenomenon
P-50 blood gas
p53 oncogene
p53 protein
p53 tumor suppressor gene
pg (picogram)
pH scale
pH, urine
PHA (phytohemagglutinin)
PHA antigen
PHA assay
Phaeoannellomyces
Phaeoannellomyces elegans
Phaeoannellomyces werneckii
Phaeococcomyces
phage, beta
phage typing of organisms
phagocyte
phagocytic cell immunocompetence profile
phagocytic cells
phagocytic index
phagocytic stellate cell
phagocytosis
phalangeal bone
phalangeal cell
phalangeal joint
phalanx (pl. phalanges)
phantom aneurysm
phantom limb
phantom pregnancy
PharmChek sweat patch drug detection system
pharyngeal aponeurosis
pharyngeal arch
pharyngeal artery
pharyngeal canal
pharyngeal gland
pharyngeal orifice of auditory tube
pharyngeal ostium of auditory tube
pharyngeal plague
pharyngeal plexus
pharyngeal pouch
pharyngeal tonsil
pharyngitis
  atrophic
  exudative
  follicular
  gangrenous
  hypertrophic

pharyngitis *(continued)*
  phlegmonous
  streptococcal
pharyngoconjunctival fever
pharyngoconjunctival fever virus
pharyngoesophageal sphincter
pharyngopalatine arch
pharynx
  laryngeal part of
  nasal part of
  oral part of
phase
  catagen
  follicular
  inadequate luteal
  luteal
  proliferative
  secretory
  telogen
phase-contrast
phase-defect, luteal
Phaseolus vulgaris
phase reactants
phenacetin
phenacetin test in urine
phenanthridium dye
phenol/chloroform method
phenol (carbolic acid) poisoning
phenolphthalein test
phenol red test
phenolsulfonphthalein (PSP) test for kidney function (also, phenol red)
phenoltetrachlorophthalein test for liver function
phenomenon (pl. phenomena)
  Anderson
  aqueous-influx
  blood-influx
  booster (on TB test)
  Bordet-Gengou
  Cushing
  Danysz

phenomenon *(continued)*
  dawn
  Debré
  Denys-Leclef
  d'Herelle
  embolic
  fall-and-rise
  first-set
  Gengou
  glass-rod
  halisteresis
  Hamburger
  Hektoen
  Houssay
  Koch
  Koebner
  LAK (lymphokine-activated killer) cell
  Lewis hydrophagocytosis
  Liacopoulos
  Liesegang
  Lucio
  Lust peroneal nerve
  Meirowsky
  Neisser-Wechsberg
  no-reflow
  peroneal nerve
  Pfeiffer
  reclotting
  Rumpel-Leede
  satellite
  Schramm
  second-set
  Somogyi
  Staub-Traugott
  Sulzberger-Chase
  Theobald Smith
  Twort-d'Herelle bacteriophagia
phenothiazine
phenotype
phenylalanine
phenylhydrazine test

phenylketonuria (PKU)
  atypical
  classic
  maternal
  transient
phenylthiocarbamoyl protein
pheochrome cell
pheochromocytoma
pheresis
phialides, flask-shaped
Phialophora bubakii
Phialophora dermatitidis
Phialophora parasitica
Phialophora pedrosoi
Phialophora repens
Phialophora richardsiae
Phialophora verrucosa
Philadelphia chromosome
Philip gland
Philippine dengue
Philippine hemorrhagic fever
Phillips 300 transmission electron microscope
philtrum
phimosis
phlebitic induration
phlebitis
phlebolith
phlebothrombosis
phlebotomus fever
phlebotomy
Phlebovirus
phlegmon
  Holz
  pancreatic
  periurethral
phlegmonous abscess
phlegmonous mastitis
phlogocyte
phlogocytosis
phloxine
phlyctenule ("flick-ten'-yule")
phoenix abscess
Phoma cruris-hominis
Phoma eupyrena
Phoma glomerata
Phoma herbarum
Phoma hibernica
Phoma oculo-hominis
phosphatase
  acid
  alkaline
  leukocyte acid
  placental alkaline (PLAP)
  prostatic acid (PAP)
  serum alkaline
phosphate
  ammonium magnesium
  amorphous
phosphate-buffered saline (PBS)
phosphate diabetes
phosphofructokinase (PFK) in erythrocytes
phosphomolybdic acid
phosphoric acid test
phosphorus (P)
phosphorus necrosis
phosphorus poisoning
phosphorylation
phosphotungstic acid
phosphotungstic acid hematoxylin (PTAH)
"phossy jaw" (osteomyelitis of maxilla and mandible)
photoallergic contact dermatitis
photoallergy
photo cell
photodermatitis
photopheresis therapy for T-cell lymphoma
photoreceptor cells
photosensitivity
phototoxic dermatitis
phrenic artery

phrenic nerve
phrenicocolic ligament
phrenicoesophageal ligament
phrenicolienal ligament
phrenicosplenic ligament
phrenoesophageal ligament
phrenoesophageal membrane
phrenogastric ligament
phrenosplenic ligament
phrygian cap deformity
phthiriasis
Phthirus pubis
phthisis (tuberculosis)
phycobiliprotein
phycoerythrin
Phycomycetes
phycomycetosis
phyllodes, cystosarcoma
phyllolith
phyma
phymatorrhysin
physaliphorous cell
physical diagnosis
physical examination
Physick pouch
physiologic atrophy
physiologic hypertrophy
physiologic jaundice
physiologic proteinuria
phytoagglutinin
phytohemagglutinin (PHA) antigen
phytophotodermatitis
pia mater
pian (yaws)
Pichinde virus
Pick body
Pick cell
Pick disease
Picker nodule
Pick inclusion body
Pick-Niemann disease
picogram (pg)
picoliter (pL)
picometer (pm)
picomole (pmol)
picornavirus
picric acid
picrocarmine stain
picroformol fixative
picro-Mallory trichrome stain
picronigrosin stain
PID (pelvic inflammatory disease)
piecemeal necrosis
piedra
Piedraia hortae
piercer tissue
Pierre Robin syndrome
pigeon-breeder's lung
pigeon-breeder's pneumonitis
pigment
- anthracotic
- bile
- blood
- blotchy clumping of
- endogenous
- exogenous
- fatty
- hematogenous
- hemosiderin-like
- hepatogenous
- lipid
- malarial
- melanotic
- respiratory
- retinal
- visual
- wear and tear

pigmental degeneration
pigmentary atrophy
pigmentary degeneration
pigmentation
pigment cell of skin
pigment cirrhosis
pigmented epidermis

pigmented hair epidermal nevus
pigmented hairy nevus
pigmented lesion (melanotic)
pigmented melanocytic proliferation
pigmented mole
pigmented nevus
pigmented purpuric lichenoid dermatitis
pigmented villonodular synovitis
pigmentosa, retinitis
pilar cyst
pilar sheath
pile, sentinel
piles (hemorrhoids)
pillar
pillar cells of Corti
pillar of fauces, anterior
pillowlike consistency
piloleiomyoma
pilomatricoma
pilonidal cyst
pilonidal fistula
pilonidal sinus
pilosebaceous follicle
pilosebaceous unit
pilus (pl. pili)
Pincus test
pine wood test for indole
pineal body
pineal cells
pineal cyst
pineal gland
pineal hormone
pinealocyte
pinealocytoma
pinealoma
pineal teratoma
pineal ventricle
pineapple test for butyric acid in stomach
pineocytoma
ping-pong bone
pink eye
pink stria
pink urine
pinna
pinocyte
pinocytic mouth
pinocytosis
pinta
pinta fever
pinworm
pinworm infestation
pinworm preparation
PIP (proximal interphalangeal) joint
pipe bone
piperidine cleavage
pipestem artery
pipestem cirrhosis
pipestem fibrosis
pipestem stool
pipet (pipette)
pipette
Piria test for tyrosine
Pirie bone
piriform
piriform sinus
Piry virus
pisiform articulation
pisiform bone
pisiform bone articulation
pisiform joint
pisocuneiform articulation
pisohamate ligament
pisometacarpal ligament
pisotriquetral joint
pisounciform ligament
pisouncinate ligament
pit
  anal
  articular
  auditory
  central
  colonic
  costal

pit *(continued)*
  cutaneous
  gastric
  postanal
pit of stomach
pitted subcapsular surface
pitted surface
Pittsburgh pneumonia
pituicytes
pituitary cyst
pituitary dwarfism
pituitary failure
pituitary gigantism
pituitary gland
pituitary gonadotropic hormone
pituitary hormone
pituitary, hyperplasia of
pituitary sinusoid
pityriasis alba
pityriasis alba atrophicas
pityriasis capitis
pityriasis circinata
pityriasis, lichenoid
pityriasis lichenoides et varioliformis acuta (PLEVA)
pityriasis linguae
pityriasis maculata
pityriasis nigra
pityriasis rosea
pityriasis rotunda
pityriasis rubra
pityriasis rubra pilaris
pityriasis sicca (dandruff)
pityriasis versicolor (tinea versicolor)
pityrodes, alopecia
Pityrosporum
Pityrosporum orbiculare
PIVKA-II levels
pivot articulation
pivot joint
pixielike facial features
PiZZ alpha antitrypsin
PKU (phenylketonuria)
pL (picoliter)
placenta
  abnormal adherence of
  accessory
  adherent
  annular
  battledore
  bilobate
  chorioallantoic
  chorioamniotic
  cirsoid
  deciduate
  Duncan
  fetal
  fundal
  horseshoe
  incarcerated
  kidney-shaped
  maternal
  nondeciduate
  panduriform
  retained
  Schultze
  third-trimester
  velamentous
  villous
placenta accreta
placenta increta
placenta percreta
placenta previa
  central
  complete
  incomplete
  lateral
  marginal
  partial
  total
placenta protein
placental alkaline phosphatase (PLAP)
placental disk
placental grade

placental lactogen hormone
placental membrane
placental polyp
placental transfusion
placental villi
placental zone
placode, dorsolateral
plague
  ambulatory
  black
  bubonic
  hemorrhagic
  lung
  meningeal
  pharyngeal
  pneumonic
  pulmonic
  septicemic
  white
plague bacillus
plague meningitis
plane
  auriculo-infraorbital
  axiolabiolingual
  axiomesiodistal
  bite
  coronal
  datum
  eye-ear
  facial
  first parallel pelvic
  fourth parallel pelvic
  Frankfort
  Frankfort horizontal
  frontal
  horizontal
  interspinous
  median
  sagittal
  subcostal (SCP)
  supracristal (SCP)
  transpyloric

plane *(continued)*
  transtubercular (TTP)
  transumbilical (TUP)
plane joint
plane of fifth intercostal space
plantar
plantar aponeurosis
plantar arch
plantar artery
plantar calcaneocuboid ligament
plantar calcaneonavicular ligament
plantar cuboideonavicular ligament
plantar cuneocuboid ligament
plantar cuneonavicular ligament
plantar ligament
plantar metatarsal ligament
plantaris aponeurosis
planus, lichen
PLAP (placental alkaline phosphatase)
plaque
  argyrophil
  arteriosclerotic
  atheromatous
  bacteriophage
  calcific
  cutaneous
  dental
  eczematous
  fibromyelinic
  fibrous
  flat
  gastrointestinal
  Hollenhorst
  Hutchinson
  iliac
  infiltrating
  Lichtheim
  neuritic
  Peyer
  pleural
  Randall
  Redlich-Fisher miliary

plaque *(continued)*
  rock-hard
  senile
  yellowish-gray
plaque of glial fibrils as repair material
plaquing
plasma
  antihemophilic
  barium sulfate-absorbed
  blood
  celite-absorbed
  citrated
  consisting of
    dissolved gases
    electrolytes
    nutrients
    proteins
    wastes
    water
  fresh normal
  normal human
  oxalate
  pooled
  salt
  seminal
  supernatant
  true
plasma assay
plasma bicarbonate
plasmablast
plasma buffer
plasma cell (plasmacyte)
plasma cell granuloma
plasma cell hepatitis
plasma cell leukemia
plasma cell mastitis
plasma cell myeloma
plasma cell pneumonia
plasma cell pneumonitis (PCP)
plasma clotting factor
plasmacyte
plasmacytic infiltrate
plasmacytic leukemia
plasmacytoma
plasmacytosis
plasma fraction
plasma hemoglobin
plasma labile factor
plasma lactic acid
plasma leaks from capillaries and venules
plasma lipid
plasma lipoprotein level
plasma membrane
plasmapheresis
plasma pool
plasma protein
plasma protein fibrinogen
plasma protein fraction
plasma proteins
plasma renin activity (PRA)
plasmarrhexis
plasma stain
plasma thromboplastin component (PTC)
plasma volume
plasmid
  conjugative
  F
  oligomeric
  R
plasminogen
plasminogen activator inhibition (PAI) assay
plasmocyte
Plasmodium
plasmodium embolism
Plasmodium falciparum
Plasmodium malariae
Plasmodium ovale
Plasmodium vivax
plastic clot
plastic induration
plasticine

plastic pleurisy
plastic plug
plastic section stain
plastic trocar plug
plate
  agar
  alar
  anal
  auditory
  axial
  basal
  base
  blood
  bone
  bony
  budding
  cardiogenic
  cell
  chorionic
  clinoid
  cloacal
  cortical
  cough
  cribriform
  cutis
  end
  epiphyseal
  epiphyseal cartilage
  equatorial
  ethmovomerine
  frontal
  growth
  hilar
  liver cell
  streak
  tarsal
platelet-activating factor
platelet adhesion test
platelet aggregation
platelet aggregation inhibitor
platelet antibody
platelet count (thrombocyte count)
platelet-derived growth factor
platelet distribution width (PDW)
platelet factor
platelet function
  abnormal
  impaired
platelet indices
platelet metamorphosis
platelet-poor blood (PPB)
platelet-poor plasma (PPP)
platelet protein
platelet-rich plasma (PRP)
platelet, Thrombosphere synthetic
platelike cell
platypelloid pelvis
Plaut bacillus
pleiotropic gene
pleocytosis of cerebrospinal fluid
pleomorphic cell
pleomorphic lymphoma
pleomorphism
Plesiomonas shigelloides (formerly *Aeromonas shigelloides*)
pleura (pl. pleurae)
  biopsy of
  cervical
  costodiaphragmatic recess of
  diaphragmatic
  mediastinal
  mesothelioma of
  parietal
  visceral
pleuracentesis
pleural calculus
pleural canal
pleural cavity
pleural cupola
pleural effusion fluid
pleural fibroma
pleural fluid
pleural plaque
pleural recess

pleural reflection
  costal
  mediastinodiaphragmatic
  sternal
  vertebral
pleural space
pleural tuberculosis
pleurisy
  acute
  adhesive
  blocked
  cholesterol
  chronic
  chyliform
  chylous
  circumscribed
  costal
  diaphragmatic
  diffuse
  double
  dry
  encysted
  exudative
  fibrinous
  hemorrhagic
  ichorous
  indurative
  interlobular
  latent
  mediastinal
  metapneumonic
  plastic
  primary
  proliferating
  pulmonary
  pulsating
  purulent
  sacculated
  secondary
  serofibrinous
  serous
  single

pleurisy *(continued)*
  suppurative
  typhoid
  visceral
pleuritic pneumonia
pleuritis
pleurodynia, epidemic
pleurogenic pneumonia
pleurolith
pleuropericardial canal
pleuroperitoneal canal
pleuropericardial effusion
pleuroperitoneal membrane
pleuropneumonia
pleuropneumonia-like organism
  (PPLO)
plexiform
plexus (pl. plexuses)
  abdominal aortic
  aortic
  Auerbach
  Auerbach mesenteric
  autonomic
  axillary
  basilar
  biliary
  brachial
  cardiac
  cavernous
  celiac
  cervical
  choroid
  ciliary ganglionic
  coccygeal
  colic
  colonic myenteric
  common carotid
  coronary
  cystic
  deep
  deferential
  enteric

plexus *(continued)*
- facial
- femoral
- gastric
- gastroesophageal variceal
- hemorrhoidal
- hepatic nerge
- hypogastric
- inferior mesenteric
- intermesenteric
- lymph
- Meissner
- nerve
- pampiniform
- pharyngeal
- presacral
- prostatic venous
- rectal
- sacral
- solar
- submucosal venous
- superficial
- superior hypogastric
- superior mesenteric
- uterovaginal
- vaginal
- vascular
- vertebral
- vesical
- vesical venous

pliable tissue
plica semilunaris (semilunar fold)
plicae circulares (circular folds)
plicae transversales (transverse folds)
PLP (parathyroid hormonelike protein)
plug
- epithelial
- keratin
- meconium
- mucus
- plastic
- skin

plug of mucous membrane
Plugge test for phenol
plugging, follicular
plump nuclei
plunging goiter
plural pregnancy
pluripotential cell
pm (picometer)
PML (progressive multifocal leukoencephalopathy)
PMN (polymorphonuclear leukocyte)
pmol (picomole)
pneumatic bone
pneumatic cell
pneumococcal meningitis
pneumococcal myocarditis
pneumococcal pneumonia
pneumococcus nephritis
Pneumococcus
pneumoconiosis
pneumocystiasis
pneumocystis pneumonia
Pneumocystis carinii pneumonia (PCP)
pneumocytosis
pneumonia (see also *pneumonitis*)
- abortive
- acute
- acute eosinophilic
- alcoholic
- allergic
- amebic
- anthrax
- apex
- apical
- aspiration
- atypical
- atypical bronchial
- atypical interstitial
- bacterial
- bilious
- bronchial
- bronchiolitis obliterans organizing

pneumonia *(continued)*
Buhl desquamative
capillary
caseous
catarrhal
central
cerebral
cheesy
chronic
chronic eosinophilic
classic interstitial
cold agglutinin
community-acquired
consolidative
contusion
Corrigan
Cryptococcus neoformans
deglutition
delayed resolution of
desquamative
desquamative interstitial (DIP)
double
Eaton agent
embolic
endogenous lipoid
eosinophilic
ephemeral
Escherichia coli (*E. coli*)
exogenous
fibrinous
fibrous
Friedländer
fungal
gangrenous
giant cell
granulomatous
gray hepatization stage of
Haemophilus influenzae
Hecht
hypersensitivity
hypostatic
incomplete resolution of

pneumonia *(continued)*
indurative
infantile
influenzal virus
inhalation
interstitial
interstitial plasma cell
intrauterine
irradiation
Klebsiella
Legionella
lipoid
lobar
lobular
lymphoid interstitial
massive
metastatic
migratory
Mycoplasma
mycoplasmal
necrotizing
nonbacterial
nosocomial
obstructive
oil-aspiration
parenchymatous
passive
pertussoid eosinophilic
Pittsburgh
plague
plasma cell
pleuritic
pleurogenetic
pleurogenic
pneumococcal
pneumocystis
Pneumocystis carinii (PCP)
postobstructive
postoperative
post-traumatic
primary atypical
Proteus

pneumonia *(continued)*
  protozoal
  Pseudomonas
  purulent
  red hepatization stage of
  rheumatic
  rickettsial
  secondary
  segmental
  septic
  staphylococcal
  streptococcal
  Streptococcus
  subacute allergic
  superficial
  suppurative
  terminal
  toxemic
  toxic
  traumatic
  tuberculous
  tularemic
  typhoid
  unresolved
  vagus
  varicella
  viral
  wandering
  white
  woolsorter's
pneumonic plague
pneumonitis (see also *pneumonia*)
  acid aspiration
  acute interstitial
  aspiration
  bacterial
  chemical
  cholesterol
  chronic
  congenital rubella
  cytomegalovirus
  early
pneumonitis *(continued)*
  granulomatous
  hypersensitivity
  interstitial
  interstitial plasma cell
  lipoid
  lymphocytic interstitial
  malarial
  manganese
  Mycoplasma (mycoplasmal)
  pigeon-breeder's
  plasma cell (PCP)
  pneumocystis
  radiation
  staphylococcal
  trimellitic anhydritic
  uremic
  ventilation
pneumonocyte
  granular
  membranous
pneumonolipoidosis
pneumonolysis
pneumonomelanosis
pneumonomoniliasis
pneumonomycosis
pneumonophthisis
pneumorenal syndrome
pneumosepticemia
pneumosilicosis
pneumothorax
Pneumovirus
PNH (paroxysmal nocturnal
  hemoglobinuria) cell
PNH cell
PO_2 (partial pressure of oxygen in
  arterial blood)
podocyte
Pohl test for globulins
poikilocyte
poikilocyte in peripheral blood
poikilocytosis

poikiloderma
point
  Addison
  alveolar
  apophysary
  apophyseal
  auricular
  Boas
  cardinal
  Chauffard
  cold-rigor
  congruent
  craniometric
  Desjardins
  dorsal
  end
  Hartmann
  Lanz
  Mackenzie
  McBurney
  midinguinal
  Munro
  Ramond
  Robson
  Sudeck
pointed condyloma
Poirier gland
Poirier space
Poiseville space
poisoning
  acidic salts
  alcohol
  arsenic
  bacterial food
  benzene
  carbon monoxide
  chemical
  chloroform
  copper
  cyanide
  dinitrophenol
  fluoride
poisoning *(continued)*
  food
  heavy metal
  hydrogen sulfide
  insecticide
  lead
  mercury
  mushroom
  naphthalene
  nitrogen oxides
  organophosphate
  petroleum distillates
  phenol
  phosphorus
  shellfish food
  snake venom
  thallium
  tobacco
  zinc
poison ivy dermatitis
poison oak dermatitis
poison sumac dermatitis
pokeweed mitogen
polar cell
polar cushion (Polkissen)
polarity, cell
polarization
polarized light
polarizing microscope
pole
  abapical
  cephalic
  frontal
  germinal
  inferior
  superior
  temporal
poles of organ
poles of vessels
poliomyelitis
poliomyelitis virus
poliovirus

Pollacci test for urine albumin
pollens, inhaled
polyacrylamide gel
polyalveolar lobe
polyarteritis nodosa (PAN)
polyarthritis, migratory
polyaxial joint
polychromatic cell
polychromatophil cell
polychromatophilic normoblast
polychrome methylene blue stain
polychrome stain
polycystic kidney
polycystic ovary
polycystic ovary syndrome
polycyte
polycythemia
polycythemia vera
polyethylene glycol (PEG)
polygonal cell
polygonal chromophobe cell
polyhedral cell
polymastia
polymer
polymerase chain reaction (PCR)
polymer fume fever
polymerization
polymorphic fungi
polymorphocellular
polymorphocyte
polymorphonuclear infiltrate of dermis
polymorphonuclear leukocyte (PMN)
polymyalgia rheumatica
polymyositis, primary idiopathic
polymyositis-dermatomyositis
polyneuritis, acute idiopathic
polynuclear
Polyomavirus, polyomavirus
polyp
- adenomatous
- benign
- bleeding

polyp *(continued)*
- bronchial
- cardiac
- cellular
- cervical
- choanal
- colon
- colonic
- cystic
- dental
- endometrial
- fibrinous
- fibroepithelial
- gastric
- gelatinous
- Hopmann
- hydatid
- hyperplastic
- inflammatory
- juvenile
- laryngeal
- lipomatous
- lymphoid
- metastatic
- mucous
- multiple
- myomatous
- nasal
- osseous
- pedunculated masses of
- placental
- polypoid adenocarcinoma
- pulp
- regenerative
- retention
- sessile
- sigmoid
- single
- uterine
- vascular
- villous

polyp stalk

polypeptide
gastric inhibitory (GIP)
glucose-dependent
insulinotropic (GIP)
islet amyloid (IAPP)
pancreatic (PP)
parathyroid-like
vasoactive intestinal (VIP)
polypeptide antigen
polypeptide chain
polyphrenic gene
polyplastic cell
polypoid mass
polyposis
familial
familial adenomatous (FAP)
familial intestinal
gastric
multiple intestinal
polypropylene line
polyptychic gland
"polys" (slang for polymorphonuclear leukocytes)
polysaccharide
polytene chromosome
polythelia
polyuria
polyvinylidene difluoride membrane
Pompe disease
Pongola virus
pons
Pontamine sky blue stain
Pontiac fever
pontine
pontine artery
pontine cistern
pool
abdominal
bile acid
blood
plasma
pooled plasma
pooling, vallecular
poorly differentiated adenocarcinoma
poorly differentiated carcinoma
popliteal artery
porencephaly
pores of Kohn
Porges-Meier flocculation test for syphilis
porokeratosis
poroma
porphobilinogen (PBG)
porphyria
acute
acute intermittent (AIP)
congenital
congenital erythropoietic (CEP)
cutaneous hepatic
erythrohepatic
erythropoietic
hepatic
hepatoerythropoietic (HEP)
symptomatic
variegate (VP)
porphyria cutanea tarda (PCT)
porphyrin
porphyrinemia
porphyrins in blood and urine
porphyrinuria
Porphyromonas asaccharolytica
portacaval anastomosis
porta hepatis
portal canal
portal cirrhosis
portal hypertension
portal lobule
portal pyemia
portal space
portal-systemic anastomotic area
portal system of veins
portal triad
portal vascular bed
portal vein

portal venous system
portal zone
Porter test for excess of uric acid
portion, intramural
port-wine nevus
port-wine stain
positive
  false
  gram
  Nitrazine
  Rh
positive charge
positive control
positive stain
positive test for occult blood
positive whiff
Posner test for albumin
"post" (postmortem examination)
postanal pit
postcoital bleeding
postcoital test
postcricoid area
postcricoid web
posterior abdominal wall
posterior alveolar artery
posterior annular ligament of wrist
posterior auricular artery
posterior auricular nerve
posterior auricular vein
posterior border of lung
posterior cell
posterior cerebral artery
posterior chamber
posterior clinoid process
posterior communicating artery
posterior cricoarytenoid ligament
posterior cruciate ligament
posterior cusp
posterior dental artery
posterior ethmoidal air cell
posterior ethmoidal sinus
posterior femoral cutaneous nerve
posterior fontanelle
posterior fornix of vagina
posterior fossa meningioma
posterior humeral circumflex artery
posterior inferior cerebellar artery
posterior intercostal artery
posterior interosseous artery
posterior intraoccipital joint
posterior layer of rectus sheath
posterior ligament of head of fibula
posterior ligament of incus
posterior ligament of knee
posterior longitudinal ligament
posterior mediastinum
posterior meniscofemoral ligament
posterior muscle, serratus
posterior occipitoaxial ligament
posterior pancreaticoduodenal artery
posterior papillary muscle
posterior recess of ischiorectal fossa
posterior rectus sheath
posterior sacroiliac ligament
posterior sacrosciatic ligament
posterior scapular artery
posterior scrotal artery
posterior semicircular canal
posterior spinal artery
posterior sternoclavicular ligament
posterior superior alveolar artery
posterior surface of pancreas
posterior surface of prostate
posterior synechiae
posterior talofibular ligament
posterior talotibial ligament
posterior tibial artery
posterior tibiofibular ligament
posterior tibiotalar ligament
posterior triangle
posterior uveitis
posterior vagal trunk
posterior wall
posterolateral fontanelle

posterolateral sclerosis
postfebrile neuritis
postganglionic fiber, unmyelinated
post-heparin lipolytic activity test
posthepatitic cirrhosis
posthitis
postinfectious myelitis
postinflammatory hypopigmentation
postinflammatory leukoderma
postischemic acute renal failure
postmenopausal atrophy
postmenopausal bleeding
postmenopausal osteoporosis
postmenopausal syndrome
postmenopausal women
postmortem clot
postmortem delivery
postmortem examination ("post")
postmortem hypostasis
postmortem livedo
postmortem lividity
postmortem pustule
postmortem rigidity
postmortem suggillation
postmortem thrombus
postmortem tubercle
postmortem wart
postmyocardial infarction pericarditis
postnecrotic cirrhosis
postobstructive pneumonia
postocular optic neuritis
postoperative diagnosis
postoperative infection
postoperative pneumonia
postoperative pressure alopecia
postpartum alopecia
postpartum hemorrhage
postpartum hypertension
postpartum pituitary necrosis
postpericardiotomy pericarditis
postprandial blood-sugar level,
  two-hour
postprandial glucose
postprandial lipemia
postprandial test
postprimary tuberculosis
post-radiation change
postrenal azotemia
postrenal proteinuria
postsphenoid bone
post-term pregnancy
post-transfusion hepatitis
post-traumatic atrophy of bone
post-traumatic osteoporosis
post-traumatic pericarditis
post-traumatic pneumonia
postural proteinuria
postvaccinal myelitis
postvertebral muscle
"post" (postmortem exam)
potassium (K)
potassium bichromate
potassium dichromate
potassium ferricyanide
potassium hydroxide (KOH)
potassium hydroxide (KOH) solution
potassium iodide test
potassium-losing nephritis
potassium metabisulfite
potassium permanganate
potential space
Pott abscess
Pott aneurysm
Pott disease
pouch
  antral
  apophyseal
  blind
  branchial
  Broca pudendal
  celomic
  deep perineal
  Denis Browne
  Douglas rectouterine

pouch *(continued)*
- endodermal
- gastric
- Hartmann
- haustral
- Heidenhain
- hepatorenal
- hypophysial
- ileoanal
- ileocecal
- jejunal
- Kock
- Morison
- paracystic
- pararectal
- paravesical
- pendulous
- pharyngeal
- Physick
- Prussak
- Rathke
- rectal
- rectouterine
- rectovaginal
- rectovaginouterine
- rectovesical
- renal
- Seessel (note: 2 e's, 2 s's)
- superficial inguinal
- superficial perineal
- ultimobranchial
- uterovesical
- vesicoureterine
- water-filled
- Zenker

pouchlike
pouch of Douglas
pounds per square inch (psi, p.s.i.)
Poupart ligament, shelving edge of
pour plate
Powassan virus
powder burn
power
- high (microscope)
- low (microscope)
- scanning

poxvirus (also, pox virus)
PPB (platelet-poor blood)
PP cell
PPD skin test
PRA (plasma renin activity)
PRA (progesterone receptor assay)
Prague pelvis
preampullary portion of bile duct
pre-B cell
precancerous dermatitis
precancerous lesion
precipitates (KPs), keratic
precipitation
precipitation reaction
precipitation test
precipitin
precipitin test
Precision-G handheld blood glucose test
precision of laboratory test
Precision Q-I-D handheld blood glucose test
preclinical diabetes
precocious sexual development
precursor cell
predator damage
predilection
predisposing factor
predominant
prefollicle cell
preganglionic fiber
preganglionic sympathetic fibers
pregangrenous
pregnancy
- abdominal
- aborted ectopic
- ampullar
- bigeminal

pregnancy *(continued)*
- broad ligament
- cervical
- combined
- compound
- cornual
- ectopic
- extrauterine
- fallopian
- false
- heterotopic
- hydatid
- hysteric
- interstitial
- intraligamentary
- intraperitoneal
- membranous
- mesenteric
- molar
- multiple
- mural
- nervous
- ovarian
- ovarioabdominal
- oviductal
- parietal
- phantom
- plural
- post-term
- prolonged
- pseudointraligamentary
- sarcofetal
- sarcohysteric
- spurious
- stump
- toxemia of
- tubal
- tuboabdominal
- tuboligamentary
- tubo-ovarian
- tubouterine
- twin

pregnancy *(continued)*
- uteroabdominal
- uterotubal

pregnancy cell
pregnancy diabetes
pregnancy gland
pregnancy test
pregnanetriol test
pregnenolone test
pregranulosa cell
prehyalin
prehyoid gland
preileal appendix
preinterparietal bone
Preisz-Nocard bacillus
prekallikrein
preliminary diagnosis
premalignant neoplasm
premammary abscess
premature alopecia
premature birth
premaxillary bone
premeasured reagent
premenstrual edema
premolar tissue
prenatal diagnosis
prenatal genetic diagnosis
prenatal sex determination
preoccipital notch
preoperative diagnosis
prepancreatic artery
prepapillary bile duct
preparation
- cytospin
- impression
- KOH (potassium hydroxide)
- LE cell
- Nuclepore prep
- sickle cell
- tissue

prepatellar bursitis
preperitoneal fat

preperitoneal space
prepuce of clitoris
preputial gland
prepyloric antrum
prepyloric sphincter
prepyloric vein
prerenal azotemia
prerenal proteinuria
presacral plexus
presacral space
presegmental artery
presphenoid bone
pressure alopecia
pressure atrophy
pressure cooker technique
pressure epiphysis
pressure, intrathoracic
pressure necrosis
pressure-type groove
pressure-volume loop
prestyloid recess
presumptive diagnosis
pre-T cell
preternatural anus
pretibial edema
pretibial fever
prevertebral artery
prevertebral ganglia
Prevotella bivia
Prevotella disiens
Prevotella intermedia
Prevotella loeschii
Prevotella melaninogenica
Prevotella oralis
Prevotella oris
Preyer test
prickle cell
prickle-cell layer of epidermis
primary aldosteronism
primary amyloidosis
primary atypical pneumonia
primary biliary cirrhosis
primary cartilaginous joints
primary center of ossification
primary disease
primary embryonic cell
primary hematuria
primary hypertension
primary idiopathic polymyositis
primary irritant dermatitis
primary lesion
primary lymphoma of central nervous system
primary malignancy
primary metabolism
primary methemoglobinemia
primary multiple myositis
primary myeloid metaplasia
primary pleurisy
primary progressive cerebellar degeneration
primary pyoderma
primary ramus
primary tuberculosis
prime movers
primipara (para 1)
primitive aorta
primitive cell
primitive gland
primitive granulosa cell
primitive reticular cell
primitive wandering cell
primordial cell
primordial cyst
primordial follicle
primordial germ cell
primordium
principal artery of pterygoid canal
principal artery of thumb
principal bronchus
principal cell
principal diagnosis
prion protein
pro time (prothrombin time)

proaccelerin
proactivator, C_3
probe patent
Probe Tech II
procedure
  diagnosis
  HPV genotyping
  immunoblot
  Northern blot (NB)
  Southern blot (SB)
  Western blot (WB)
process
  accessory
  acromial
  alar
  alveolar
  apical
  articular
  ascending
  auditory
  basilar
  calcaneal
  caudate
  ciliary
  clinoid
  cochleariform
  condyloid
  conoid
  coracoid
  costal
  dendritic
  ensiform
  ethmoidal
  falciforn
  fibroplastic
  frontal
  frontonasal
  frontosphenoidal
  transverse
  uncinate
  vertebral spinous
  xiphoid
processing of tissue specimen
process of fat, digital
process of maxilla, alveolar
process of pancreas, uncinate
process of vertebra, articular
proconvertin (Factor VII)
proctitis
production antibody
productive nephritis
products of conception
proerythroblasts in marrow
profile
  antigenic
  biochemical
  chemistry
  executive
  lipid
  liver
  phagocytic cell immunocompetence
  test
  thyroid
  20-channel chemistry
  urethral pressure
profuse sweat
progenitalis, herpes
progenitor
progestational endometrium
progestational hormone
progestational pattern
progesterone
progesterone hormone
progesterone receptor assay (PRA)
proglottid
prognosis, grave
programmed cell death
progranulocyte
progressive choroidal atrophy
progressive degeneration
progressive emphysematous necrosis
progressive multifocal leuko-
  encephalopathy (PML)
progressive muscular atrophy

progressive muscular dystrophy
progressive neural muscular atrophy
progressive ossifying myositis
progressive spinal muscular atrophy
progressive staining
progressive subcortical atrophy
progressive systemic sclerosis
progressive unilateral facial atrophy
progressive visual impairment
proinsulin
projectile horn
projection, enamel
prokaryotic cell
prolactin
prolactin anterior pituitary hormone
prolactin cell
prolactin hormone (hPRL)
prolactin-inhibiting factor
prolactin-inhibiting hormone
prolactin–insulin stimulation test
prolactin-releasing factor
prolactin-releasing hormone
prolactin, serum
prolactoliberin hormone
proliferans, retinitis
proliferating astrocytes
proliferating by mitosis
proliferating pleurisy
proliferation
  bony
  cellular
  fibroplastic
  nodular
  papillary
  pigmented melanocytic
proliferation of amastigotes in dermal cells
proliferation of fibroblasts
proliferation of fibrous tissue
proliferative dermatitis
proliferative endometrium
proliferative glomerulitis
proliferative glomerulonephritis
proliferative inflammation
proliferative myositis
proliferative pattern
proliferative periostitis
proliferative stage
proliferative synovitis
prolonged bleeding from wounds
prolonged pregnancy
prolymphocyte
prominent nucleus
prominent scalene tubercle
promontory
promyelocyte
promyelocytic anemia
pronormoblast
pronounced dead
proparathyroid hormone
properdin test
proper ligament of ovary
properitoneal fat
properitoneal flank stripe (on x-ray)
propidium iodide
Propionibacterium acnes (formerly *Corynebacterium acnes*)
Propionibacterium avidum
Propionibacterium freudenreichii
Propionibacterium granulosum
Propionibacterium jensenii
propionic acid
propria
  lamina
  substantia
  tunica
prorubricyte
prosector
prospective recipient
prostaglandin test
prostate
  adenocarcinoma of
  apex of
  inferolateral surfaces of

prostate *(continued)*
  lateral lobe of
  lymph vessels of
  median lobe of
  posterior surface of
prostate chip
prostate gland
prostate specific antigen (PSA)
prostatic abscess
prostatic acid phosphatase (PAP)
prostatic adenocarcinoma
prostatic calculus (pl. calculi)
prostatic capsule
prostatic carcinoma
prostatic concretion
prostatic cyst
prostatic duct
prostatic fluid
prostatic hyperplasia
prostatic malignancy
prostatic shaving
prostatic sinus
prostatic urethra
prostatic venous plexus
prostatitis
  acute
  chronic
Protargol
protection test
protective layer of fat
protective protein
protein
  abnormal mitochondrial
  acute phase
  acyl carrier
  alcohol-soluble
  amyloid A (AA)
  androgen binding (ABP)
  antitumor
  antiviral (AVP)
  autologous
  bacterial

protein *(continued)*
  bacterial cellular
  Bence Jones
  binding
  bone morphogenetic
  carrier
  cationic
  CD14 membrane
  c-erb
  cerebrospinal fluid
  C4 binding
  c-myc
  coagulated
  complete
  compound
  conjugated
  constitutive
  cord
  C-reactive (CRP)
  CSF (cerebrospinal fluid)
  deficiency
  denatured
  derived
  desmoplakin
  DNA tumor virus
  encephalitogenic
  fibrillar
  fibrous
  floating
  foreign
  G
  glial fibrillary acidic (GFAP)
  globular
  GM activator
  guanyl-nucleotide-binding
  heat shock
  Hektoen, Kretschmer, and Welker
  heterologous
  HIV
  homologous
  immune
  incomplete

protein *(continued)*
- insoluble
- integral
- intrinsic
- iodized
- iron-sulfur
- leukocyte adhesion (LAP)
- M
- macrophage inflammatory
- maintenance
- MCP-1 (monocyte chemoattractant)
- metabolism, disorders of
- microtubule-associated (MAP)
- mutant
- myelin basic (MBP)
- myeloblastic
- myeloma
- myofilament
- native
- neurofilament triplet
- neutrophil activating (NAP)
- non-heme iron
- nonspecific
- odorant binding
- p53
- parathyroid hormonelike (PLP)
- partial
- peripheral
- phenylthiocarbamoyl
- placenta
- plasma
- platelet
- prion
- protective
- pS2
- purified placental
- R
- racemized
- receptor
- retinol-binding (RBP)
- S100
- serum

protein *(continued)*
- serum amyloid A (SAA)
- simple
- sphingolipid activator (SAP)
- staphylococcal A
- stimulatory (SP1)
- strong silver
- structure
- synthetic
- Tamm-Horsfall
- thyroxine-binding (TBP)
- total
- transport
- troponin T
- uncoupling
- unwinding
- urinary
- vitamin D-binding (DBP)
- water-soluble
- whole
- Z-
- zinc finger

protein A
proteinaceous
proteinase, cysteine
proteinase enzyme
proteinase K
protein C
protein C deficiency
protein C inhibitor (PCI)
protein concentration of spinal fluid, total
protein electrophoresis
proteinemia, Bence Jones
protein factor
protein hyaline
protein hydrolysate
protein in spinal fluid
protein in urine
proteinosis
- lipoid
- pulmonary alveolar

protein phosphatase
protein-rich fluid
protein S (*not* S protein)
protein shell of virus particle
protein test
proteinuria
  accidental
  adventitious
  athletic
  Bence Jones
  colliquative
  dietetic
  effort
  emulsion
  enterogenic
  essential
  false
  febrile
  functional
  gestational
  globular
  gouty
  hematogenous
  intermittent
  isolated
  light-chain
  lordotic
  mixed
  nephrogenous
  nonisolated
  orthostatic
  overflow
  palpatory
  paroxysmal
  physiologic
  postrenal
  postural
  prerenal
  pyogenic
  regulatory
  renal
  serous

proteinuria *(continued)*
  transient
  true
proteinuria praetuberculosa
proteolytic enzyme
proteose test
Proteus
Proteus hydrophilus
Proteus inconstans subgroup B
Proteus mirabilis
Proteus morganii
Proteus Ox-19 antibody
Proteus Ox-2 antibody
Proteus Ox-K antibody
Proteus penneri
Proteus pneumonia
Proteus rettgeri
Proteus vulgaris
Proteus zenkeri
prothrombin
prothrombin consumption test (PCT)
prothrombin-proconvertin test
prothrombin test
prothrombin time (pro time, PT)
  one-stage (Quick)
  two-stage modified
    (Ware and Seegers)
prothrombin time ratio
protocol, GTC/silica beads
Protocult test
proto-oncogene
protoplasm
protoporphyrin
protozoa
protozoal myocarditis
protozoal pneumonia
protruded disk
protruding
protuberant
proudflesh
Proust space
Providencia

Providencia alcalifaciens
Providencia rettgeri
Providencia stuartii
provisional anatomic diagnosis
Prower-Stuart factor
proximal clot
proximal interphalangeal joint
proximal muscles
proximal part of dorsal pancreatic duct
proximal phalanges
proximal radioulnar articulation
proximal radioulnar joint
proximal tibiofibular joint
proximally
prurigo ("itch")
  Besnier
  Hebra
  melanotic
  nodular
  summer p. of Hutchinson
prurigo actinic
prurigo aestivalis (also, estivalis)
prurigo agria
prurigo chronica multiformis
prurigo ferox
prurigo gestationis
prurigo infantilis
prurigo mitis
prurigo simplex
pruritic eruption
pruritic urticarial papules of pregnancy
pruritus
  aquagenic
  essential
  senile
  symptomatic
  uremic
pruritus aestivalis (summer itch)
pruritus ani
pruritus at site of skin invasion (ground itch)
pruritus balnea (bath itch)
pruritus hiemalis
pruritus scroti
pruritus vulvae
Prussak pouch
Prussak space
Prussian blue stain
pS2 protein
PSA (prostate specific antigen)
psammoma body
psammomatous meningioma
psammous
Pseudallescheria boydii
pseudoatrophoderma colli
pseudobacillus
pseudobacterium
pseudocartilage
Pseudochaetosphaeronema larense
pseudochancre redux
pseudocholinesterase (PCHE)
pseudocoarctation
pseudocowpox virus
pseudocyst
  adrenal
  pancreatic
  pulmonary
pseudodiverticulum
pseudoepitheliomatous hyperplasia
pseudofollicular salpingitis
pseudofolliculitis
pseudogout, calcium pyrophosphate crystals in
pseudo-Gaucher cell
pseudogranulomatous aggregations of cells
pseudohermaphroditism
pseudohypertrophic muscular atrophy
pseudohypertrophy
pseudohyphae
pseudohypoparathyroidism
pseudointraligamentary pregnancy
pseudokeloidal band
pseudolymphoma

pseudomelanosis
pseudomembrane
pseudomembranous enterocolitis
pseudomembranous gastritis
pseudomembranous inflammation
pseudometaplasia
Pseudomonas
Pseudomonas acidovorans (formerly *Comamonas terrigena*)
Pseudomonas aeruginosa
Pseudomonas alcaligenes
Pseudomonas cepacia
Pseudomonas diminuta
Pseudomonas fluorescens
Pseudomonas-like bacteria
Pseudomonas mallei
Pseudomonas maltophilia
Pseudomonas paucimobilis
Pseudomonas pickettii
Pseudomonas pneumonia
Pseudomonas pseudoalcaligenes
Pseudomonas pseudomallei
Pseudomonas putida
Pseudomonas putrefaciens
Pseudomonas stutzeri
Pseudomonas testosteroni
pseudomucinous
pseudomyxoma peritonei
pseudo-osteomalacic pelvis
pseudopalisade formation
pseudopalisading
pseudoparenchyma
pseudophakic
pseudoplatelet
pseudopod
pseudopolyp
pseudoproteinuria
pseudopyogenic granuloma
pseudorabies virus
pseudosac
pseudosarcoma
pseudostoma
pseudostone
pseudostratification
pseudostratified columnar epithelium
pseudostratified epithelium
pseudostratified nuclei
pseudotubercle
pseudotuberculosis
pseudotumor cerebri
pseudotumor, inflammatory
pseudounipolar cell
pseudovacuole
pseudoxanthoma cell
pseudoxanthoma elasticum
psi, p.s.i. (pounds per square inch)
psi factor
psittacosis
psoas abscess
psoas fascia
psoas gap
psoas major muscle
psoas margin
psoas muscle
psoas muscle abscess
psoas shadow
psorelcosis
psorenteritis
psoriasis
  circinate
  diffused
  discoid
  exfoliative
  generalized pustular p. of Zambusch
  guttate
  gyrate
  inverse
  nummular
  ostraceous
  palmar
  pustular
  seborrheic
psoriasis geographica

psoriasis inveterata
psoriasis orbicularis
psoriasis punctata
psoriasis rupioides
psoriasis spondylitica
psoriasis universalis
PSP (phenolsulfonphthalein) test for kidney function (also, phenol red)
pS2 protein
PT (prothrombin time, pro time)
PTAH (phosphotungstic acid-hematoxylin) stain
PTC (plasma thromboplastin component)
pterion
pterygoid artery
pterygoid bone
pterygoid canal
pterygoid plate
pterygoid plexus
pterygoid process
pterygomandibular ligament
pseudomandibular raphe
pterygomaxillary fissure
pterygopalatine canal
pterygopalatine fossa
pterygopalatine ganglion
pterygospinal ligament
PTT (partial thromboplastin time)
p24 antigen
ptyocrinous cell
pubes
pubic arch
pubic artery
pubic bone
pubic hair line
pubic itching
pubic ligament
pubic louse
pubic ramus
pubic symphysis
pubic tubercle
pubis (slang for os pubis)
  mons
  pecten
  Phthirus
  ramus of
  symphysis
pubocapsular ligament
pubocervical ligament
pubococcygeal line
pubococcygeal muscle
pubofemoral ligament
pubo-obturator area
puboprostatic ligament
puborectalis loop
puborectalis muscle
pubovaginalis muscle
pubovesical ligament
puckered
Puchtler-Sweat stain
pudendal artery
pudendal canal
pudendal cleft
pudendal nerve
pudendal vein
pudendal vessel
puerperal fever
puerperal mastitis
puerperal osteomalacia
pulled tendon
pulmoaortic canal
pulmonale, cor
pulmonary alveolar proteinosis
pulmonary alveolus
pulmonary artery
pulmonary artery aneurysm
pulmonary cirrhosis
pulmonary congestion
pulmonary consolidation
pulmonary edema
pulmonary embolism
pulmonary emphysema
pulmonary endothelial cell

pulmonary epithelial cell
pulmonary excretion of carbon dioxide
pulmonary fibrosis
pulmonary function
pulmonary gas exchange
pulmonary gases
pulmonary hypertension
pulmonary infarct(ion)
pulmonary ligament
pulmonary macrophage
pulmonary nerve
pulmonary orifice
pulmonary osteoarthropathy
pulmonary parenchyma
pulmonary pleurisy
pulmonary retention of carbon dioxide
pulmonary segment
pulmonary stenosis
pulmonary tissue–blood barrier
pulmonary trunk, bifurcation of
pulmonary tuberculosis
pulmonary valve
pulmonary valvular leaflet
pulmonary venous–systemic air embolism
pulmonary vein
pulmonic plague
pulmonic valve
pulmonis, apex
pulp
  coronal
  dead
  dental
  dentinal
  devitalized
  digital
  enamel
  red
  splenic
  white
pulp abscess
pulp canal
pulp cavity
pulp chamber
pulpar cell
pulpitis, hyperplastic
pulposus, nucleus
pulp polyp
pulsating metastases
pulsating pleurisy
pulse (pl. pulses)
pulseless disease
pulsion diverticulum
pultaceous
pumped-dye laser
punch biopsy
punch, cylindrical
punctate hemorrhage
punctate infiltrate
punctate keratotic lesion
puncture
  arterial
  cisternal
  fingerstick
  lumbar (LP)
puncture diabetes
puncture ulcer
puncture wound
pupil (pupillae), dilator
pupillary zone
Purdy test for albumin
purified placental protein
Purkinje cell
Purkinje corpuscle
Purkinje fiber
purplish discoloration of skin
purplish rash
purpura
  acute vascular
  allergic
  anaphylactoid
  factitious
  fibrinolytic
  Henoch-Schönlein (Shoenlein)

purpura *(continued)*
- hyperglobulinemic
- idiopathic thrombocytopenic (ITP)
- immune thrombocytopenic
- iodic
- nonthrombocytopenic
- psychogenic
- Schönlein-Henoch (Shoenlein)
- thrombocytopenic (TP)
- thrombotic thrombocytopenic (TTP)
- Waldenström

purpura angioneurotica
purpura annularis telangiectodes
purpura fulminans
purpura hemorrhagica
purpura nervosa
purpura pulicans
purpura pulicosa
purpura rheumatica
purpura senilis
purpura simplex
purpura urticans
purpuric bleeding
purpuric cutaneous eruption
purpurinuria
purulence
purulent discharge
purulent exudate
purulent inflammation
purulent lesion
purulent material
purulent meningitis
purulent otitis media
purulent pancreatitis
purulent pericarditis
purulent pleurisy
purulent pneumonia
purulent salpingitis
purulent sinusitis
purulent subarachnoid exudate
purulent synovitis
purulosanguineous pus
pus
- anchovy sauce
- blue
- blue-green
- burrowing
- cheesy
- collagen
- creamy
- curdy
- discrete yellow masses in
- green
- ichorous
- laudable
- sanious

pus cell
pus corpuscle
pus-forming bacteria
pus in pleural cavity
pustular eruption
pustular exanthem and enanthem
pustular psoriasis
pustule
- acneiform
- multiloculated
- postmortem
- spongiform
- unilocular

pustules in lash follicles
putamen
Putnam-Dana syndrome
putrefaction of gases
putrefactive changes in dead body
putrefy
putrescence
putrescent
putrid
putty kidney
Puumala virus
Puusepp reflex
pyelocaliceal
pyelocaliectasis
pyelocalyceal

pyelocystitis
pyelolymphatic
pyelonephritic kidney
pyelonephritis
  acute
  ascending
  chronic
  descending
  hematogenous
  xanthogranulomatous
pyeloureterectasis
pyelovenous
pyemesis
pyemia
  cryptogenic
  portal
pyemic abscess
pyesis
pyknosis
pyknotic nucleus
pylephlebitis
pyloric antrum
pyloric antrum cardiacum
pyloric artery
pyloric canal
pyloric channel
pyloric gland
pyloric mucosa
pyloric orifice
pyloric outlet
pyloric ring
pyloric sphincter
pyloric stenosis
pyloroduodenal junction
pylorostenosis
pylorus (pl. pylori)
pyocele
pyocephalus, circumscribed
pyochezia
pyocin
pyococcus
pyocolpocele
pyocolpos
pyocyanic
pyocyanogenic
pyocyst
pyocystis
pyocyte
pyoderma
  chancriform
  primary
  secondary
pyoderma gangrenosum
pyoderma vegetans
pyodermatitis
pyodermatosis
pyogen
pyogenesis
pyogenic bacteria
pyogenic fever
pyogenic granuloma
pyogenic infection of sweat glands
pyogenic meningitis
pyogenic organism
pyogenic proteinuria
pyogenous
pyohemothorax
pyoid
pyometra
pyometritis
pyomyositis
pyonephritis
pyonephrolithiasis
pyonephrosis
pyo-ovarium
pyopericarditis
pyopericardium
pyoperitoneum
pyoperitonitis
pyophysometra
pyopneumocholecystitis
pyopneumohepatitis
pyopneumoperitoneum
pyopneumoperitonitis

pyopneumothorax, subphrenic
pyopoiesis
pyopoietic
pyopyelectasis
pyorrhea
pyorrhea alveolaris
pyosalpingitis
pyosalpingo-oophoritis
pyosalpinx
pyosemia
pyosepticemia
pyosis, Manson
pyostomatitis vegetans
pyramid
pyramidal bone
pyramidal cell
pyramidal decussation
pyramidal eminence
pyramidal tract
Pyramidon test for occult blood in urine
pyridoxilated stroma-free hemoglobin (SFHb)
pyriform (piriform) sinus
pyrogen, endogenous
pyrogenicity
pyrogenic proteins
pyroglobulin
pyrosis
pyrrol blue stain
pyrrol cell
pyruvic acid
pyuria

Q, q

Q band
Q-banding stain
Q-b band
Q fever
Qiaex bead
QNS (quantity not sufficient)
Q-Prep staining system
quadrant
  left lower (LLQ)
  left upper (LUQ)
  left upper outer
  right lower (RLQ)
  right upper (RUQ)
  right upper outer
quadrate ligament
quadrate lobe of liver
quadrate muscle
quadriceps artery of femur
quadrigeminal cistern
quadrilateral bone
qualitative
qualitative analysis
quantitative
quantitative analysis
quantity not sufficient (QNS)
quantum
Quaranfil virus
quartan fever
quartan malaria
quenching of fluorescence intensity
Quervain disease
Queyrat, erythroplasia of
Quick prothrombin test
Quick test
QuickVue Chlamydia test
quiescent cell
quinacrine fluorescent method of staining
Quincke edema
Quincke meningitis
quinine
quinine carbacrylic resin test for gastric anacidity
Quinlan test for bile
quinsy
quotidian malaria

R, r

Raabe test for albumin
rabbit stool
rabies
rabies-like viruses
rabies virus
Rabuteau test for hydrochloric acid in urine
RA (ragocyte) cell
racemized protein
racemose aneurysm
racemose gland
rachitic pelvis
rachitis
rad (radiation absorbed dose)
radial artery
radial bone
radial carpal artery
radial cells of Mueller
radial collateral ligament
radial groove
radial immunodiffusion (RID)
radial neck groove
radial sclerosing lesion
radial sigmoid notch
radial styloid
radiant energy
radiate ligament
radiate sternocostal ligament
radiation
  diagnostic
  ionizing
  ultraviolet
radiation absorbed dose (rad)
radiation cell change
radiation colitis
radiation cystitis
radiation dermatitis
radiation gastritis
radiation necrosis
radiation neuritis
radiation pneumonitis
radiation therapy
radical
  free
  biliary
  intrahepatic
  tertiary
radicular abscess
radicular artery
radicular neuritis
radicular odontoma
radiculitis
radioactive chromium
radioactive cobalt

radioactive iodide uptake test
radioactive iodinated serum albumin (RISA) test
radioactive isotope
radioactively tagged
radioallergosorbent test (RAST)
radiocarpal articulation
radiocarpal joint
radiocarpal ligament
radiocarpal portal
radioceptor assay
radiodermatitis
radiohumeral articulation
radiohumeral joint
radioimmunoassay (RIA)
  direct
  indirect
radioimmunosorbent test (RIST)
radioisotopically tagged antihuman antibody
radiolunotriquetral ligament
radioneuritis
radioscaphocapitate ligament
radioscapholunate ligament
radioulnar articulation
radioulnar joint, articular disk of distal
radioulnar ligament, anterior
radium
radius, annular ligament of
ragocyte
raised flap
Raji cell
Raji cell assay
rales, basilar
Ralfe test for acetone in urine
Rambourg chromic acid-phosphotungstic acid stain
Rambourg periodic acid-chromic methenamine-silver stain
rami (pl. of ramus)
Ramon flocculation test
Ramón y Cajal stain
Ramond point
Ramsay Hunt syndrome
Ramularia
ramus (pl. rami)
  dorsal
  dorsal primary
  inferior pubic
  ischiopubic
  pubic
  ventral
  ventral primary
ramus bone
ramus communicans
  gray
  white
ramus of ischium, ascending
ramus of os pubis, ascending
RANA (rheumatoid-associated nuclear antigen)
Randall plaque
Randolph test for peptones in urine
random blood glucose
random blood sugar
range
  normal
  reference
  therapeutic
ranine artery
Ranke complex
Rankine scale
Ranson pyridine silver stain
Rantzman test
Ranvier node
raphe
  abdominal
  amniotic
  anococcygeal
  anogenital
  longitudinal
  median
  palpebral
  penile

raphe *(continued)*
  pterygomandibular
  scrotal
  tendinous
raphe anococcygea
raphe corpus callosi
raphe palati
raphe penis
raphe pharyngis
rapid absorption of dietary glucose
rapid flow cytometry assay
rapid mucin stain
rapid plasma reagin (RPR) test
rapid serum amylase test
Rapoport differential ureteral catheterization test
Rappaport lymphoma classification
Rasmussen aneurysm
ras oncogenes
rash
  butterfly
  lilac
  maculopapular
  malar
  purplish
RAST (radioallergosorbent test)
rate
  erythrocyte sedimentation (ESR)
  glomerular filtration (GFR)
  mitotic
  sed (sedimentation)
  sedimentation
  Westergren sedimentation
rat-bite fever
Rathke pouch
ratio
  A/G (albumin/globulin)
  BUN/creatinine
  cytoplasmic
  cytoplasmic/nuclear
  erythroid/myeloid
  international normalized (INR)

ratio *(continued)*
  inversion of
  inversion of A/G
  lecithin/sphingomyelin (L/S)
  leukocyte/erythrocyte
  M/E (myeloid/erythroid)
  nuclear/cytoplasmic
  prothrombin time
  reversal
  reversal of A/G
  T4/T8
  T_4/TBG (thyroxine/thyroxine-binding globulin)
rat-mite dermatitis
RAV (Rous-associated virus)
ray, medullary
Raynaud phenomenon
R band
R-banding stain
R-b band
RBC (red blood cell)
RBC/hpf (red blood cells per high-power field)
RB1 tumor suppressor gene
RBP (retinol-binding protein)
RCA (right coronary artery)
RDW (red cell distribution width)
reabsorbed
reabsorption of aqueous humor
reactant
  acute phase
  phase
reaction
  acetowhite
  acid base
  allergic
  antigen-antibody
  Arias-Stella
  Bence Jones
  biochemical
  chromaffin
  colorless

reaction *(continued)*
  diffuse fibrotic
  fibrotic
  focal fibrotic
  foreign body
  Forssman
  glial
  hemolytic
  hypersensitivity
  inflammatory
  insulin
  leukemoid
  nitroprusside
  nodular fibrotic
  polymerase chain (PCR)
  precipitation
  sunburn-like
  transfusion
  urine
  white-graft
reactive airways disease (RAD)
reactive cell
reactive hyperplasia
reactive mesothelial cell
reagent
  ninhydrin
  premeasured
reagin
Rebuck skin window test
recanalization
recanalized area
recanalized occlusion
receptor
  acetylcholine
  adrenergic
  alpha-adrenergic
  aortic
  B cell antigen
  beta-adrenergic
  cholinergic
  epidermal growth factor (EGFR)
  estrogen
receptor *(continued)*
  low-density lipoprotein (LDL)
  progesterone
  T cell antigen (TCR)
receptor protein
recess
  attic
  cecal
  cerebellopontine
  cochlear
  costodiaphragmatic
  costomediastinal
  duodenojejunal
  epitympanic
  hepatorenal
  ileocecal
  inferior duodenal
  intersigmoid
  paraduodenal
  peritoneal
  pleural
  prestyloid
  retrocecal
  retroduodenal
  splenorenal
  subphrenic
  superior duodenal
recessive gene
recess of ischiorectal fossa
recess of pleura, costodiaphragmatic
recipient
  prospective
  transfusion
  universal
recipient cells
recipient serum
reciprocal reception, articulation by
reciprocal transfusion
reciprocal translocation
Recklinghausen, canal of
Recklinghausen disease of bone
reclotting phenomenon

recombinant antihemophilic factor
recombinant DNA
recombinant hemoglobin (rHb1.1)
recombinant human erythropoietin (rhEPO)
recombinant tissue plasminogen activator (rtPA, rt-PA)
recruitable collaterals
rectal ampulla
rectal artery
rectal fold
  inferior transverse
  superior transverse
rectal mucosa
rectal muscle cuff
rectal nerve
rectal plexus
rectal polyp
rectal pouch
rectal prolapse
rectal shelf
rectal stricture
rectal stump
rectal valve
rectal vault
rectal vein
rectosigmoid carcinoma
rectosigmoid junction
rectouterine fold
rectouterine pouch
rectovaginal fistula
rectovaginal pouch
rectovaginal septum
rectovaginouterine pouch
rectovesical fistula
rectovesical pouch
rectovesical septum
rectum, ampulla of
rectus abdominis muscle
rectus sheath
recurrent abortion
recurrent aphthous stomatitis
recurrent bleeding
recurrent canal
recurrent embolism
recurrent interosseous artery
recurrent intravascular thrombosis
recurrent laryngeal nerve
recurrent radial artery
recurrent ulnar artery
red algae
red atrophy
red blood cell (pl. cells) (RBC, rbc)
  fragility of
  hemolyzed
  nucleated
  packed
  urinary
red blood cell cholinesterase level
red blood cell count
red blood cell fragility
red blood cell indices
red blood cell mass
red blood cell precursor
red blood cells per high-power field (RBC/hpf)
"red cell" (slang for red blood cell)
red cell adherence test
"red count" (slang for red blood cell count)
red cell clot
red cell distribution width (RDW)
red cell indices
red cell survival, ^{51}Cr
red cell volume
red degeneration of uterine leiomyoma
red hepatization stage of pneumonia
red induration
Redlich-Fisher miliary plaque
red marrow
redness of bone
redness of skin
redox equilibrium
red phenolsulfonphthalein test

red pulp
red pulp of spleen
red test
reduced hemoglobin
reducing substance in stool
reducing sugar
reduction deformity
reduction division
reduplication, chromosomal abnormality of
reduplication of a kidney
reduplication of a ureter
redwater fever
Reed cells
Reed-Sternberg cell
Reese-Ellsworth classification of retinoblastoma
Rees test for albumin
re-excreted
reference laboratory
reference range
reflected
reflected inguinal ligament
reflected light
reflecting edge of ligament
reflection
- costopleural
- hepatoduodenal-peritoneal
- hepatoduodenoperitoneal
- mediastinodiaphragmatic pleural
- peritoneal
- sternal pleural
- vertebral pleural

reflex
- abdominal
- abdominocardiac
- accommodation
- acquired
- acromial
- adductor
- anal
- arc

reflex *(continued)*
- auricular
- cardiac
- costal arch
- crossed
- deltoid
- depressor
- digital
- dorsum of foot
- dorsum pedis
- elbow
- epigastric
- erector spinal
- esophagosalivary
- external oblique
- eye-closure
- facial
- faucial
- femoral
- finger-thumb
- flexor
- forced grasping
- fundus
- gag
- gastrocolic
- gastroileac
- involuntary
- Moro startle
- nasolabial
- nasomental
- neck
- neck righting
- nociceptive
- nostril
- obliquus
- oculoauricular
- oculocardiac
- oculocephalogyric
- oculopharyngeal
- oculopupillary
- oculosensory
- oculovagal

reflex *(continued)*
- open loop
- Oppenheim
- opticofacial winking
- orbicularis
- orbicularis oculi
- orbicularis pupillary
- orienting
- palatal
- palatinc
- palmar
- palm-chin
- palmomental
- paradoxical pupillary
- patellar
- patelloadductor
- pathologic
- pectoral
- penile
- perianal
- periosteal
- peristaltic
- peritoneointestinal
- pharyngeal
- phasic
- Philippson
- pilomotor
- Pilitz
- placing
- plantar
- platysmal
- postural
- pressor
- Preyer
- proprioceptive
- psychic
- psychocardiac
- psychogalvanic
- pulmonocoronary
- pupillary
- Puusepp
- quadriceps

reflex *(continued)*
- quadrupedal extensor
- radial
- rectal
- red
- regional
- Remak
- renointestinal
- renorenal
- retrobulbar pupillary
- reversed pupillary
- Riddoch mass
- righting
- Roger
- rooting
- Rossolimo
- Ruggeri
- Saenger
- scapular
- scapulohumeral
- Schäffer (Schaeffer)
- scratch
- scrotal
- segmental
- senile
- sexual
- shot-silk
- simple
- skin
- skin pupillary
- Snellen
- sole
- somatointestinal
- spinal
- stapedial
- startle
- static
- statotonic
- stepping
- Stookey
- stretch
- Strümpell (Struempell)

reflex *(continued)*
- sucking
- superficial
- supinator longus
- supraorbital
- suprapatellar
- suprapubic
- supraumbilical
- swallowing
- tapetal light
- tarsophalangeal
- tendon
- testicular compression
- threat
- Throckmorton
- tibioadductor
- toe
- tonic neck
- trained
- triceps
- triceps surae
- trigeminus
- ulnar
- unconditioned
- urinary
- vagus
- vascular
- vasopressor
- vertebra prominens
- vesical
- vesicointestinal
- vestibular
- vestibulo-occular
- virile
- visceral
- viscerocardiac
- visceromotor
- viscerosensory
- viscerotrophic
- voluntary
- von Mering
- water-silk

reflex *(continued)*
- Weiss
- Westphal pupillary
- withdrawal
- zygomatic

reflex inguinal ligament
refract
refracted light
refractile
refractile medium
refraction, angle of
refractive index
Regan isoenzyme
Regaud fixative
regeneration
regeneration of damaged tissues
regenerative polyp
region
- abdominal
- anal
- ankle
- axillary
- buccal
- calcaneal
- deltoid
- epigastric
- femoral
- frontal
- gluteal
- hypochondriac
- hypogastric
- inguinal
- lumbar
- paraumbilical
- perianal
- scapular
- suprapubic
- umbilical
- urogenital

regional enteritis
regional ileitis
regional lymph nodes

registry, tumor
regressive staining
regular connective tissue
regulator gene
regulatory peptide
regulatory proteinuria
regurgitant fraction
regurgitation
Rehberg test
Reichert canal
Reichl test for proteins
Reil ansa
Reil band
Reinke crystals
Reinke space
Reinsch test for heavy metals
Reiter complement fixation test
  for syphilis
Reiter syndrome
rejection
  acute cellular renal
  acute renal
  cellular
  chronic
  first-set
  hyperacute
  second-set
  transplant
  vasculitic
relapsing febrile nodular nonsuppurative panniculitis
relapsing fever
relapsing malaria
relative lymphocytosis
relative molecular mass
relaxation factor
relaxin
release of fluid into intercellular tissues
releasing factor (RF)
releasing hormone (RH)
remittent fever
remittent malaria
remnant, gastric
remnant of ductus arteriosus
remnant of processus vaginalis
remodeling process
renal abscess
renal agenesis
renal amino acid diabetes
renal amyloidosis
renal artery
renal artery dilatation
renal atrophy
renal calix (pl. calices)
renal calyces
renal calyx
renal capsule
  fatty
  fibrous
renal cell carcinoma
renal cholesterol embolism
renal column
renal cortex
renal cyst
renal degeneration
renal diabetes
renal disease
renal dwarfism
renal edema
renal excretion of hydrogen ion
renal failure
renal fascia
renal fat
renal function test
renal glycosuria
renal hematuria
renal hilum
renal hilus
renal hypertension
renal impression on liver
renal infarction
renal insufficiency
renal labyrinth
renal medulla

renal nerve
renal obstruction
renal osteitis fibrosa
renal osteodystrophy
renal papilla
renal parenchyma
renal pelvis
renal plasma flow (RPF) test
renal pouch
renal proteinuria
renal pyramids
renal rickets
renal shutdown
renal sinus
renal sodium
renal tuberculosis
renal tubular acidosis
renal tubular degeneration
renal tubular epithelial cast (RTE cast)
renal tubular necrosis
renal tubular osteomalacia
renal tubule
renal vein
renal vessel
Rendu-Osler-Weber disease
reniform pelvis
renin (*not* rennin)
renin hormone
rennin test (not renin)
renovascular hypertension
Renshaw cells
REO (respiratory enteric orphan) virus
reovirus
repair
  cellular
  fracture
  process
  wound
repair in inflammation
repair of fracture
repair or bridging of defects with
  fibrous scar tissue
reparative
replacement bone
replacement fibrosis
replicate
replication
report
  cytologic
  gross
  laboratory
  macroscopic
  pathology
repressor gene
reproducibility
reptilase test for blood clotting time
requisition
resection
  limit of
  line of
  margin of
  transurethral
reserve cell
reservoir, chromatin
residential cell
residual abscess
residual capacity
residual flaccid paralysis
residual stool
resilient
resin
resistance
resistance factor
resistance-inducing factor
resistance-transfer factor
resorbed
resorcinol–hydrochloric acid test for
  fructose
resorption, bone
resorption of calcium
respirator brain
respiratory acidosis
respiratory alkalosis
respiratory apparatus

respiratory area of nose
respiratory arrest
respiratory bronchiole
respiratory capacity
respiratory depression
respiratory distress
respiratory disturbance of acid-base balance
respiratory droplets
respiratory epithelium
respiratory failure
respiratory lobule
respiratory metabolism
respiratory nodule
respiratory obstruction
respiratory paralysis
respiratory pigment
respiratory syncytial disease
respiratory syncytial virus (RSV)
respiratory system
respiratory virus
response, desmoplastic
Response GM handheld device to test granulocyte count
rest (mass of cells)
resting cell
resting wandering cell
restructured cell
results of fracture
resurrection bone
resuscitation, artifacts of
retained dead fetus
retained placenta
retained products of conception
retained root
rete (pl. retia)
rete mirabile
rete pegs of epidermis
rete ridges
rete testis
retention cyst
retention defect
retention meal
retention of carbon dioxide, pulmonary
retention polyp
reticular cell
reticular colliquation
reticular connective tissue
reticular dermis
reticular fiber
reticular layer
reticulated bone
reticulated tissue
reticulin stain
reticulocyte
reticulocyte count
reticulocytosis
reticuloendothelial cell
reticuloendothelial organ
reticuloendotheliosis
reticulohistiocytic granuloma
reticulohistiocytosis
reticulonodular pattern
reticulosis
reticulum
- agranular
- Chiari
- cistern of endoplasmic
- Ebner
- endoplasmic
- granular endoplasmic
- sarcoplasmic
- stellate
- trabecular endoplasmic
- vesicle of endoplasmic

reticulum cell
reticulum cell sarcoma
retina
- amacrine cells of
- capillary microaneurysms of
- central artery of
- coarctate
- deeply pigmented lesions in
- detached

retina *(continued)*
  leopard
  necrotic lesions in
  pigmentary degeneration of
  shot-silk
  tessellated
  tigroid
  watered-silk
retinaculum, caudal
retinal artery
retinal cone
retinal degeneration
retinal detachment
retinal dysplasia
retinal ganglion cells, degeneration of
retinal pigment
retinal rod
retinal tumor
retinitis pigmentosa
retinitis proliferans
retinoblastoma
retinoblastoma hereditary human cancer
retinol-binding protein
retraction clot
retraction, stromal
retroauricular nodes
retrobulbar abscess
retrobulbar optic neuritis
retrocecal abscess
retrocecal appendix
retrocecal recess
retrocolic appendix
retrocostal artery
retroduodenal artery
retroduodenal recess
retroesophageal subclavian artery
retroflexed uterus
retroverted uterus
retrograde degeneration
retrograde metamorphosis
retroileal appendix
retrolental fibroplasia
retromammary mastitis
retromolar gland
retropancreatic tunnel
retroperitoneal cavity
retroperitoneal fibrosis
retroperitoneal organ
retroperitoneal region
retroperitoneal space
retroperitoneum
retropharyngeal abscess
retropubic space
retrorectal lymph node
retrotonsillar abscess
retrovascular goiter
retrovirus
Retzius
  ligament of
  line of
  space of
  system of
  vein of
Retzius space
Reuss test for atropine
Reverdin needle
reversal of A/G ratio
reversal of ratio
reverse triiodothyronine (rT_3) test
Rex-Cantli-Serege line
Reye syndrome
Reynolds test for acetone
Reynold lead citrate
rhabdoid
rhabdomyolysis
rhabdomyoma
rhabdomyosarcoma
rhabdovirus
rhagiocrine cell
Rh (Rhesus)
Rh antibody
Rh antigen
Rh blocking

Rh blood system
Rh blood type
rheumatic atrophy
rheumatic endocarditis
rheumatic fever
rheumatic granuloma
rheumatic myocarditis
rheumatic pericarditis
rheumatic pneumonia
rheumatoid (rheumatology) panel
rheumatoid arthritis
rheumatoid arthritis test
rheumatoid-associated nuclear antigen (RANA)
rheumatoid factor (RF)
rheumatoid myositis
rheumatoid nodule
rheumatoid spondylitis
rheumatology panel
Rh factor
Rhinocladiella aquaspersa
rhinoscleroma bacillus
Rhinosporidium seeberi
Rhinovirus, rhinovirus
Rhizoctonia
Rhizoctonia solani
Rhizomucor pusillus
Rhizopus
Rhizopus arrhizus
Rhizopus microsporus
Rhizopus nigricans
Rhizopus rhizopodiformis
Rhizopus stolonifer
Rh negative
Rh negative blood type
rhodopsin
Rhodotorula
Rhodotorula rubra
rhomboid
rhomboid ligament
Rh positive
Rh positive blood type
Rh test
rhubarb test in urine
rhus dermatitis
RIA (radioimmunoassay)
rib
  angle of
  bicipital
  bifid
  cervical
  facet for head of
  false
  first
  floating
  fused
  head of
  inferior margin of superior
  lumbar
  neck of
  notching of
  periosteum of
  shaft of
  superior
  superior margin of inferior
  true
  tubercle of
  typical
  vertebrocostal
  vertebrosternal
ribbon stool
riboflavin test
ribonucleoprotein particle
ribosome
ribovirus
rib shears, Gluck
rib tubercle
rice-water stool
Richter syndrome
rickets, renal
ricketts
Rickettsia
Rickettsia akari
Rickettsia australis

Rickettsia conorii
Rickettsia mooseri
Rickettsia prowazekii
Rickettsia rickettsii
Rickettsia sibirica
Rickettsia tsutsugamushi
Rickettsia typhi
rickettsiae
rickettsial infection
rickettsial myocarditis
rickettsial pneumonia
rickettsialpox
RID (radioimmunodiffusion)
rider's bone
rider's tendon
ridge
  alveolar
  apical ectodermal
  basal
  bicipital
  buccocervical
  buccogingival
  bulbar
  cutaneous
  dental
  epidermal
  epipericardial
  ganglion
  genital
  sagittal
  supraorbital
riding embolism
Riedel lobe
Riedel struma
Rieder cell
Rieder cell leukemia
Riegler test for albumin
Rift Valley fever virus
right atrium
right auricle
right border of heart
right colic artery
right colic (or colonic) flexure
right colon
right coronary artery (RCA)
right crus (pl. crura)
right dominant coronary artery
right gastric artery
right gastroepiploic artery
right gutter
right heart
right hemisphere
right lobe of liver
right lower quadrant (RLQ)
right shift on WBC count
right-sided pneumonia
right triangular ligament
right upper outer quadrant
right upper quadrant (RUQ)
right ventricle of heart
rigid canal
rigidity
  muscle
  nuchal
  postmortem
rigor mortis
rim degeneration
Rimini test
rim of fascia
Rindfleisch cell
ring
  abdominal
  amnion
  anorectal
  benzene
  Cabot
  choroidal
  ciliary
  common tendinous
  conjunctival
  crural
  distal esophageal
  external
  femoral

ring *(continued)*
fibrinocartilaginous
fibrous
Fleischer-Kayser
ilioinguinal
iliopsoas
inguinal
internal abdominal
internal inguinal
intrahaustral contraction
Kayser-Fleischer
Ochsner
pyloric
Schatzki
sphincter contraction
superficial inguinal
Waldeyer
ring abscess
ringbone, false
ring chromosome
Ringer's solution
ring ligament
ring of esophagus, B
ring precipitin test
ring-shaped cluster
ring test for antibiotic activity
ring test for protein
ring-wall lesion
ringworm (tinea corporis)
ringworm of groin
ringworm of scalp
ringworm of skin
Riolan, arc of
Riolan bone
RISA (radioactive iodinated serum albumin) test
risk factor
RIST (radioimmunosorbent test)
Ritter disease
Rivinus canal
Rivinus gland
riziform
RLQ (right lower quadrant)
RNA (ribonucleic acid)
RNA tumor virus
RNA virus (ribovirus)
Rnase
RNAzolB method of RNA extraction
Ro (SS-A) autoantibody
Robert ligament
robertsonian translocation
Roberts test for albumin
Robinson index
Robinson-Kepler test for adrenocortical insufficiency
Robson point
Rochalimaea
Rochalimaea henselae
Rochalimaea quintana
Rocio virus
rock-hard plaque
rocking microtome
Rocky Mountain spotted fever
rod
Auer
basal
Corti
germinal
gram-negative
gram-positive
retinal
rod cell of retina
rod neutrophil
rod nuclear cell
rod-shaped granule
rodent ulcer
Rohon-Beard cell
Rokitansky-Aschoff sinus
Rokitansky pelvis
Rolando cell
Rolando zone
roll of erythrocytes
rolled margin
Romaña sign

Romanovsky blood stain
Ronchese test for ammonia in urine
roof of abdomen
root
  anatomical
  cochlear
  cranial
  dental
  facial
  lingual
  motor
  nerve
  palatine
  retained
  sensory
  spinal
  ventral
root abscess
root canal of tooth
root cell
rooting reflex
root of lung
root of mesentery
root of penis
ropy bile
rose bengal radioactive (^{131}I) test
rose bengal test for liver function
Rose-Bradford kidney
Rosenbach-Gmelin test for bile pigment
Rosenmüller fossa
Rosenmüller gland
Rosenthal canal
Rosenthal degeneration
Rosenthal fibers in astrocytomas
Rosenthal test for blood in urine
roseola
roseola infantum
rose spot
rosette formation
rosette-forming cell
rosette, Homer-Wright
rosette test
Rose-Waaler agglutination test for rheumatoid factor
Rosin test for indigo red
Ross-Jones test
Ross River fever
Ross River virus
rostrum (pl. rostra)
Rotalex
rotary joint
rotary microtome
rotator cuff tear
rotavirus
rotavirus antigen
rotavirus DNA virus
rotavirus in stool specimen
Rotex cutting biopsy needle
Rothera nitroprusside test for ketone bodies
Rothera test for acetone
Roth spot
Rouget bulb
Rouget cell
roughened epithelium
roughening
rough texture
rouleau (pl. rouleaux)
rouleaux formation
round cell
round cell sarcoma
round ligament, artery of
round ligament of elbow joint
round ligament of femur
round ligament of liver
round ligament of uterus
rounded keratin inclusions
roundworm, human intestinal
Roughton-Scholander apparatus
Rous-associated virus (RAV)
Rous sarcoma
Rous sarcoma virus (RSV)
Roussin test

Rous test for hemosiderin
Rous virus
route, collateral
Roux-en-Y jejunal limb
Roux stain
Rowntree and Geraghty test
R plasmid
R protein
RPR (rapid plasma reagin) test for syphilis
RSV (respiratory syncytial virus)
RSV (Rous sarcoma virus)
RTE (renal tubular epithelium)
RTE cast
rubbery consistency
rubbery gray mass
rubbery nodule
rubbery texture
rubella
rubella HI (hemagglutination inhibition) test
rubella titer
rubella virus
rubeola
rubescent
rubifacient
Rubivirus
Rubner test for carbon monoxide in blood
Rubner test for lactose or glucose in urine
rubor
rubriblast (red blood cell precursor)
rubricyte
rudimentary bone
ruga (pl. rugae)
rugal pattern
rugate
Ruge solution
Ruhemann test for uric acid in urine
rule of nines
rumble (bowel sounds)
Rumpel-Leede phenomenon
Rumpel-Leede test
Rumpel-Leede tourniquet
Runeberg disease
runner's knee
runny stool
ruptured aneurysm
ruptured appendix
ruptured disk
ruptured fallopian tube
ruptured follicle
ruptured hernia
ruptured intraperitoneal viscus
ruptured membranes
ruptured perineum
ruptured spleen
rupture of congenital aneurysm
rupture, spo ntaneous
RUQ (right upper quadrant)
rushes (bowel sounds), peristaltic
Russell body
Russian autumn encephalitis virus
Russian spring-summer encephalitis virus
rust-colored papule
Rust disease
rusty sputum
Ruttan and Hardisty test for blood
Rye histopathologic classification of Hodgkin disease

S, s

SA (sinoatrial) node
SA virus (simian virus SV5)
SAA (serum amyloid A) protein
Saathoff test for fat in stools
saber shin
Sabin-Feldman dye test
Sabouraud agar
Sabouraud culture medium
sabra dermatitis
sac
  abdominal
  air
  allantoic
  alveolar
  amniotic
  anal
  aneurysmal
  aortic
  chorionic
  conjunctival
  cupular blind
  dental
  embryonic
  endolymphatic
  fluid-filled
  gestational
  greater peritoneal

sac *(continued)*
  hernial
  lacrimal
  lesser peritoneal
  pericardial
  peritoneal
  thecal
  wide-mouth
saccharimeter test
Saccharomyces cerevisiae
sacciform kidney
saccular aneurysm
saccular gland
sacculated pleurisy
sacculation
sacculocochlear canal
sacculoutricular canal
Sachs bacillus
Sachsse test for glucose in urine
Sachs-Tay disease (also, Tay-Sachs)
Sacks-Libman endocarditis
sacral artery
sacral bone
sacral canal
sacral foramina
sacral meningocele
sacral nerve

sacral parasympathetic outflow
sacral plexus
sacral promontory
sacral vertebra
sacred bone
sacroabdominoperineal
sacrococcygeal joint
sacrococcygeal junction
sacrococcygeal symphysis articulation
sacrococcygeal symphysis joint
sacrodural ligament
sacrogenital fold
sacroiliac articulation
sacroiliac joint
sacroiliac ligament
sacrospinous ligament
sacrotuberous ligament
sacrovertebral angle
sacrum
  alae of
  assimilation
  cornua of
  promontory of
  scimitar
  tilted
sacrum and coccyx articulation
sacrum and coccyx joint
saddle articulation
saddle embolus
saddle joint
safranin
sagittal fontanelle
sagittal limb
sagittal plane
sagittal ridge
sagittal section
sagittal suture
sago-grain stool
Sahli-Nencki test for lipolytic activity of pancreas
Sainte-Marie method of alcoholic fixation and paraffin embedding
saint (see *St.*)
Saint triad
Sakaguchi test for arginine
Saksenaea vasiformis
Sala cell
salicylate
salicylic acid
salicylic acid test
saline solution
Salinem infection
Salisbury common cold virus
saliva
salivary gland
salivary gland atrophy
salivary gland hormone
salivary gland stone
salivary gland tumor
salivary gland virus
salivary stone
Salkowski and Schipper test for bile pigments
Salkowski-Ludwig test for uric acid
Salkowski test
salmon-patch hemorrhage
salmonella food poisoning
salmonella osteomyelitis
Salmonella
Salmonella arizonae
Salmonella choleraesuis
Salmonella enteritidis
Salmonella typhi
salmonellosis
salpingitis
  chronic interstitial
  follicular
  gonococcal
  hemorrhagic
  interstitial
  pseudofollicular
  purulent
  tuberculous
salpingo-oophorectomy

salt (pl. salts)
  bile
  bone
  inorganic
  mercuric
salt-losing defect
salt-losing nephritis
salt plasma
sampling, endometrial
S&A (sugar and acetone)
sandal strap dermatitis
sand, brain
sandfly fever–Naples virus
sandfly fever–Sicilian virus
sandfly fever virus
sandpaper gallbladder
Sandrock test for thrombosis
Sandström gland
sand test for bile and hemoglobin in urine
sanguineous fluid
sanguineous infiltration
sanguinopurulent
sanguinoserous
sanguinoseropurulent
sanious pus
San Joaquin Valley fever
Saõ Paulo fever
Santorini canal
Santorini, duct of
Santorini labyrinth
Santorini ligament
SAP (sphingolipid activator protein)
saphenous artery
saphenous opening
saphenous vein
saponification
Sappey ligament
Sarastro-2000 confocal scanning microscope
sarcofetal pregnancy
sarcogenic cell
sarcohysteric pregnancy
sarcoid, Boeck
sarcoidosis, hepatic
sarcolemma
sarcoplasmic reticulum
sarcoma
  Abernethy
  alveolar soft part
  ameloblastic
  angiolithic
  botryoid
  endometrial stromal
  Ewing
  fascicular
  giant cell
  giant cell monstrocellular
  granulocytic
  immunoblastic
  Jensen
  juxtacortical osteogenic
  Kaposi
  leukocytic
  lymphatic
  medullary
  mixed cell
  multiple idiopathic hemorrhagic
  myelogenic
  myeloid
  neurogenic
  osteogenic
  periosteal
  reticulum cell
  round cell
  Rous
  spindle cell
  synovial
  telangiectatic osteogenic
sarcomere
sarcophagic syndrome
sarcoplasm
sarcoplasmic matrix
sarcoplasmic reticulum

Sarcoptes scabiei
satellite abscess
satellite cell of skeletal muscle
satellite, chromosome
satellite lesion
satellite metastasis
satellite phenomenon
satellite structure
satellite virus
satellitism
satellitosis
saturated solution
saturation index (SI) of bile
saturation recovery technique
saturnine nephritis
saucerize
saucer-like crusts of favus
Saundby test for blood in stool
sausage finger
sawtooth configuration
saw-toothed acanthosis
saw-toothed gland
scabbard trachea
scab of exudate
scabies
scalded skin syndrome
scale (pl. scales)
  absolute
  absolute temperature
  Baumé
  Bloch
  Celsius
  centigrade
  coma
  extensive shedding of
  Fahrenheit
  French
  gray
  hardness
  interval
  Karnofsky
  Kelvin
scale *(continued)*
  pH
  Rankine
  Sörensen
  temperature
  Zubrod
scale formation
scalelike cell
scalene tubercle, prominent
scalenus anterior
scalenus anterior muscle
scalenus medius
scalenus minimus
scaling
  dry
  greasy
  moist
scalloped
scalp hair
scalp infection
scalp, occipital
scaly dermatosis
scaly erythematous dermatitis
scaly erythematous patches of face
scaly erythematous patches of scalp
scanning power
scant cellularity
scant discharge
scanty cytoplasm
scaphoid abdomen
scaphoid bone
scaphoid facet
scaphoid fossa
scaphoid waist
scapholunate joint
scapholunate ligament
scaphotrapezoid trapezial (STT) joint
scapula (pl. scapulae)
scapula bone
scapular artery
scapular circumflex artery
scapular region

scapuloclavicular articulation
scapuloclavicular joint
scapulohumeral
scar
  astroglial
  excised
  flank
  keloid
  postnecrotic
  surgical
  traumatic
scar formation
scarification test
scarified duodenum
scarlatina
scarlatinal nephritis
scarlet fever
scarlet red
Scarpa
  canal of
  fascia of
  ligament of
Scarpa fascia
Scarpa triangle
scarring
  hypertrophic
  keloid
  peritoneal
  postnecrotic
scarring alopecia
scarring of cornea
scarring of uterine tube
scar tissue
scar tissue reaction
SCAT (sheep cell agglutination test)
scavenger cell
Scedosporium apiospermum
S cell
SCFA (short chain fatty acid)
Schäffer-Fulton stain (Schaeffer)
Schäffer test for nitrites in urine
Schalfijew test
Schällibaum solution
Schamberg dermatitis
Scharlach R
Schatzki ring
Schaudinn fixative
Schaumann body
Scherer test
Scheuermann disease
Schick test
Schiff reagent
Schiff solution
Schilder disease
Schiller test for cervical cancer
Schilling band cell
Schilling monocytic leukemia
Schilling test
schindylesis (wedge-and-groove joint) articulation
schindylesis articulation
schindylesis joint
schistocyte (keratocyte)
Schistosoma
Schistosoma haematobium
Schistosoma japonicum
Schistosoma mansoni
schistosome dermatitis
schistosomiasis, cutaneous
Schivoletto test for hydrochloric acid in urine
Schlatter-Osgood disease
Schlemm canal
Schlemm ligaments
Schlesinger test for urobilin
Schlichter test
Schmitz bacillus
Schmorl bacillus
Schmorl ferric-ferricyanide reduction stain
Schmorl node
Schmorl nodule
Schmorl picrothionin stain
Schönbein test for blood

Schönberg-Albers disease
 (also, Schoenberg)
Schönlein-Henoch purpura (Schoenlein)
Schramm phenomenon
Schroeder test for urea
Schüffner dots (Schueffner)
Schüller (Schueller)
Schüller-Christian-Hand disease
Schüller gland
Schulte test for proteins
Schultze cell
Schultze placenta
Schultze test
Schultz stain
Schumm test
Schwalbe space
Schwann cell
Schwann, sheath
schwannoma, vestibular
sciatic artery
sciatic foramen (pl. foramina)
 greater
 lesser
sciatic nerve, companion artery of
sciatic neuritis
sciatic notch
 greater
 lesser
scirrhous carcinoma of breast
scirrhous lesion
scirrhous tumor
SCLC (small cell lung carcinoma)
sclera (pl. sclerae)
scleral canal
sclerenchyma cell
sclerocorneal junction
sclerodactyly
scleroderma antibody
scleromyxedema
sclerosing hemangioma
sclerosing hepatic carcinoma (SHC)
sclerosing inflammation
sclerosing myeloma
sclerosing nonsuppurative osteomyelitis
sclerosing osteitis
sclerosis
 amyotrophic lateral
 combined
 focal glomerular
 gastric
 Mönckeberg
 multiple
 posterolateral
 progressive systemic
 tuberous
 valvular
sclerosis of brain
sclerosis of pubic bones
sclerotic bone
sclerotic degeneration
sclerotic kidney
sclerotic vein
scoliotic pelvis
Scopulariopsis brevicaulis
score, Gleason
Scotch tape technique
Scott solution
scraping
 conjunctival
 fungal
 skin
 surgical
 vesical
scratch test
screen
 fluorescent
 Glucola
 Monospot
 strep
 TORCH
 toxicology
screening test
screening, toxicology
screw joint

scroll bones
scrotal artery
scrotal raphe
scrotal swelling
scrotal vein
scrotum, lymphatics of
scrub typhus
scurvy
scutulum (pl. scutula)
scutum
scybalous stools
SDS (sodium dodecyl sulfate)
Se (selenium)
seabather's eruption
sea-blue histiocyte
seal-fin deformity
seatworm
sebaceous cyst
sebaceous gland
sebaceous nevus
seborrhea
seborrhea corporis
seborrheic dermatitis
seborrheic eczema
seborrheic keratosis
sebum
sec (second)
second (sec)
secondary aldosteronism
secondary amyloidosis
secondary anemia
secondary biliary cirrhosis
secondary cartilaginous joint
secondary center of ossification
secondary degeneration
secondary diabetes
secondary disease
secondary hypertension
secondary infection
secondary metabolism
secondary methemoglobinemia
secondary myeloid metaplasia
secondary pleurisy
secondary pneumonia
second-look laparotomy
second-set phenomenon
secretin test
secretion
  cytocrine
  gastric acid
  nasal
  nasopharyngeal
  serous
  thin
  vaginal
  watery
secretor
secretor factor
secretory cell
secretory endometrium
secretory epithelium
secretory granule
secretory phase
secretory stage
section
  abdominal
  celloidin
  cesarean
  coronal
  cross-
  cryostat
  deep
  fresh frozen
  frontal
  frozen
  longitudinal
  paraffin
  perineal
  permanent
  Pitres
  plastic
  representative
  Saemisch
  sagittal

section *(continued)*
  semithin
  serial
  serosal
  serous fluid
  serpiginous
  step
  transverse
  ultrathin
sectioning a block of tissue
sectioning of tissue specimen
secundipara (para 2)
"sed rate" (slang for erythrocyte sedimentation rate)
sediment
  amorphous
  urinary
sedimentation rate ("sed rate")
seeding, peritoneal
Seessel pouch (2 e's, 2 s's)
"seg" (slang for segmented neutrophil)
segment
  apical
  apicoposterior
  bronchopulmonary
  cardiac
  liver
  pulmonary
  vaterian
segmental artery
segmental bronchi
segmental colonic resection
segmental demyelination
segmental necrotizing glomerulonephritis
segmental neuritis
segmental neuropathy (demyelination)
segmental pneumonia
segmental resection
segmental zone
segmented cell
segmented neutrophil ("seg")
"segmenter" (slang for segmented neutrophil)
segregation analysis
SeHCAT (selenium-labeled homocholic acid conjugated with taurine) test
Seidel test for inositol
seizure
Seldinger needle
selective stain
selenium (Se)
self-limited inflammatory response
Selivanoff test
sella turcica
Seller stain
semen
semen analysis (sperm count)
semicircular canal
semiformed stool
semilunar bone
semilunar fold
semilunar ganglion artery
semilunar lobule
semilunar-shaped fold
semilunar valve, aortic
seminal cell
seminal colliculus
seminal fluid
seminal gland
seminal plasma
seminal vesicle
seminiferous tubule
seminoma
semiquantitative test
semisolid material
semisolid sebaceous debris
semisolid stool
semisynthetic
semithin section
Semliki Forest virus
Semunya virus
Sendai virus

Senear-Usher disease
senile arteriosclerosis
senile atrophy
senile cataract
senile degeneration
senile hemangioma
senile keratosis
senile lentigo
senile myocarditis
senile myocardium
senile nephrosclerosis
senile osteomalacia
senile osteoporosis
senile plaque
senile pruritus
senile vaginitis
senilis
  arcus
  circus
senna test in urine sensitivity
sensitivity index
sensitivity of laboratory test
sensitized cell
sensory cell
sensory fiber
sensory ganglion
sensory root
sentinel cell
sentinel fold
sentinel gland
sentinel loop
sentinel lymph node
sentinel pile
Seoul virus
separator tube
Sephadex
sepsis
  catheter
  gram-negative
  incarcerated
  intestinal
  intra-abdominal (IAS)
sepsis *(continued)*
  oral
  puerperal
sepsis syndrome
septa (pl. of septum)
septal artery of nose
septal bone
septal cartilage
septal cell
septal cirrhosis, diffuse
septal cusp
septal defect
septal mucosa
septal panniculitis
septal papillary muscle
septal tissue
septal wall
septate uterus
septic abortion
septic arthritis
septic embolism
septic embolus
septicemia
  meningococcal
  viral
septicemic abscess
septicemic plague
septic fever
septic infarct
septic myocarditis
septic necrosis
septic pneumonia
septic pulmonary embolism
septic shock
septic splenitis
septic wound
septomarginal band
septomarginal trabecular
septicopyemia
  cryptogenic
  metastatic
  spontaneous

septum (pl. septa)
  alveolar
  anal intermuscular
  aortic
  aortopulmonary
  bulbar
  cartilaginous
  crural
  distal bulbar
  femoral
  fibroelastic
  gingival
  interatrial
  interventricular
  nasal
  rectovaginal
  rectovesical
septum pellucidum (translucent)
septum secundum
sequela (pl. sequelae)
sequence analysis
Sequential Multiple Analyzer (SMA)
Sequential Multiple Analyzer plus Computer (SMAC)
sequestered disk
sequestrum
Sereny test to determine invasiveness of bacteria
serial cardiac isoenzymes
serial CK enzyme study (also, CPK)
serial dilutions
serial hemoglobin
serially sectioned
serial sections
seroculture
serocystic
serofibrinous inflammation
serofibrinous pleurisy
serologic cross-reactivity
serologic markers for hepatitis
serologic test(ing)
serologic test for syphilis (STS)
serologic titer
"serology" (slang for serologic test for syphilis or lues)
seromucous cell
seromucous gland
seromuscular layer
seronegative
seroplastic inflammation
seropositive
serosa (serous membrane)
serosal cyst
serosal puckering
serosal section
serosal surface
serosanguineous discharge
serosanguineous fluid
serosanguinopurulent
serotonin test
serotype
serous adenocarcinoma
serous atrophy
serous cell
serous cystadenocarcinoma
serous cystadenoma
serous cystoma
serous effusion
serous exudate
serous fluid
serous gland of tongue
serous infiltration
serous inflammation
serous ligament
serous membrane (serosa)
serous meningitis
serous otitis
serous pericardium
serous pleurisy
serous proteinuria
serous secretion
serous synovitis
serovar
serpentine aneurysm

serpentine appendix
serpiginous ulceration
serrate bone
Serratia
Serratia liquefaciens
Serratia marcescens
Serratia rubidaea
serratus anterior muscle
serratus posterior inferior muscle
serratus posterior superior muscle
Serres gland
Sertoli cell
serum
  acidified
  acute
  aged normal
  antivenomous
  convalescent
  donor
  Löffler
serum albumin
serum alkaline phosphatase
serum amylase
serum amylase level
serum bactericidal activity test
serum bilirubin
serum chloride
serum cholesterol
serum electrolytes
serum gamma-glutamyl transpeptidase (SGGT)
serum glutamic-oxaloacetic transaminase (SGOT) (now AST)
serum glutamic-pyruvate transaminase (SGPT) (now ALT)
serum hemoglobin
serum hepatitis
serum hepatitis (SH) antigen
serum leucine aminopeptidase (SLAP)
serum lipase
serum marker
serum neuritis
serum neutralization test
serum osmolality
serum prolactin
serum protein
serum protein electrophoresis
serum recipient
serum sickness
sesamoid bone
sessile hydatid
sessile papule
sessile polyp
seton wound
set point
sex cell
sex chromatin analysis
sex chromatin mass
sex factor
sex hormone
sex-linked recessive trait
sexual development, precocious
sexual gland
sexually transmitted disease (STD)
Seyderhelm solution
Sézary cell
SFHb (pyridoxilated stroma-free hemoglobin)
Sgambati reaction test
SGGT (serum gamma-glutamyl transpeptidase)
SGOT (serum glutamic-oxaloacetic transaminase) (now AST)
SGPT (serum glutamic-pyruvate transaminase) (now ALT)
shadow cell
shaft
shaft of rib
shaggy aorta
shaggy pericardium
shake test
shallow funnel
shallow mucosal ulcers
shank bone (tibia)

shape
  boat
  oval
  sickle
  spherical
shaped spindle
sharp, intermittent pain
Sharpey fiber
shave biopsy
SHb (sulfhemoglobin)
SHC (sclerosing hepatic carcinoma)
sheath
  carotid
  caudal
  common synovial flexor
  crural
  dentinal
  dural
  extensor carpi ulnaris
  fascial
  femoral
  fenestrated
  fibrous
  myelin
  nerve
  pilar
  rectus
  Schwann
  tendon
sheathing canal
sheath ligament
sheath of artery
Sheehan syndrome
sheep cell agglutination test (SCAT)
sheep red blood cells (sRBC)
sheet, areolar
sheetlike connection
sheetlike tendon
shelf
  buccal
  dental
  mesocolic
shelf *(continued)*
  palatine
  rectal
shellfish, contaminated
shell vial
shelving edge of Poupart ligament
S, hemoglobin (*not* S hemoglobin)
shield, embryonic
shift to the left on WBC count
shift to the right on WBC count
shifting dullness
Shiga bacillus
Shiga-Kruse bacillus
Shigella
Shigella boydii
Shigella dysenteriae
Shigella flexneri
Shigella sonnei
shin bone
shingles (herpes zoster)
shirt-stud abscess
shock
  anaphylactic
  electrical
  hemorrhagic
  hypovolemic
  septic
shock absorption
shock kidney
shock syndrome, toxic
Shorr trichrome
short bone
short chain fatty acid (SCFA)
short ciliary artery
short gastric artery
short palpebral fissures
short root
short stature
shortening lifespan
shortening of muscle
shot-silk retina
shotty lymph node

shoulder articulation
shoulder bone
shoulder joint
shoulder-girdle neuritis
shoulder muscles
"shower" of emboli
shrinkage and cavitation of basal
  ganglia
shrinkage of cells
shriveled or pitted surface
shrunken eye
shuleri articulation
shuleri joint
shunt, AV (arteriovenous)
SI (saturation index) of bile
Sia test for macroglobulinemia
sialic acid, lipid-associated (LASA)
sialolithiasis
sialorrhea
sialosyl-Tn
"sibilous" (see *scybalous stool*)
Sibson groove
Sicard-Cantelouble test
sicca, keratoconjunctivitis
sickle cell
sickle cell anemia
sickle cell disease
sickle cell hemoglobin
sickle cell preparation
sickle cell test
sickle cell trait
Sickledex test for hemoglobin S
Sicklequik rapid screening test
sickle shape
sickle-shaped erythrocytes
sickling
sickling test
sickness
  African sleeping
  serum
sideroblast
sideroblastic anemia
siderocyte
siderophage
siderophilin
sidewall, pelvic
SIDS (sudden infant death syndrome)
Siebold and Bradbury test for salicylic
  acid in urine
sieve bone
SIF, SRIF (somatotropin releasing-
  inhibiting factor)
sigma factor
sigmoid artery
sigmoid colon
sigmoid curve
sigmoid flexure
sigmoid fold
sigmoid kidney
sigmoid mesocolon
sigmoid notch of radius
sigmoidovesical fistula
sigmoid sinus
Sigmund gland
sign
  fronding
  Nikolsky
  Romana
  Winterbottom
signet-ring cell
signet-ring cell carcinoma
signet ring pattern
SIH (somatotropin release-inhibiting
  hormone)
silane-coated slide
Silastic band
silent gallstone
silhouette, cardiovascular
siliceous earth
silicosis
silicotic granuloma
silk suture
silo filler disease
silver (Ag)

silver cell
silver-fork deformity
silver nitrate
silver protein stain
silver stool
silver test for glucose in urine
Silverman needle
Simbu virus
simian immunodeficiency virus (SIV)
simian virus 40 (SV40)
simian virus SV5
Simmonds disease
Simonart band
Simonart ligament
Simplate
simple articulation
simple atrophy
simple columnar epithelium
simple cuboidal epithelium
simple epithelium
simple gland
simple goiter
simple inflammation
simple joint
simple obesity
simple protein
simple squamous epithelium
simplex, herpes
Simplexvirus
Sims test
Sindbis virus
singer's nodule
Singh-Vaughn-Williams arrhythmia classification
single-breath diffusing capacity of lung ($DLCO_{SB}$)
single human leukocyte antigen
single phase
single pleurisy
single ventricle
sinilis arch
sinoatrial node
sinus
  anal
  aortic
  Aschoff-Rokitansky
  barber's pilonidal
  basilar
  carotid
  cervical
  circular
  coccygeal
  coronary
  costomediastinal
  cranial
  dermal
  dural
  ethmoidal
  frontal
  Guérin
  lymph node
  marginal
  medullary
  oblique pericardial
  paranasal
  pilonidal
  piriform
  prostatic
  pyriform (piriform)
  renal
  Rokitansky-Aschoff
  sphenoidal
  thin-walled venous
  thrombosis of a venous
  transverse pericardial
  valve of coronary
  venous
sinus histiocytosis
sinus hyperplasia
sinus of epididymis
sinusitis
sinusoid
  hepatic
  pituitary

sinusoidal capillary
sinusoidal lymphocyte
SISI (small increment sensitivity index)
Sister Joseph nodule
sitosterolemia
situ, in
situs inversus viscerum
situs perversus
situs solitus
situs transversus
SIV (simian immunodeficiency virus)
Siwe-Letterer disease
6-phosphatase-glucose
6-phosphate dehydrogenase-glucose
65-2A6 monoclonal antibody
Sjögren antibody
Sjögren syndrome
skein cell
skeletal abnormalities
skeletal defects
skeletal deformity
skeletal muscle
skeletal muscle fiber
skeletal muscle, striated
skeletomuscular system
skeleton
  appendicular
  articulated
  axial
  cardiac
  fibrous
  gill arch
  visceral
Skene glands
skin
  abnormal whiteness of
  absence of pigment from
  biopsy of
  color and consistency of
  deciduous

skin *(continued)*
  elastic
  keratinized
  microabscess of
  perianal
  premature wrinkling of
  purplish discoloration of
  redness of
  ringworm of
  stretchability of
  thin
  yellow discoloration of
skin crease
skin laceration
skin lesion
Skinny needle
skin pigment, reduced
skin puncture test for Behçet syndrome
skin slip
skin tag
skin test
skin window test
skull bone
skullcap
skull-type joint
slant, agar
SLAP (serum leucine aminopeptidase)
"slapped cheek" erythema
SLE (systemic lupus erythematosus)
slender body habitus
slender elongated cell
slide
  gelatin-chrome
  organosilane-coated glass
  preparation of
  silane-coated
  Superfrost/Plus Fisherbrand glass
  urine dip
slide clumping factor test
slide coagulase test
slide test
sliding microtome

slime fungus
sling muscle fibers
sling, volar ulnar
slipped intervertebral disk
slipped tendon
slit-scan measurement
slough
sloughing
slow virus
sludge
  bile
  biliary
  blood
  gallbladder
sludged blood
slurry of stool
SMA (smooth muscle antibody)
SMA (Sequential Multiple Analyzer)
SMAC ("smack") (Sequential Multiple Anayzer plus Computer) analyzer
SMA-6 chemistry panel*
  BUN
  chloride
  creatinine
  glucose
  potassium
  sodium
SMA-12 chemistry panel*
  bilirubin
  BUN
  calcium
  chloride
  cholesterol
  creatinine
  glucose
  phosphorus
  potassium
  sodium
  total protein
  uric acid

*The tests included may vary from lab to lab. The tests listed here are an example.

SMA-20 chemistry panel*
  albumin
  alkaline phosphatase
  ALT
  AST
  bilirubin
  BUN
  calcium
  chloride
  cholesterol
  creatinine
  direct bilirubin
  glucose
  iron
  LDH
  phosphorus
  potassium
  sodium
  total protein
  triglycerides
  uric acid
small B-cell lymphoma
small bowel
small canal of chorda tympani
small cardiac vein
small cell carcinoma
small cell lung carcinoma (SCLC)
small cell osteosarcoma
small cleaved cell
small cleaved cell lymphoma
small eye muscle
small granule cell
small gut
small increment sensitivity index (SISI)
small intestine
small intestine gland
small lymphocytic lymphoma
small noncleaved cell lymphoma
smallpox (variola)
smallpox-like disease
small round cell carcinoma
small round cell infiltrate

Sm antigen
SMAP (systemic mean arterial pressure)
smear (see also *stain, test*)
  AFB (acid-fast bacillus)
  air-dried
  alimentary tract
  bacteriologic
  blood
  bronchoscopic
  buccal
  buffy coat
  cervical
  cul-de-sac
  cytologic
  endocervical
  endometrial
  eosinophil
  fast
  feces
  FGT (female genital tract) cytologic
  fungal
  lateral vaginal wall
  lower respiratory tract
  malaria
  nasal
  oral
  pancervical
  PAP (Papanicolaou)
  peripheral
  peripheral blood
  pus
  sputum
  stool
  Tzanck
  urine
  vaginal
  VCE (vagina, ectocervix, endocervix)
  wet
smear immersed in fixative
smear sprayed with fixative
smear test
smegma bacillus
Smith test for bile pigments
smoker's lung
smoker's palate
smooth muscle
smooth-muscle antibody (SMA)
smooth-muscle hypertrophy
smooth texture
smudge cell
snake venom poisoning
snakelike
snap-frozen
SNOMED (Standard Nomenclature of Medicine)
Snook reticulum stain
snuff box, anatomical
soaplike material
socket
socket joint
SOD (superoxide dismutase)
sodium
sodium bicarbonate
sodium bisulfite
sodium chromate ^{51}Cr sterile solution
sodium dodecyl sulfate (SDS)
sodium hydroxide
sodium test
sodium thiosulfate
sodoku (spirillary rat-bite fever)
Soemmering crystalline
Soemmering ligament
softening of bone
soft palate
soft papilloma
soft spot, capitate
soft stool
soft tissue
solar cheilitis
solar degenerative change
solar dermatitis
solar elastosis

solar irradiation
solar keratosis
solar lentigo
solar plexus
Soldaini test for glucose in urine
Solera test for thiocyanates
solid matrix
solid ovarian teratoma
solid-phase extraction tube
solid teratoma
solid tissue specimen
solitary bone cyst
solitary cells of Meynert
solitary glands of large intestine
solitary glands of small intestine
solitary lesion
solitary lymph node
solitary myeloma
solitary nodule
solubility screening test for sickle cell hemoglobin
solution (see also *fixative*, *stain*)
  acid alcohol
  alcoholic
  anticoagulant heparin
  aqueous
  astringent
  Bouin
  buffered
  Burow
  DAKO target retrieval
  Depex mounting
  Drabkin
  Flemming
  formalin
  formol-Zenker
  Gilson
  Gowers
  half-normal
  Hamdi
  Ham F-10
  Hayem

solution *(continued)*
  heparin lock flush
  Hollande
  iodine topical
  lactated Ringer
  Lugol
  mordant
  normal
  Orth
  pyridoxilated stroma-free hemoglobin
  Ringer
  Ruge
  saline
  saturated
  Schällibaum
  Seyderhelm
  sodium chromate ^{51}Cr sterile
  stroma-free hemoglobin
  TAC (tetracaine, epinephrine, and cocaine)
  Toison
  Zamboni
  Zenker fixative
somatic artery
somatic cell
somatic death
somatic nerve
somatic tissue
somatomedin-C polypeptide hormone
somatostatin cell
somatotropic hormone (STH)
somatotropin release-inhibiting hormone (SIH)
somatotropin-releasing factor (SRF)
somatotropin-releasing hormone (SRH)
somatotropin releasing–inhibiting factor (SRIF, SIF)
Somogyi effect
Somogyi phenomenon
Sondermann canal
S100 protein

sonicator
Sonne-Duval bacillus
Sonnenschein test
sorbent
Sörensen scale
sore, Oriental
sorehead (filarial dermatosis)
Soret band
sorter, fluorescence-activated cell
(FACS)
SOS gene
sounds, bowel
South American blastomycosis
Southern blot (SB) analysis
Southern blot test
Southern blotting
soy bean test for urease
sp. (species)
space
alveolar dead
anatomical dead
antecubital
apical
axillary
Baros
Berger
Bogros
Böttcher
Bowman
Burns
capsular
cartilage
Chassaignac
Cloquet
Colles
corneal
Cotunnius
dead
Disse
epidural
episcleral
epitympanic

space *(continued)*
filtration
Fontana
gingival
Henke
His
intercellular
intercostal
Kiernan
Kretschmann
Kuhnt
Lesgaft
Magendie
Malacarne
Meckel
Mohrenheim
Nuel
Parona
perineal
perisinusoidal
peritoneal
plane of fifth intercostal
Poiseuille
potential
preperitoneal
presacral
Proust
Prussak
Reinke
retroperitoneal
retropubic
Retzius
Schwalbe
subperitoneal
suprahepatic
supralevator
Tarin
Tenon
tissue
Traube semilunar
Trautmann triangular
vesicovaginal

space *(continued)*
  Virchow-Robin
  Waldeyer
  Westberg
  zonular
space of Mall, periportal
space of Poirier
space of Retzius
spade finger
spaghetti-like tangles of basophilic connective tissue fibers
spastic
spasticity
spasticity and rigidity, muscular
spatula, Ayre
specialized cell
species (sp.)
specific gravity, decreased in:
  diabetes insipidus
  ingestion or infusion of fluid
  renal failure
specific gravity, increased in:
  acute glomerulonephritis
  congestive heart failure
  dehydration
  diabetes mellitus with glycosuria
  toxemia
specific gravity test
specific gravity, urinary
specific inflammation
specificity of laboratory tests
specimen
  autopsy
  biopsy
  blood
  catheterized
  clean-catch urine
  clean-voided urine
  dimensions of
  fingerstick
  first-voided urine
  gross description

specimen *(continued)*
  histologic
  identification
  laboratory
  midstream urine
  processing of tissue
  sectioning of tissue
  solid tissue
  stool
  surgical
  tissue
  24-hour urine
speck finger
speckled appearance
speckled fluorescence
speckled pattern
speckling with fine dots
spectrophotometric test
spectrophotometry
S peptide
sperm
  donor
  frozen
  motile
  washed
sperm penetration assay
sperm allergy
sperm antibody
sperm motility study
sperm washing
spermatic abscess
spermatic artery
spermatic cord
spermatid
spermatogenesis
spermatogenic cell
spermatogenic granulomatous orchitis
spermatozoa
sperm cell
S-phase fraction
sphenoethmoidal recess
sphenoid biopsy

sphenoid bone
sphenoid cell
sphenoid fontanelle
sphenoid mucosa
sphenoidal ridge
sphenoidal roof of nasal cavity
sphenoidal sinus
sphenoidal turbinated bone
sphenomandibular ligament
spheno-occipital joint
sphenopalatine artery
sphenopalatine canal
sphenopalatine foramen
sphenopalatine ganglia
sphenopalatine vein
sphenopharyngeal canal
sphenoturbinal bone
spherical shape
spherocytosis, hereditary
spheroid or spheroidal (ball-and-socket)
spheroid articulation
spheroid joint
spheroplast
Spiegler test
Spielmeyer swelling
sphincter
  antral
  basal
  bicanalicular
  Boyden
  canalicular
  choledochal
  colic
  cricopharyngeal
  duodenal
  duodenojejunal
  external anal
  extrinsic
  first duodenal
  hypertensive lower esophageal
  Hyrtl
  inferior esophageal

sphincter *(continued)*
  lower esophageal (LES)
  Lutkens
  Nélaton
  O'Beirne
  pancreatic duct
  pancreaticobiliary
  pharyngoesophageal
  prepyloric
  pyloric
  upper esophageal (UES)
sphincter contraction ring
sphincter of anal canal, involuntary
sphincter of bile duct
sphincter of hepatopancreatic ampulla
sphincter of Oddi
sphincter urethral muscle
sphincteric mechanism
sphingolipid activator protein (SAP)
sphingomyelin
sphingomyelin accumulation in liver
  and spleen
sphingomyelinase deficiency
sphingomyelin in marrow histiocytes,
  accumulation of
spiculated
spicule
spider angioma (pl. angiomata)
spider cell
spider hemangioma
spider nevus (pl. nevi)
spider-web clot
Spiegler test for albumin
spillage of tumor cells
spina bifida cystica
spina bifida occulta
spinach stool
spinal artery of Adamkiewicz
spinal canal
spinal cord
spinal cord tissue
spinal defect

spinal degeneration
spinal fluid
  bloody
  cloudy
  frankly purulent
  glucose level of
  milky
  protein in
  total protein concentration of
spinal ganglion
spinal marrow
spinal meninges
spinal meningitis
spinal meningocele
spinal muscular atrophy
spinal nerve
spinal neuron
spinal part of accessory nerve
spinal roots
  C1-7 (cervical)
  Co. 1 (coccygeal)
  L1-5 (lumbar)
  S1-5 (sacral)
  T1-12 (thoracic)
spinal stenosis
spinal tap
spindle
  aortic
  cleavage
spindle cell
spindle cell nevus
spindle cell sarcoma
spindle colonic groove
spindle-shaped cell
spindle-shaped fibroblasts replacing osteoblasts
spindle-shaped incision
spindle-shaped structure
spine
  alar
  anterior superior iliac
  anteroposterior iliac

spine *(continued)*
  cervical (C)
  dorsal (D)
  iliac
  ischial
  lumbar (L)
  lumbosacral (LS)
  posterior column of
  posterior-inferior
  sacral (S)
  thoracic (T)
  thoracolumbar
spine cell
spinelike projection
spinnbarkeit
spinoglenoid ligament
spinothalamic tract
spinous processes, vertebral
spiral artery
spiral band of Gosset
spiral canal of cochlea
spiral canal of modiolus
spiral fashion
spiral fold
spiral fracture
spiral joint
spiral ligament of cochlea
spirals, Curschmann
spiral-shaped bacteria
spiral wound
spirillary rat-bite fever
Spirillum
Spirillum minus
spirochetal myocarditis
spirochete
spironolactone test
Spiro test
Spitz nerve
splanchnic artery
splanchnic nerve
splanchnomegaly
splatter

spleen
  accessory
  dccp purple
  floating
  function
  inflammation
  long axis of
  red pulp of
  soft
  white pulp of
spleen tip
splenic abscess
splenic artery
splenic atrophy
splenic capsule
splenic cell
splenic congestion
splenic engorgement
splenic flexure
splenic hilum
splenic hyperplasia
splenic hypertrophy
splenic notch
splenic parenchyma
splenic pulp
  red
  white
splenic-renal angle
splenic tissue
splenic vein
splenic vessel
splenitis, acute septic
splenium
splenocolic ligament
splenogastric omentum
splenoid gland
splenomegaly
splenoportal hypertension
splenorenal anastomosis
splenorenal angle
splenorenal ligament
splenorenal recess
splint bone
split brain
split-brain syndrome
split gene
split-renal function test
splitting bone
spoke bone
Spondweni virus
spondylitis
  ankylosing
  rheumatoid
  tuberculous
spondylolisthesis
spondylolisthetic pelvis
sponge kidney
spongiform degeneration of gray matter
spongiform encephalopathy
spongiform leukodystrophy
spongiform pustule
spongioblast
spongiosis
spongiosum penis, corpus
spongy bone
spongy degeneration of central nervous system
spongy degeneration of white matter
spongy urethra
spontaneous abortion
spontaneous bacterial myositis
spontaneous rupture
spore stain
Sporothrix schenckii
sporotrichosis
Sporotrichum schenckii
spot
  blue
  café au lait
  capitate soft
  coffee-colored
  cotton-wool
  germinal

spot *(continued)*
- Koplik
- red
- rose
- soft
- violet
- white

spot test for infectious mononucleosis
spout, ileal
Sprengel deformity
spring ligament
S protein (*not* protein S)
sprue
spur, calcaneal
spur cell (acanthocyte)
spur-cell anemia
spurious meningocele
spurious pregnancy
Spurr medium
Sputasol
sputum (pl. sputa)
- albumoid
- blood-tinged
- bloody
- gelatinous
- globular
- grayish
- green
- icteric
- moss-agate
- mottled
- nummular
- opalescent
- prune-juice
- reddish brown
- rusty
- yellow

sputum aeroginosum
sputum cruentum
sputum in rounded disks
SQ (subcutaneous)
squama alveolaris
squamate
squamocellular
squamocolumnar junction
squamocolumnar mucosal junction
squamo-occipital bone
squamous alveolar cell
squamous bone
squamous cell
squamous cell carcinoma
squamous cell carcinoma of cervix
squamous cell carcinoma of digestive tract
squamous cell carcinoma of lung
squamous cell carcinoma of penis
squamous cell carcinoma of skin
squamous cell carcinoma of uterine cervix
squamous cell carcinoma of vagina
squamous cell carcinoma of vocal cord
squamous epithelial cell
squamous epithelium
squamous intraepithelial lesion
squamous metaplasia of bronchus
squamous metaplasia of cervix
squamous-type bone
squeeze, tussive
sRBC (sheep red blood calls)
sRBC and phenylethyl alcohol
SS-A antibody
SS-B antibody
SSPE (subacute sclerosing panencephalitis)
stab (neutrophil)
stab cell
stable factor (Factor VII)
stab wound
staff cell
stage
- end-
- menstrual
- proliferative
- secretory

staghorn calculus
staging
  cancer
  Dukes
  FIGO
  malignancy
  malignant melanoma
  metastasis
  neoplasm
  tumor
staging of tumor, TNM
  T (primary tumor)
  N (regional nodes)
  M (metastasis)
stagnation mastitis
stagnation of urine
Stahr gland
stain (see also *method*, *solution*)
  acetic acid
  acid
  acid alcohol
  acid-fast
  acid-fast bacilli (AFB)
  acid fuchsin
  acid phosphatase
  Alcian blue
  alizarin
  alpha-naphthol esterase
  alum-carmine
  Alzheimer
  ammoniacal silver
  ammonium silver carbonate
  amyloid
  aniline blue
  argentaffin
  auramine-rhodamine
  auramine-rhodamine fluorescent
  auramine rhodamine fluorochrome
  azocarmine
  azure
  basic
  basic fuchsin

stain *(continued)*
  Best
  Best carmine
  Betke-Kleihauer
  Biebrich scarlet
  Bielschowsky
  blue aniline
  Bodian
  Bowie
  Brown-Brenn Gram
  Brown-Hopp tissue Gram
  Bullard hematoxylin
  Cajal gold sublimate
  Cajal trichrome
  carbolfuchsin
  carmine
  Celani method
  Congo red
  contrast
  counter
  cresyl blue
  cresyl blue brilliant
  cresyl fast violet
  crystal violet
  Dane and Herman keratin
  Darrow red
  Davenport
  Del Rio Hortega method
  Delafield
  Delafield hematoxylin
  Dieterle
  Dieterle silver
  differential
  DOPA (dihydroxyphenylalanine)
  double
  Ehrlich acid hematoxylin
  Ehrlich neutral
  Ehrlich triacid
  elastic (elastin)
  elastica-van Gieson
  elastic fibers
  electron

stain *(continued)*
- eosin
- eosin azure
- eosin-phloxine
- fast blue
- fast green
- fast red
- ferric ammonium sulfate
- ferric chloride
- Feulgen
- Feulgen method
- Fite-Faraco
- F method
- Fontana-Masson
- Fontana methenamine-silver
- Foot reticulum
- Fouchet reagent
- fuchsin
- Gallego method
- gentian orange
- gentian violet
- Giemsa
- Giemsa-Wright
- Gill hematoxylin
- Gimenez
- GMS (Gomori methenamine-silver)
- gold
- gold chloride
- Golgi method
- Gomori aldehyde fuchsin
- Gomori methenamine-silver (GMS)
- Gomori-Takamatsu
- Gram
- Gridley
- Grocott-Gomori methenamine-silver nitrate
- Grocott methenamine-silver
- H&E (hematoxylin and eosin)
- Hale iron
- Hanks
- Hansel
- Harris hematoxylin

stain *(continued)*
- heavy-metal
- Heidenhain iron hematoxylin
- Heinz body
- hemalum
- hematoxylin
- hematoxylin and eosin (H&E)
- hematoxylin-malachite green–basic fuchsin
- hematoxylin-phloxine B
- Hirsch-Peiffer
- Hiss capsule
- Holmes silver nitrate
- Holzer method
- Hortega neuroglia
- Hucker-Conn
- hydrochloric acid
- immunofluorescent
- immunoperoxidase
- India ink
- India ink capsule
- indigo carmine
- intravital
- iodine
- iron
- iron hematoxylin
- Isamine blue
- Janus green B
- Jenner method
- Jones kidney
- Kasten fluorescent Feulgen
- Kernechtrot
- Kinyoun
- Kinyoun acid-fast
- Kinyoun carbolfuchsin
- Kleihauer-Betke
- Kluver-Barrera
- Kossa (von Kossa)
- Kronecker
- Langeron iodine
- Laquer
- lead hydroxide

stain *(continued)*
- Leder
- Leifson flagella
- Leishman
- Lendrum phloxine-tartrazine
- Lepehne-Pickworth
- Levaditi
- Levine alkaline Congo red method
- Lillie
- Lillie allochrome connective tissue
- Lillie azure-eosin
- Lillie ferrous iron
- Lillie sulfuric acid Nile blue
- lipoid
- Lison-Dunn
- lithium carbonate
- lithium-carmine
- Löffler (Loeffler)
- Löffler caustic
- Lorrain Smith
- Lugol
- Luna-Ishak
- Luna modification of Bodian
- Luxol fast blue
- Macchiavello
- MacNeal tetrachrome blood
- malachite green
- Malbin-Sternheimer
- Maldonado-San Jose
- Mallory aniline blue
- Mallory-Azan
- Mallory collagen
- Mallory hemofuchsin
- Mallory iodine
- Mallory iron
- Mallory phloxine
- Mallory phosphotungstic acid–hematoxylin
- Mallory trichrome
- Mallory triple
- Mancini iodine technique
- Mann methyl blue–eosin

stain *(continued)*
- Marchi method
- Masson argentaffin
- Masson–Fontana ammoniacal silver
- Masson trichrome
- Maximow
- May-Grünwald
- May-Grünwald-Giemsa
- Mayer
- Mayer mucicarmine
- meconium
- metachromatic
- methyl green–pyronin
- methyl violet
- methylene blue
- Michaelis
- Milligan trichrome
- Mowry colloidal iron
- MSB trichrome
- mucicarmine
- mucin
- multiple
- myeloperoxidase
- Nakanishi
- naphthol-ASD chloroacetate esterase
- naphthol green B
- naphthol yellow S
- Nauta
- negative
- Neisser
- neutral
- neutral red
- Nicolle
- Nile blue fat
- ninhydrin-Schiff
- Nissl
- Nobel
- nuclear
- nuclear fast red
- oil red O
- orange G

stain *(continued)*
- orcein
- Orth
- osmic acid
- osmium tetroxide
- oxalic acid
- Padykula-Herman
- Paget-Eccleston
- panoptic
- PAP (Papanicolaou)
- Pappenheim
- paracarmine
- Paragon
- PAS (periodic acid-Schiff)
- Perdrau method
- periodic acid-Schiff (PAS)
- Perls Prussian blue
- peroxidase
- phloxine
- phosphomolybdic acid
- phosphotungstic acid
- phosphotungstic acid-hematoxylin (PTAH)
- picrocarmine
- picro-Mallory trichrome
- picronigrosin
- plasma
- plasmatic
- plastic section
- polychrome
- polychrome methylene blue
- Pontamine sky blue
- port-wine
- positive
- potassium metabisulfite
- potassium permanganate
- protoplasmic
- Protargol
- Prussian blue
- PTAH (phosphotungstic acid-hematoxylin)
- Puchtler-Sweat

stain *(continued)*
- pyrrol blue
- Q-banding
- quinacrine fluorescent method
- Rambourg chromic acid–phosphotungstic acid
- Rambourg periodic acid–chromic methenamine–silver
- Ramón y Cajal stain
- Ranson pyridine silver
- rapid mucin
- R–banding
- reticulin
- reverse Giemsa method
- Romanowsky
- Romanowsky blood
- Roux
- safranin
- scarlet red
- Schaeffer–Fulton
- Scharlach R
- Schiff solution
- Schmorl ferric–ferricyanide reduction
- Schmorl picrothionin
- Schultz
- Scott solution
- selective
- Seller
- Shorr trichrome
- silver
- silver nitrate
- silver protein
- Snook reticulum
- sodium bicarbonate
- sodium bisulfite
- sodium hydroxide
- sodium thiosulfate
- spore
- Sternheimer–Malbin
- Stirling modification of Gram
- Sudan

stain *(continued)*
Sudan black
Sudan black B fat
Sudan III
supravital
Taenzer
Takayama
telomeric R–banding
tetrachrome
thioflavine T
thionin
Tilden
Tizzoni
T method
T-staining method
Toison
toluidine blue
trichrome
Truant auramine-rhodamine
trypsin G-banding
tumor
Turnbull blue
Unna
Unna-Pappenheim
Unna-Taenzer
uranium nitrate
uranyl acetate
urate crystals
van Ermengen
van Gieson
Verhoeff
Verhoeff elastic
vital
von Kossa
von Kossa calcium
Warthin-Starry
Wayson
Weigert
Weigert-Gram
Weigert iron hematoxylin
Weigert-Pal method
Weil

stain *(continued)*
Weil myelin sheath
Wilder reticulum
Williams
Wirtz-Conklin spore
Wright
Ziehl-Neelsen
Ziehl-Neelsen acid-fast

stainable iron

staining (see also *stain*)
acid-fast
bipolar
differential
double
fluorescent
intravital
multiple
negative
polar
postvital
preagonal
progressive
regressive
relief
simple
substantive
supravital
telomeric
terminal
T method
triple
vital

staining antibody

staining of tissue sections

stalk
allantoic
body
polyp

standard, calibration

standard cell

Standard Nomenclature of Medicine (SNOMED)

standard serologic test for syphilis (STS)
standing plasma test
Stanley bacillus
Stanley cervical ligament
stapedial artery
stapes bone
staph sepsis
staphyline gland
staphylococcal myocarditis
staphylococcal pericarditis
staphylococcal pneumonia
staphylococcal pneumonitis
staphylococcal protein A
staphylococcal scalded skin syndrome
staphylococcus
Staphylococcus albus
Staphylococcus aureus
Staphylococcus auricularis
Staphylococcus capitis
Staphylococcus cohnii
Staphylococcus epidermidis
Staphylococcus haemolyticus
Staphylococcus hominis
Staphylococcus pyogenes
Staphylococcus saccharolyticus
Staphylococcus saprophyticus
Staphylococcus warneri
Staphylococcus xylosus
staphyloma
star cell
starch granules
starch-iodine test
starch test
Stargardt macular degeneration
starry-sky pattern
star-shaped cell
starvation acidosis
starvation diabetes
stasis
  circulatory
  venous
stasis dermatitis
stasis gallbladder
stasis cirrhosis
stat (statim)
stat test
stature, abnormally increased
status asthmaticus
status post
Staub-Traugott phenomenon
STD (sexually transmitted disease)
steady state diffusing capacity of lung ($DLCO_{SS}$)
steamy appearance
steatorrhea
Stein-Leventhal syndrome
stellar nevus
stellate abscess
stellate cell
stellate cells of cerebral cortex
stellate cells of liver
stellate configuration
stellate ganglia
stellate granuloma
stellate ligament
stellate pattern
stellate reticulum
stem cell
stem cell assay
stem cell marrow harvesting
Stenella araguata
stenosis
  aortic valve
  arterial
  bowel
  bronchial
  cardiac valvular
  cervical
  esophageal
  mitral
  pulmonary
  pyloric
  spinal

Stensen canal
Stensen duct
step section
stephanofiliariasis
stercoraceous abscess
stercoral abscess
stereospecific enzyme
stereotactic biopsy
sterile lancet
sterile abscess
sterile hyphae
sterile meningitis
sterility
sternal angle
sternal articulation
sternal joint
sternal pleural reflection
Sternberg cell
Sternberg giant cell
Sternberg-Reed cell
sternebra (pl. sternebrae)
Sterneedle tuberculin test
Sternheimer-Malbin stain
sternoclavicular articulation
sternoclavicular joint, articular disk of
sternoclavicular ligament
sternocleidomastoid artery
sternocleidomastoid muscle
sternocostal articulation
sternocostal hiatus
sternocostal joint
sternocostal junction
sternomanubrial junction
steroid diabetes
steroid fever
steroidogenic diabetes
Stirling modification of Gram stain
St. Louis encephalitis
St. Louis encephalitis virus
Stock test
Stokvis test
Stoll test
stoma
stomach
  aberrant umbilical
  antrum of
  bilocular
  canal of
  cardia of
  cardiac
  cascade
  convex border of
  coronary artery of
  cup-and-spill
  distal blind
  dumping
  greater curvature of
  hourglass
  leather bottle
  lesser curvature of
  miniature
  Pavlov
  pit of
  scaphoid
  sclerotic
  thoracic
  trifid
  upside-down
  waterfall
  water-trap
stomach bed
stomach calculus
stomach fundus
stomatitis
  allergic
  aphthous
  bismuth
  catarrhal
  gonococcal
  gonorrheal
  herpetic
  infectious
  lead
  membranous

stomatitis *(continued)*
- mercurial
- mycotic
- nonspecific
- recurrent aphthous
- syphilitic
- trophical
- ulcerative
- uremic
- vesicular
- Vincent

stomatitis exanthematica
stomatitis medicamentosa
stomatitis nicotina
stomatitis scarlatina
stomatitis scorbutica
stomatitis venenata
stomatocyte
stone (also, calculus, gallstone)
- barrel-shaped
- bile duct
- biliary tract
- bilirubinate
- black faceted
- bladder
- blue
- bosselated
- calcium bilirubinate
- chalk
- common bile duct (CBD)
- cholesterol
- cystine
- gallbladder
- intrahepatic
- intraluminal
- kidney
- lung
- metabolic
- noncalcified
- renal
- residual
- salivary

stone *(continued)*
- skin
- staghorn
- struvite
- tear
- ureteric
- urinary
- vein
- womb

stonelike mass
stone mole
stool
- acholic
- bilious
- black tarry
- bloody
- brown
- bulky
- caddy (dark, sandy mud)
- caliber of
- clay-colored
- color and caliber
- consistency of
- currant jelly
- dark
- dark-green
- diarrhea
- fatty
- flattened
- floating
- foamy
- formed
- foul-smelling
- frank blood in
- frequency of
- green
- guaiac-negative
- guaiac-positive
- hard
- heme-negative
- heme-positive
- impacted

stool *(continued)*
- lienteric
- light gray
- liquid
- loose
- mahogany-colored
- malodorous
- maroon-colored
- melenic
- mucoid
- mucous
- mushy
- nonbloody
- occult blood in
- oily
- pale
- pea soup
- pelleted
- pencil-like
- pipe-stem
- rabbit
- reducing substance in
- residual
- ribbon
- rice-water
- runny
- sago-grain
- scybalous
- semiformed
- semisolid
- silver
- slurry of
- soft
- spinach
- tarry black
- undigested food in
- unformed
- watery
- white fatty

stool color
stool consistency
stool culture
stool for occult blood
stool for ova and parasites (O&P)
stooling
stool osmotic gap
stool smear
stool specimen
stool urobilinogen
storage disease
store (pl. stores)
- hepatic glycogen
- glycogen
- iron
- liver iron

storiform
straddling embolism
straight-chain fatty acid
straight sinus
straight tubule
strand, complementary
strangulated bowel
strangulation of hernia
strap cell
straplike connection
straplike muscle
strap muscle
Strassburg test for bile acids in albumin-free urine
stratification
stratified clot
stratified columnar epithelium
stratified cuboidal epithelium
stratified epithelium
stratified squamous epithelium
stratified squamous mucosa
stratified squamous submucosa
stratified transitional epithelium
stratographic analysis
straw itch
strawberry gallbladder
strawberry hemangioma
strawberry nevus
strawberry tongue

straw-colored fluid
straw-colored urine
streak
streaking, atheromatous
streak plate
Streeter band
strep (slang for streptococcus)
strep screen
strep throat
streptavidin-biotin peroxidase complex
streptavidin-horseradish peroxidase
streptobacillary rat-bite fever
Streptobacillus moniliformis
streptococcal antigen
streptococcal disease of newborn
streptococcal enzyme hyaluronidase
streptococcal pharyngitis
streptococcal pneumonia
streptococcus
  alpha-hemolytic
  anhemolytic
  beta-hemolytic
  gamma-hemolytic
  hemolytic
  group A beta-hemolytic (GABHS)
  nonhemolytic
Streptococcus acidominimus
Streptococcus aecium
Streptococcus agalactiae
Streptococcus anginosus
Streptococcus avium
Streptococcus bovis
Streptococcus constellatus
Streptococcus durans
Streptococcus equi
Streptococcus equinus
Streptococcus equisimilis
Streptococcus faecalis
Streptococcus faecium
Streptococcus intermedius
Streptococcus M antigen
Streptococcus milleri
Streptococcus mitis
Streptococcus morbillorum
Streptococcus mutans
Streptococcus pneumoniae
Streptococcus pyogenes
Streptococcus salivarius
Streptococcus sanguis
Streptococcus uberis
Streptococcus viridans
Streptococcus zooepidemicus
Streptomyces
Streptomyces paraguayensis
Streptomyces somaliensis
Streptozyme serologic test
stretchability of skin
stria (pl. striae)
  acoustic
  auditory
  brown
  dermal
  pink
striate artery
striated cardiac muscle
striated muscle
striated skeletal muscle
striation, basal
striations
striatonigral degeneration
string cell carcinoma
stringency
stringent factor
stringy mucous exudate
strip
stripe, properitoneal flank
striped muscle
stripped
stripper, vein
stroke
stroma
  abnormally scanty
  connective-tissue
  desmoplastic

stroma *(continued)*
  endometrial
  fibrofatty
  fibrous
  fibrovascular
  nonmalignant
  ovarian
  periductal
  synovial
stroma-free hemoglobin solution
stromal ganglion
stromal hemorrhage
stromal invasion
stromal necrosis
stromal retraction
strong silver protein
strong trichrome staining method
Strongyloides stercoralis
strongyloidiasis
Strong bacillus
structural lesion
structure
  biliary
  cord
  denture-supporting
  elongated
  glandular
  hollow
  organoid
  satellite
  subcutaneous
structure of cell
structure protein
struma ovarii
struma, Riedel
strumous abscess
Strümpell (Struempell)
Strümpell-Leichtenstern encephalitis
Strümpell-Marie disease
Struthers
  arcade of
  ligament of
Struve test for blood in urine
struvite
STS (serologic test for syphilis)
STT (scaphotrapezoid trapezial) joint
Stuart factor
Stuart medium
Stuart-Prower factor
study
  serial CK enzyme
  sperm motility
stump
  appendiceal
  cervical
  duodenal
  gastric
  limb
  rectal
stump pregnancy
stunned myocardium
stunting of growth
stupor
stye
styloglossus muscle
stylohyoid ligament
styloid, radial
stylomandibular ligament
stylomastoid foramen
stylomaxillary ligament
Stypven time test
subacromial bursitis
subacute allergic pneumonia
subacute atrophy of liver
subacute bacterial endocarditis
subacute combined degeneration of spinal cord
subacute granulomatous thyroiditis
subacute hepatitis
subacute hepatic necrosis
subacute inflammation
subacute myelitis
subacute myoendocarditis
subacute necrotic myelitis

subacute nephritis
subacute nodular migratory panniculitis
subacute sclerosing panencephalitis (SSPE)
subacute thyroiditis
subadventitial fibrosis
subaponeurotic abscess
subarachnoid cistern
subarachnoid exudate
subarachnoid hemorrhage
subarachnoid space
subareolar abscess
subauricular gland
subcapsular
subcarinal node
subcecal appendix
subchronic atrophy of liver
subclavian artery
subclavian loop
subclavian vein
subclinical diabetes
subclinical infection
subcostal artery
subcostal muscle
subcostal nerve
subcostal plane (SCP)
subcu (subcutaneous)
subculture
subcutaneous (SQ, subcu)
subcutaneous annulus
subcutaneous connective tissue
subcutaneous emphysema
subcutaneous fascia
subcutaneous fat
subcutaneous fat necrosis
subcutaneous inflammation
subcutaneous layer
subcutaneous nodule
subcutaneous pannus
subcutaneous structure
subcutaneous tissue
subcutaneous wound
subcutis
subdeltoid bursitis
subdiaphragmatic abscess
subdural abscess
subdural clot
subdural effusion
subdural hematoma, encapsulated
subdural hemorrhage
subdural space
subendocardial
subepicardial myocarditis
subepidermal abscess
subepithelial
subfascial abscess
subgaleal abscess
subhepatic abscess
subhepatic area
subhepatic cecum
subintimal fibrosis
subjacent
sublingual artery
sublingual gland
sublingual salivary gland
subluxation of lens
submammary mastitis
submandibular duct
submandibular ganglion
submandibular gland
submandibular lymph node
submandibular node
submandibulary salivary gland
submassive hepatic necrosis
submassive pulmonary embolism
submaxillary artery
submaxillary gland
submaxillary glandular artery
submental artery
submental lymph node
submucosa
submucosal venous plexus
submucous leiomyoma
submuscular

subpectoral abscess
subperiosteal abscess
subperitoneal fatty areolar tissue
subperitoneal space
subphrenic abscess
subphrenic pyopneumothorax
subphrenic recess
subpubic angle
subsartorial canal
subscapular abscess
subscapular angle
subscapular artery
subserosa
subserosal fibrosis
subserosal hemorrhage
subserosal layer
substance
  amorphous ground
  anterior pituitary-like
  basophil
  beta
  cement
  central gray
  chromophil
  cortical
  exophthalmos-producing
  ground
  lipoid
  medullary
  Nissl
substantia nigra (black substance)
substantia propria (proper substance)
substernal goiter
substitution bone
substrate
subtalar articulation
subtalar joint
subungual
subungual abscess
subungual melanoma
subunit
subvesical duct
subxiphoid
succulent
succumb
sucking wound
Sucquet-Hoyer canal
sucrose hemolysis test
sucrose lysis test
sucrose test
suction artifact
suction pipette
Sudan black
Sudan black B fat stain
sudanophilic leukodystrophy
Sudan III (oil red O)
sudden cardiac death
sudden infant death syndrome (SIDS)
Sudeck atrophy
Sudeck point
sudoriferous gland
sudoriparous abscess
SUDS (Single Use Diagnostic System)
suffocative goiter
sugar
  blood
  brain
  differential
  fasting blood
  random blood
  reducing
  threshold
  two-hour postprandial
  urine
sugar and acetone (S&A)
sugar-icing liver
suggillation, postmortem
Suipoxvirus (swinepox virus)
sulcal artery
sulcus (pl. sulci)
sulfate, keratan
sulfhemoglobin
sulfhemoglobinemia
sulfosalicylic acid turbidity test

sulfur granules
sulfuric acid
sulfur test for protein
Sullivan test for cysteine
Sulzberger-Chase phenomenon
summer prurigo
sunburn-like reaction
sunlight radiation
superciliary arch
superficial abscess
superficial brachial artery
superficial cardiac dullness
superficial cell
superficial cervical artery
superficial dorsal sacrococcygeal ligament
superficial epigastric artery
superficial external pudendal artery
superficial fascia
superficial iliac circumflex artery
superficial inguinal lymph node
superficial inguinal pouch
superficial inguinal ring
superficial layer, fatty
superficial lymph vessel
superficial necrosis
superficial palmar arch artery
superficial plexus
superficial perineal artery
superficial perineal pouch
superficial petrosal artery
superficial pneumonia
superficial posterior sacrococcygeal ligament
superficial pustular perifolliculitis
superficial spreading melanoma
superficial temporary artery
superficial transverse metacarpal ligament
superficial transverse metatarsal ligament
superficial transverse perineal muscle
superficial volar arch artery
superficial volar artery
Superfrost/Plus Fisherbrand glass slide
superimposed
superior alveolar artery
superior articular artery of knee
superior articular process
superior border of heart
superior bronchus
superior cerebellar artery
superior cistern
superior colliculi
superior costotransverse ligament
superior deep cervical lymph node
superior demifacet
superior duodenal fold
superior duodenal recess
superior epigastric artery
superior gluteal artery
superior gluteal vessel
superior hemorrhoidal artery
superior hypogastric plexus
superior intercostal artery
superior labial artery
superior laryngeal artery
superior ligament of epididymis
superior ligament of incus
superior ligament of malleus
superior lobe
superior lobe bronchus
superior longitudinal muscle of tongue
superior margin of inferior rib
superior meatus
superior mediastinum
superior mesenteric artery
superior mesenteric ganglion
superior mesenteric plexus
superior mesenteric vein
superior nasal concha
superior orbital fissure
superior pancreaticoduodenal artery
superior pelvic aperture

superior phrenic artery
superior pole
superior profunda artery
superior pubic ligament
superior pulmonary vein
superior radioulnar joint
superior rectal artery
superior rectal vein
superior rib, inferior margin of
superior sagittal sinus
superior thoracic aperture
superior thoracic artery
superior thyroid artery
superior tibial articulation
superior tibiofibular joint
superior transverse rectal fold
superior transverse scapular ligament
superior turbinated bone
superior tympanic artery
superior ulnar collateral artery
superior vena cava
superior vesical artery
supermedial surface
supernatant
supernatant plasma
supernumerary bone
supernumerary kidney
supernumerary nipple
superoxide dismutase (SOD)
supply
  motor
  nerve
supporting cell
suppressor cell
suppressor gene tumor
suppressor T cell
suppuration, frank
suppurativa, hidradenitis
suppurative infection
suppurative mastitis
suppurative nephritis
suppurative pleurisy
suppurative pneumonia
supraceliac aorta
supraciliary canal
supraclavicular lymph node
supraclavicular nerve
supraclinoid aneurysm
supracolic compartment
supracristal plane (SCP)
supraduodenal artery
suprahepatic abscess
suprahepatic caval cuff
suprahepatic space
suprahepatic vena cava
suprahyoid aponeurosis
suprahyoid artery
suprainterparietal bone
supralevator space
supranuclear lesion
supraoccipital bone
supraoptic anastomosis
supraoptic canal
supraorbital artery
supraorbital canal
supraorbital ridge
suprapharyngeal bone
suprapleural membrane
suprapubic region
suprarenal artery
suprarenal gland
suprarenal impression
suprascapular artery
suprascapular ligament
suprasellar meningioma
supraspinous ligament
suprasternal bone
supratrochlear artery
supravaterian duodenum
supravital stain
supravital staining of blood specimen
supreme nasal concha
supreme turbinated bone
sural artery

surface
  acromial articular
  anterolateral
  anteromedial
  articular
  articulating
  arytenoidal articular
  auricular
  axial
  basal
  buccal
  calcaneal articular
  carpal articular
  cerebral
  colic
  costal
  cuboidal articular
  denture basal
  denture foundation
  denture impression
  denture occlusal
  denture polished
  diaphragmatic
  distal
  facial
  fibular
  fibular articular
  gastric
  glenoid
  mucous
  occlusal
  posterior
  supermedial
surface biopsy
surface epithelium
surface mucous cells of stomach
surface of heart
  diaphragmatic
  sternocostal
surface of liver bed
surfactant
surfactant protein A concentration
surfer's knee
surfer's knot
surfer's nodule
surgery, Mohs
surgical margin
surgical neck
surgical scar
surgical scraping
surgical specimen
surgical wound
surveillance, medical
susceptibility test
suspensory ligament
suspensory muscle of duodenum
sustentacular cell of ear
sustentacular cell of testis
Sutter blood group
Sutton nevus
sutural bones
sutural ligament
suture (fibrous joint)
  coronal
  cranial (joint)
  dentate
  ethmoidolacrimal
  ethmoidomaxillary
  false
  frontal
  frontoethmoidal
  frontolacrimal
  frontomaxillary
  frontonasal
  frontozygomatic
  lambdoid
  metopic
  sagittal
suture joint
suture line
Suzanne gland
SVR (systemic vascular resistance)
swab, throat
swaged needle

swallowing center
swallowing mechanism
swan-neck deformity
sweat
  bloody
  blue
  drenching
  fetid
  green
  night
  phosphorescent
  profuse
sweat chloride
sweat electrolytes
sweat gland
sweat test
sweep, duodenal
Sweet disease
swelling (see also *edema*)
  ankle
  arytenoid
  brain
  Calabar
  capsular
  cloudy
  fugitive
  genital
  glassy
  hunger
  Kamerun
  labial
  labioscrotal
  Neufeld capsular
  scrotal
  Soemmering crystalline
  Spielmeyer
  tropical
swimmer's dermatitis
swimmer's ear
swimmer's itch
swimming pool granuloma
swine influenza virus
swinepox virus
swirls and tangles
swordfish test
sycosis nuchae
sylvian aqueduct
Sylvius, aqueduct of
Symmers fibrosis
symmetric
symmetrical distribution
symmetry
sympathetic abscess
sympathetic fibers, preganglionic
sympathetic formative cell
sympathetic ganglion
sympathetic hormone
sympathetic nerve
sympathetic ophthalmia
sympathetic system
sympathetic trunk
sympathicotropic cell
sympathochromaffin cell
symphysis cartilaginous joint
symphysis pubis
symptomatic porphyria
symptomatic pruritus
synapse
  axoaxonic
  axodendritic
  electrotonic
synarthrodial joint
synarthrosis articulation
synarthrosis joint
synchondrosis articulation
synchondrosis, cranial
synchondrosis joint
synchronous multicentric osteosarcoma
syncope
syncytial knot
syncytial meningioma
syncytium
  circular
  horseshoe-shaped

syncytium formation
syndesmosis
syndesmosis joint
syndrome
  acquired immune deficiency (AIDS)
  adrenogenital
  antiphospholipid
  aortic arch
  aplastic anemia
  autoerythrocyte sensitization
  Banti
  Barré-Guillain
  Behçet
  Bloom
  carcinoid
  Chédiak-Steinbrinck-Higashi
  Churg-Strauss
  Conn
  CREST
  Crigler-Najjar
  CRST
  crush
  Curtis–Fitz-Hugh
  Cushing
  dengue shock
  double-crush
  Down
  Dresbach
  Dubin-Johnson
  dumping
  dysplastic nevus
  Ehlers-Danlos
  Ellison-Zollinger
  empty sella
  Fanconi
  fetal alcohol
  Fitz-Hugh–Curtis
  fragile X
  Friderichsen-Waterhouse
  Goodpasture
  Gougerot-Blum
  Griscelli

syndrome *(continued)*
  Guillain-Barré
  Hantavirus pulmonary (HPS)
  hemolytic-uremic
  Henoch-Schönlein (Schoenlein)
  Hurler
  hyper-IgE
  inherited malformation
  Job
  Johnson-Dubin
  Klinefelter
  Leventhal-Stein
  Lichtheim
  Li-Fraumeni (LFS)
  locked-in
  Lutembacher
  malabsorption
  Mallory-Weiss
  Marfan
  Meigs
  Mikulicz
  mucocutaneous lymph node
  Najjar-Crigler
  nephrotic
  nutritional deficiency
  Omenn
  paraneoplastic
  Pierre Robin
  pneumorenal
  polycystic ovary
  postmenopausal
  Putnam-Dana
  Reiter
  Reye
  sarcophagic
  scalded skin
  sepsis
  Sheehan
  Sjögren
  staphylococcal scalded skin
  Stein-Leventhal
  testicular feminization

syndrome *(continued)*
  toxic shock
  Treacher Collins
  Turner
  Waterhouse-Friderichsen
  Weiss-Mallory
  Wiskott-Aldrich
  Zollinger-Ellison
syndrome of fever, urticaria, and joint inflammation due to allergy
synechia (pl. synechiae)
synergic
synergist
synostosis
synovia
synovial articulations of cranium
synovial cell
synovial fluid
synovial fluid differential count
  clasmatocytes
  lymphocytes
  monocytes
  polymorphonuclear cell
  synovial cell
  unclassified
synovial fluid lactic acid
synovial frost
synovial gland
synovial joint
synovial ligament
synovial-like
synovial lining
synovial membrane
synovial osteochondromatosis
synovial sarcoma
synovitis
  local
  localized nodular
  pigmented villonodular
  purulent
  serous
  villonodular
synovium, hyperplastic
synthase
synthesis of ammonia
synthetic azo dye
synthetic protein
syphilis
  congenital
  serologic test for (STS)
  tertiary
  VDRL test for
syphilitic abscess
syphilitic aneurysm
syphilitic aortitis
syphilitic arteritis
syphilitic chancre
syphilitic cirrhosis
syphilitic fever
syphilitic leukoderma
syphilitic meningitis
syphilitic myelitis
syphilitic myocarditis
syphilitic necrosis
syphilitic nephritis
syphilitic neuritis
syphilitic osteochondritis
syphilitic periarteritis
syphilitic stomatitis
syringobulbia
syringomyelia
system
  alimentary
  articular
  automatic nervous
  bulbosacral
  cardiovascular
  caudal neurosecretory
  cell-free
  central nervous
  cerebrospinal
  chromaffin
  circulatory
  colloid

system *(continued)*
- conducting
- craniosacral
- cytochrome
- dermal
- dermoid
- digestive
- endocrine
- esthesiodic
- excretory
- exterofective
- extrapyramidal motor
- female reproductive
- gamma motor
- genital
- genitourinary
- glandular
- haversian
- hemolymphatic
- intrahepatic duct
- lymphatic
- male reproductive
- nervous

system *(continued)*
- parasympathetic
- portal
- portal venous
- respiratory
- sympathetic
- venous

systematized nevus
Système International (SI) units
systemic and topical hypothermia
systemic effects
systemic fungal infection
systemic lesion
systemic lupus erythematosus (SLE)
systemic mean arterial pressure (SMAP)
systemic mycosis
systemic necrotizing vasculitis
systemic vascular resistance (SVR)
systemic vein
systemic zygomycosis
system of Retzius
Szabo test

T, t

T (temperature)
T (tesla)
T_3 (triiodothyronine)
T_4 (thyroxine, tetraiodothyronine)
TA (therapeutic abortion)
TAC (tetracaine, epinephrine, and
  cocaine) solution
Tacaribe virus
tachypnea
tactile cell
taenia (also, tenia)
Taenia saginata
Taenia solium
taeniae of Valsalva
Taenzer stain
tag
  skin
  toe
  wrist
tagged antibody, fluorescently
tagged, radioactively
Tahyna virus
tail bone
tail of epididymis
tail of pancreas
Takayama stain
Takayasu disease
tall columnar epithelium
talocalcaneal articulation
talocalcaneal ligament
talocalcaneonavicular articulation
talocalcaneonavicular joint
talocrural articulation
talocrural joint
talonavicular articulation
talonavicular joint
talonavicular ligament
talotibial ligament, anterior
talus bone
Tamiami virus
Tamm-Horsfall mucoprotein
Tamm-Horsfall protein
tamponade, cardiac
tanapox virus
T and B lymphocyte subset assay
T&C (type and crossmatch)
tangentially
tangential wound
tangles, neurofibrillary
tanned red cell (TRC)
tanning
Tanret test for albumin
tapeworm
tapeworm infestation

tapeworm segments and ova in stool
Taq Dye
target cell
target gland
target lesion
Tarin space
tarry black stools
tarsal artery
tarsal bone
tarsal canal
tarsal cyst
tarsal gland
tarsal ligament
tarsal plate
tarsal tunnel
tarsoconjunctival glands
tarsometatarsal articulation
tarsometatarsal joint
tarsometatarsal ligaments
tartaric acid
tart cell
tartrate resistant leukocyte acid phosphatase
taste bud
taste cell
TAT (thrombin-antithrombin III complex)
tattoo
Tatumella
Tatumella ptyseos
taurine test
Taylor test
Tay-Sachs disease
TB (tuberculin; tuberculosis)
TBG (thyroxine-binding globulin)
TBII (TSH-binding inhibitory immunoglobulins)
TBP (thyroxine-binding protein)
TBPA (thyroxine-binding prealbumin)
Tc (technetium)
T (thymus-dependent) cell
T (thymus-derived) cell
T cell activation marker
- CD25
- CD26
- CD69

T cell growth factor
T cell lymphoma
- convoluted
- cutaneous
- small lymphocytic

TCMI (T cell-mediated immunity)
TCPI Rapid Test for HIV
TCR (T cell antigen receptor)
T cytotoxic cell
TDA (TSH-displacing antibody)
T-dependent antigen
TdT (terminal deoxynucleotidyl transferase)
TDTH cells
teacher nodule
tear (laceration)
- full-thickness
- Mallory-Weiss
- partial-thickness

teardrop cell
teardrop-shaped erythrocyte
tear in articular cartilage
tearing of a muscle
technetium (Tc)
technetium 99m (^{99m}Tc)
technique (see also *method*, *staining*)
- PAP (peroxidase-antiperoxidase) technique for detecting antigen or antibody in tissue sections
- pressure cooker
- Scotch tape

teeth
- Hutchinson
- incisor
- milk
- primary
- secondary
- wisdom

teeth of Huschke, auditory
T effector cell
Teichmann test for blood
teichoic acid antibody
T-8 suppressor cell
tela (weblike tissue)
tela subcutanea (subcutaneous fascia)
telangiectasia
  generalized essential
  hemorrhagic
  hereditary
  hereditary hemorrhagic
  spider
  unilateral nevoid
telangiectasis
telangiectatic angioma
telangiectatic osteogenic sarcoma
telangiectatic osteosarcoma
Tellyesniczky solution
telogen phase
telomeric R-banding stain
temperate virus
temperature, basal body (BBT)
temperature scale
temporal arteritis
temporal artery
temporal bone
temporal canal
temporal fascia
temporal fossa
temporal muscle
temporal pole
temporomandibular articulation
temporomandibular joint
temporomandibular ligament
tenacious
tenderness, cervical motion (CMT)
tendineae, chordae
tendinitis
tendinous arch of pelvic fascia
tendinous band
tendinous fibers, interlacing
tendinous intersection
tendinous raphe
tendo Achillis
tendo calcaneus (calcaneal tendon)
tendon
  Achilles
  biceps
  bowed
  brachioradialis
  calcanean
  central (of diaphragm)
  central perineal
  common
  conjoined
  conjoint
  contracted
  coronary
  cricoesophageal
  Gerlach annual
  hamstring
  heel (tendo calcaneus)
  intermediate (of diaphragm)
  patellar
  pulled
  rider's
  sheetlike
  slipped
  Todaro
  trefoil
  Zinn (common tendinous ring)
tendon cell
tendon of Achilles
tendon of diaphragm, center
tendon of Hector (heel tendon)
tendon sheath
tendon sheath of ganglion
Tenon capsule
Tenon space
tenosynovitis of digital tendon sheath
tension, carbon dioxide
tension pneumothorax
tensor fasciae latae

tensor tympani muscle canal
tensor veli palatini (tensor palati)
tentative diagnosis
tentorial incisure
tentorial meningioma
tentorium cerebelli
teratocarcinoma of ovary
teratocarcinoma of testis
teratogen
teratogenic
teratology
teratoma
  cystic
  ovary
  pineal
  solid
  solid ovarian
  testis
teres, ligamentum
terminal artery
terminal bile duct
terminal bronchiole
terminal deletion
terminal deoxynucleotidyl transferase (TdT)
terminal hematuria
terminal ileum
terminal infection
terminal pneumonia
terminal sulcus
terminal ventricle of spinal cord
termination factor
territorial matrix
Terson gland
tertian malaria
tertiary radicle
tertiary syphilis
Teschen virus
tesselated retina
test (see also *smear* and *stain*)
  acetaldehyde
  acetoacetate

test *(continued)*
  acetone
  acetowhite
  acid clearance (ACT)
  acid elution (for fetal hemoglobin)
  acidification of stool
  acidified serum (for paroxysmal nocturnal hemoglobinuria)
  acid-lability
  acid perfusion
  acid phosphatase (for semen)
  acid reflux
  acid serum
  acoustic immittance
  ACTH stimulation
  activated coagulation time (ACT)
  activated partial thromboplastin time (APTT)
  Addis
  adrenocorticotropic hormone (ACTH)
  adrenocorticotropic hormone stimulation test
  agglutination
  alanine
  AlaSTAT latex allergy
  Albarran
  albumin
  aldolase
  aldosterone
  alkali denaturation
  alkaline phosphatase
  Allen
  Allen-Doisy
  Almén (for blood)
  AL patch
  alpha-fetoprotein
  ALT (alanine aminotransferase) (formerly SGPT)
  Ames assay
  amino acid nitrogen (AAN)
  aminolevulinate dehydratase

test *(continued)*
- aminolevulinic acid (ALA)
- aminopyrine breath
- ammonia nitrogen
- ammonium chloride loading
- amylase
- Anderson and Goldberger
- Anderson-Collip
- androstenedione
- angiotensin I
- angiotensin II
- anion gap
- anoxemia
- antibiotic sensitivity
- antichymotrypsin
- anticytoplasmic antibody (ACPA)
- anti-deoxyribonuclease B titer (anti-DNAse titer)
- antidiuretic hormone (ADH)
- antidiuretic hormone-water deprivation stimulation test
- anti-DNA antibodies
  - Farr
  - Ginsberg-Keiser
  - indirect fluorescence
- anti-double-stranded DNA
- antiglobulin (AGT)
- antiglobulin consumption
- antihuman globulin
- antihyaluronidase titer (AH titer)
- anti-LA/SS-B
- anti-Ro/SS-A
- anti-Sm
- anti-streptolysin-O titer (ASO titer)
- antithrombin III (AT-III)
  - amidolytic (chromogenic)
  - radioimmunodiffusion (RID)
- antitrypsin
- Apt
- argentaffin reaction
- arsenic
- arylsulfatase

test *(continued)*
- Ascoli precipitin (for anthrax)
- ascorbate-cyanide
- ascorbic acid
- aspirin tolerance
- AST (aspartate aminotransferase) (formerly SGOT)
- ASTRA profile
- atropine
- augmented histamine (of gastric function)
- autoerythrocyte sensitivity
- autohemolysis
- Autolet blood glucose
- automated reagin (ART)
- Autopath QC
- Bachman
- Bachman-Pettit
- bacteriolytic
- Bárány caloric
- basal secretory flow rate (BSFR)
- base excess
- baseline
- basophil degranulation
- battery of
- BEI (butanol-extractable iodine)
- bench
- Benedict (for glucose)
- bentiromide
- bentonite flocculation
- benzidine
- Bernstein acid perfusion
- Bernstein esophageal acid infusion
- Berson
- betazole stimulation
- Bettendorff (for arsenic)
- Bial
- bicarbonate
- bile acid breath
- bile acid tolerance
- bile acids, total
- bile esculin

test *(continued)*
- bile solubility
- bilirubin
  - conjugated
  - direct
  - indirect
  - total
- Binz (for quinine in urine)
- biuret (for serum proteins)
- bleeding time (BT)
  - Duke
  - Ivy
  - Mielke
  - Simplate
- blood (see Table, pp. 576-590)
- blood sugar
- blood volume
- bone marrow, differential count
- borderline
- Bozicevich
- breath analysis
- breath-holding
- breath hydrogen
- bromosulfophthalein (BSP)
- bromphenol
- brucellosis agglutinins
- buffy coat smear
- CA15-3 RIA
- CA 19-9 (carbohydrate antigen)
- calcitonin (hCT)
- calcitonin–calcium infusion stimulation
- calcium
  - ionized
  - total
- Calmette
- caloric
- CAMP (Christie, Atkins, and Munch-Petersen) factor
- cancer antigen 125 (CA125)
- C&S (culture and sensitivity)
- capillary fragility

test *(continued)*
- capillary resistance
- carbohydrate utilization
- carbon dioxide
  - partial pressure (PCO_2)
  - total (TCO_2)
- carbon monoxide
- carbon 13-labeled ketoisocaproate breath
- carboxyhemoglobin
- carcinoembryonic antigen (CEA)
- cardiac enzymes
- cardiac isoenzymes
- Cardiac T Rapid Assay
- carotene
- carotene absorption
- carotid sinus
- Carr-Price
- Casoni intradermal (for hydatid disease)
- Casoni skin
- catalase
- catecholamines
  - fractionated
  - free
  - plasma
  - total
  - urinary
- CEA (carcinoembryonic antigen)
- cephalin-cholesterol flocculation
- cerebrospinal fluid pressure
- cerebrospinal fluid volume
- ceruloplasmin
- CF (complement fixation)
- C-glycocholic acid breath
- “chem” (chemical profile)
- chemical
- Chemstrip bG
- chenodeoxycholic acid, total
- chenodeoxycholylglycine, conjugated
- Chick-Martin

test *(continued)*
Chlamydiazyme
chloride
cholecystokinin
cholesterol, total
cholic acid, total
cholinesterase II
chorionic gonadotropin
chromatin
chromium red blood cell
chromogenic enzyme substrate
citrate
citrulline
C lactose
Clinitest stool
clomiphene
CLOtest
clot lysis
clot retraction
clotting time
Lee-White
plasma
coagulase
coagulation factor assay
coagulation time
coccidioidin
cold pressor
cold water calorics
colloidal gold
Coloscreen Self
competitive binding assay
complement fixation (CF)
concentration (for renal function)
conglutinating complement absorption (CCAT)
Congo red (for amyloidosis)
conjunctival
contact patch
contraction stress (CST)
copper
copper-binding protein
coproporphyrin

test *(continued)*
Corner Allen
corticobinding globulin (CBG)
corticosterone
cortisol
cortisol, free
CO_2-withdrawal seizure
C-peptide
creatinine
C-reactive protein
creatine kinase (CK)
total
isoenzymes
creatinine
creatinine clearance
CSF glutamine
Cult-Dip Plus bacteriological culture
culture and sensitivity (C&S)
cutaneous
cutaneous tuberculin
cyanide
cyanide-nitroprusside
cyclic AMP
cysteine (also, cystine)
cytotropic antibody
DA pregnancy
Davidsohn differential absorption
Day
d-dimer
deferoxamine mesylate infusion
Dehio
dehydrocholate
dehydroepiandrosterone (DHEA)
dehydroepiandrosterone sulfate ($DHEA-SO_4$)
deoxycholic acid, total
11-deoxycortisol (Compound S)
11-deoxycorticosterone (DOC)
deoxyribonuclease (DNase)
deoxyuridine suppression
dexamethasone single dose overnight suppression

test *(continued)*
- dexamethasone suppression
- dextrose
- DFA-TP (direct fluorescent antibody-*Treponema pallidum*)
- diabetes
- diacetyl
- diagnostic
- Dick intracutaneous
- differential
- differential count
- differential renal function
- differential ureteral catheterization
- dihydrotestosterone (DHT)
- 1,25-dihydroxycholecalciferol assay (1,25-OH-D_3)
- dinitrophenylhydrazine
- diphtheria
- direct antiglobulin
- direct Coombs
- direct fluorescent antibody
- discontinuation
- disk-diffusion
- Donath-Landsteiner
- double glucagon
- Dragendorff (for bile)
- Ducrey intradermal
- Duke bleeding time
- D-xylose absorption
- D-xylose tolerance
- dye exclusion
- edrophonium
- ELISA titer
- Ellsworth-Howard
- eosinophil count
- E-rosette
- erythrocyte adherence
- erythrocyte count
- erythrocyte protoporphyrin (EP)
- erythrocyte sedimentation rate (ESR)
- erythropoietin

test *(continued)*
- esophageal acid infusion
- esophageal function
- estradiol
- estriol (E_3)
  - free
  - total
- estrogen receptor assay (ERA)
- estrogens, total
- estrone (E_1)
- euglobulin clot lysis
- ExacTech blood glucose meter
- executive profile
- Farber
- Farr
- fat, fecal
- fatty acid profile
- fatty acids
  - nonesterified (free)
  - total
- FDL (fluorescein dilaurate)
- fecal alpha$_1$-antitrypsin
- fecal leukocyte count
- fecal occult blood
- Felix-Weil
- fermentation
- fern
- ferric chloride
- ferritin
- ferrohemoglobin solubility
- alpha$_1$-fetoprotein
- fibrin degradation products
- fibrin lysis time
- fibrinogen
- fibrin stabilizing factor (FSF)
- FIGLU excretion
- Finn chamber patch
- Fishberg concentration
- Fishman-Doubilet
- fluorescent antibody (FA)
- fluorescent antinuclear antibody (FANA)

test *(continued)*
- fluorescent treponemal antibody (FTA)
- fluorescent treponemal antibody absorption (FTA-ABS)
- fluoride
- folate
- folate absorption
- follicle-stimulating hormone (FSH)
- follicle-stimulating hormone-releasing (FSH-RH)
- Foshay (for tularemia)
- Fouchet (for bilirubin in urine)
- fragility
- Francis
- free thyroxine index (FT_4I)
- free triiodothyronine (T_3)
- Frei intracutaneous diagnostic
- fructose challenge
- fructose loading
- fructose tolerance
- FTA-ABS (fluorescent treponemal antibody-absorption)
- function
- Gaddum and Schild
- galactose tolerance
- gastric acid
- gastric content
- gastric emptying
- gastric function
- gastric secretion rate
- gastric secretory
- gastrin
- gastrin-secretin stimulation
- gastrin stimulation
- Gastroccult
- GBIA (Guthrie bacterial inhibition assay)
- gel diffusion
- gel (double) diffusion precipitin in one or two dimensions

test *(continued)*
- gel diffusion reaction
- Geraghty
- Gerhardt (for acetoacetic acid)
- Gerhardt (for urobilin in urine)
- germ tube
- Gerrard
- GGTP liver function
- Gies biuret
- Gilchrist skin
- globulin
- glomerular selectivity (IgG/albumin clearance)
- glucagon stimulation
- glucose
- glucose oxidase paper strip
- glucose-6-phosphate dehydrogenase (G-6-PD)
- glucose tolerance (GTT)
- glucose tolerance with cortisone
- glucose, two-hour postprandial
- glutamine
- glutamyltransferase (GGT)
- glutathione reductase in erythrocytes
- glycerol, free
- glycerophosphate
- glycine
- glycogen storage
- glycolic acid
- glycosylated hemoglobin
- glycyltryptophan
- glyoxylic acid
- Gmelin
- Gofman
- gold
- gonadotropins
- Gordon
- Gothlin capillary fragility
- Graham-Cole cholecystography
- Gram stain of stool
- Gravindex pregnancy

test *(continued)*
- Gregerson and Boas
- Grigg
- Gross
- growth hormone–arginine stimulation
- growth hormone–glucagon stimulation
- growth hormone, human (hGH, somatotropin)
- growth hormone–L-dopa stimulation
- G-6-PD (glucose-6-phosphate dehydrogenase)
- guaiac (for occult blood)
- Gunning
- Gunning-Lieben
- Günzberg (Guenzberg)
- Guthrie bacterial inhibition assay (GBIA)
- Gutzeit
- Ham acidified serum
- hamatein
- Hamel
- Hammarsten
- hamster egg penetration assay
- hapten inhibition
- haptoglobin (Hp)
- Harding and Ruttan
- Harris and Ray
- Harrison spot
- Hart
- HATTS (hemagglutination treponemal test for syphilis)
- Hay
- H_2 breath
- HDL cholesterol (HDLC)
- Heaf
- heat coagulation
- heat instability
- heavy metal screening

test *(continued)*
- Heinz body
- *Helicobacter pylori* urease
- Helisal rapid blood
- Heller
- hemadsorption
- hemadsorption virus
- hemagglutination
- hemagglutination inhibition (HI, HAI)
- Hematest
- hematocrit (HCT, Hct)
- hemin (for blood)
- Hemoccult II
- hemoglobin (Hb)
- hemoglobin A
- hemoglobin A_{IC}
- hemoglobin A_2 (HbA_2)
- hemoglobin electrophoresis
- hemoglobin F
- hemoglobin H (HbH)
- HemoQuant fecal blood
- hemosiderin
- hepatic function
- Herzberg
- Hess capillary
- heterophile agglutination
- Hickey-Hare
- Hildebrandt
- Hines-Brown cold pressor
- Hinton
- Histalog
- Histalog stimulation
- histamine
- histamine flare
- histidine loading
- histoplasmin-latex
- HIVAGEN
- HIV-antibody test on blood
- HIV Blot 2•2
- Hoffmann

test *(continued)*
- Hofmeister
- Hollander
- homocystine
- homovanillic acid (HVA)
- Hooker-Forbes
- Hopkins-Cole
- Hopkins thiophene
- Hoppe-Seyler
- Horsley
- Howard
- Howell prothrombin
- Huddleson agglutination
- Huhner
- Huppert
- Huppert-Cole
- Hurtley
- hydrochloric acid
- hydrogen breath
- hydrogen peroxide
- hydroxybutyric acid
- 17-hydroxycorticosteroids (17-OHCS)
- 5-hydroxyindole acetic acid (5-HIAA)
- hydroxylamine (for glucose)
- 17-hydroxyprogesterone (17-OHP)
- hydroxyproline
- 25-hydroxyvitamin D assay (25-OH-D)
- hyperventilation
- hypoxemia
- ice water calorics
- Ilosvay
- immobilization
- immune adhesion
- immunoglobulin A (IgA)
- immunoglobulin D (IgD)
- immunoglobulin G (IgG)
- immunoglobulin G/albumin ratio
- immunoglobulin G synthesis rate
- immunoglobulin M (IgM)

test *(continued)*
- immunologic pregnancy
- immunoperoxidase
- IMViC metabolic
- indigo carmine
- indigo red
- indirect antiglobulin
- indirect Coombs
- indirect fluorescent antibody
- indirect hemagglutination
- indole
- indophenol
- inhibition
- insulin (12 hours fasting)
- insulin antibodies
- insulin and glucose suppression
- insulin clearance test
- insulin hypoglycemia
- insulin with oral glucose tolerance
- insulin tolerance
- intracutaneous
- intracutaneous tuberculin
- intradermal
- intraductal secretin (IDST)
- intraesophageal acid
- intraesophageal pH
- intrinsic factor, vitamin B_{12}
- iodine
- iodoform
- iron
- iron-binding capacity, total (TIBC)
- iron saturation
- islet cell antibody screening (ICA)
- isocitrate dehydrogenase (ICD)
- isoleucine
- isopropanol precipitation
- Ito-Reenstierna
- ^{131}I uptake (thyroid function)
- Ivy bleeding time
- Jacquemin
- Jaffe
- Johnson

test *(continued)*
- Jolles
- Jones and Cantarow urea concentration
- Jones fluorescein instillation
- Jorissen
- Kantor and Gies
- Kaplan
- Kapsinow
- Katayama
- Kentmann
- Kerner
- 17-ketogenic steroids (17-KGS)
- 17-ketosteroid (17 KS) fractions
- ketone bodies
- kidney function
- Killian
- Kirby-Bauer
- Kjeldahl
- Kleihauer acid elution
- Kleihauer-Betke
- Kleihauer-Betke acid elution
- Klimow
- Knapp
- Knott
- Kober
- Kobert
- KOH (potassium hydroxide)
- Kolmer
- Kondo
- Korotkoff
- Kossel
- Kowarsky
- Krokiewicz
- Kurzrok-Miller
- Kurzrok-Ratner
- Kveim intradermal
- lactic acid
- lactose
- lactose breath hydrogen
- Ladendorff
- lamellar body number density

test *(continued)*
- Lancefield precipitation
- Lang (for taurine)
- Lange (for acetone in urine)
- LAP (leucine aminopeptidase)
- latex agglutination
- latex fixation
- LDL cholesterol (LDLC)
- lead
- LE cell
- Lechini
- Lee
- Lee-White clotting time
- Legal
- leishmanin
- Leo
- lepromin
- Lesser
- leucine
- leukocyte adherence assay
- leukocyte bactericidal assay
- leukocyte esterase (LET)
- Levinson
- Lieben
- Lieben-Ralfe
- Liebermann
- Liebermann-Burchard
- Liebig
- limulus
- *Limulus* amebocyte lysate assay
- Lindemann
- line (for rickets)
- lipase
- lipoprotein electrophoresis
- litmus milk
- liver function (LFT)
- Loewe
- long-acting thyroid stimulating hormone (LATS)
- Lowenthal
- Lücke
- lupus band

test *(continued)*
lupus erythematosus (LE) cell
luteinizing hormone (LH)
Luttke
Lyle and Curtman
lymphocyte proliferation
lymphocyte transformation
lysozyme
Macdonald
Machado
Machado-Guerreiro
Maclagan thymol turbidity
MacLean
MacLean-de Wesselow urea concentration
MacMunn
macrophage migration inhibition
MacWilliam
magnesionitric
magnesium
magnetic susceptibility
Magpie
Malot
maltose
Mann-Whitney
Mann-Whitney-Wilcoxon
Mantoux intracutaneous tuberculin
Mantoux skin
Maréchal
Marquis
Masset
Mathews
Maumené
Mayerhofer
Mayer
Mazzotti (for onchocerciasis)
McNemer ascites
Meigs
melanin
Meltzer-Lyon
Mendel
mercury

test *(continued)*
Mester
metabisulfite (for sickle cell hemoglobin)
metanephrine, total
methanol
methionine
methyl red
methylphenylhydrazine
metratrophic
Mett
metyrapone stimulation
MHA-TP (microhemagglutination-*Treponema pallidum*)
Michailow
Micral urine dipstick
Microflow
microhemagglutination
microprecipitation
microsomal antibodies, thyroid
migration inhibitory factor (MIF)
Millard
Miller-Kurzrok
Millon
Millon-Nasse (for protein)
Mitscherlich
mixed agglutination
mixed lymphocyte culture (MLC)
Mohr
Molisch
Moloney
Mono-Diff
Monoscreen
Monospot
Monosticon Dri-Dot
Montenegro
Moore
Morelli (exudate vs. transudate)
Moretti (typhoid fever)
Moritz
Mörner
Mosenthal

test *(continued)*
- motility
- Motulsky dye reduction
- mucin clot
- Mulder
- multiple-puncture intracutaneous tuberculin
- mumps sensitivity
- Murayama
- MycoAKT latex bead agglutination
- mycologic
- myelin basic protein
- Myers and Fine
- Mylius
- myoglobin
- Nakayama
- Nencki
- Neukomm
- neutralization
- niacin (for *Mycobacterium tuberculosis*)
- Nickerson-Kveim
- ninhydrin
- Nippe
- nitrate reduction
- Nitrazine
- nitric acid
- nitric acid–magnesium sulfate
- nitrites
- nitroblue tetrazolium (NBT)
- nitrogenous compound
- nitrogen partition
- nitrogen, total
- nitropropiol
- nitroprusside
- nitroso-indole-nitrate
- Nobel
- Noguchi
- nontreponemal antigen
- normetanephrine, total
- Northern blot
- Nyiri

test *(continued)*
- Obermayer
- Obermueller cholesterol
- occult blood
- OCT (oxytocin challenge)
- oleic acid-^{131}I absorption
- Oliver
- optochin sensitivity
- Oral Fluid Vironostika HIV-1 Microelisa System
- oral lactose tolerance
- orosomucoid
- OraSure HIV-1 Oral Specimen Collection Device
- Osgood-Haskins
- osmolality
- osmolality ratio, urine/serum
- osmotic fragility
- Osterberg
- Ouchterlony
- ova and parasites (O&P)
- OvuGen
- OvuKIT
- OvuQUICK
- oxalate
- ox cell hemolysin
- oxidase
- oxygen, partial pressure (PO_2)
- oxygen saturation
- oxytocin
- Palmer acid (for peptic ulcer)
- palmin
- pancreatic function
- pancreozymin-secretin
- PAP (Papanicolaou)
- PAP (peroxidase-antiperoxidase)
- Papnet
- parathyroid hormone (PTH)
- partial thromboplastin time
- passive cutaneous anaphylaxis
- passive protection
- patch

test *(continued)*
paternity
Patterson
Paul-Bunnell
Paul-Bunnell-Davidsohn
Pavy
PBI (protein-bound iodine)
peak and trough levels
peak secretory flow rate (PSFR)
penicillinase
pentagastrin
pentagastrin gastric secretory
pentagastrin infusion
pentagastrin provocative
pentagastrin stimulated analysis
pentoses
Penzoldt
Penzoldt-Fischer
pepsin
pepsinogen (PG I)
peptide
peptone
Peria
periodic acid-Schiff (PAS)
Perls hemosiderin
peroxidase
peroxidase-antiperoxidase (PAP)
Petri
Pettenkofer
Petzetaki
pH
PharmChek sweat patch drug detection
phenacetin
phenol
phenolphthalein
phenolsulfonphthalein
phenoltetrachlorophthalein
phentolamine (for pheochromocytoma)
phenylalanine
phenylhydrazine

test *(continued)*
phenylpyruvic acid, qualitative
phosphatase
acid
alkaline
phospholipids, total
phosphoric acid
phosphorus, inorganic
Pincus
pine wood
pineapple
Piria
Pirquet cutaneous tuberculin
placental lactogen (hPL)
plasmacrit
platelet adhesion
platelet aggregation
Plugge
POA (pancreatic oncofetal antigen)
Pohl
Pollacci
polyuria
Porges-Meier flocculation (for syphilis)
porphobilinogen (PBG)
Porter
positive whiff
Posner
postcoital
post-heparin lipolytic activity
postprandial
potassium
potassium iodide
PPD skin
precipitation
precipitin
Precision-G handheld blood glucose
Precision Q-I-D handheld blood glucose
pregnancy
pregnanediol
pregnanetriol

test *(continued)*
pregnenolone
Preyer
progesterone
progesterone receptor assay (PRA)
proinsulin
prolactin (PRL)
prolactin–insulin stimulation
properdin
prostaglandins
protection
protein-bound iodine
protein, total
proteose
prothrombin
prothrombin consumption
prothrombin-proconvertin
Protocult
protoporphyrin
provocative
pseudocholinesterase (PCHE)
Purdy
Pyramidon
pyruvic acid
quantitative fecal fat
Quick prothrombin
QuickVue Chlamydia
quinine carbacrylic resin (for gastric anacidity)
Quinlan
Raabe
Rabuteau
radioactive iodide uptake
radioactive iodinated serum albumin (RISA)
radioallergosorbent (RAST)
radioimmunosorbent (RIST)
Raji cell assay
Ralfe
Ramon flocculation
Randolph
Rantzman

test *(continued)*
rapid plasma reagin (RPR)
rapid serum amylase
Rapoport differential ureteral catheterization
RAST (radioallergosorbent)
Rebuck skin window
red cell adherence
red phenolsulfonphthalein
reducing substances
Rees
Rehberg
Reichl
Reinsch
Reiter complement fixation (for syphilis)
renal function
renal plasma flow (RPF)
renin
rennin
reptilase
resorcinol–hydrochloric acid
Response GM (for granulocyte count)
Reuss
reverse triiodothyronine (rT_3)
Reynolds
Rh blocking
rheumatoid arthritis
rhubarb
riboflavin (vitamin B_2)
rice-flour breath
Riegler
Rimini
ring
ring precipitin
RISA (radioactive iodinated serum albumin)
RIST (radioimmunosorbent)
Roberts
Robinson-Kepler
Ronchese

test *(continued)*
- rose bengal
- rose bengal radioactive (^{131}I)
- Rosenbach (for bile in urine)
- Rosenbach-Gmelin
- Rosenthal
- Rose-Waaler agglutination
- Rosin
- rosette
- Ross-Jones
- Rotazyme
- Rothera
- Rothera nitroprusside (for ketone bodies)
- Rous
- Roussin
- Rowntree and Geraghty
- RPR (rapid plasma reagin)
- rubella HI (hemagglutination inhibition)
- Rubner
- Ruhemann
- Rumpel-Leede
- Ruttan and Hardisty
- Saathoff
- Sabin-Feldman dye
- saccharimeter
- Sachs-Georgi
- Sachsse
- Sahli-Nencki
- Sakaguchi
- salicylic acid
- saline continence
- Salkowski
- Salkowski and Schipper
- Salkowski-Ludwig
- sand
- Sandrock
- santonin
- SART (standard acid reflux)
- Saundby (for blood in stool)
- scarification

test *(continued)*
- S-CCK-Pz (secretin, cholecysto-kinin, pancreatozymin)
- Schaffer
- Schalfijew
- Scherer
- Schick
- Schiller
- Schilling
- Schivoletto
- Schlesinger
- Schlichter
- Schönbein
- Schroeder
- Schulte
- Schultze
- Schumm
- scratch
- screening
- secretin
- secretin-CCK stimulation
- secretin-pancreozymin
- secretin provocation
- secretin stimulation
- sediment
- sedimentation rate (sed rate)
- Seidel
- SeHCAT (selenium-labeled homocholic acid conjugated with taurine)
- selenium
- Selivanoff
- semen analysis (sperm count)
- semiquantitative
- senna
- Sereny
- serial cardiac isoenzymes
- serologic (for syphilis) (STS)
- serotonin
- serum amylase
- serum bactericidal activity
- serum iron

test *(continued)*
- serum protein
- serum protein electrophoresis
- serum neutralization
- Sgambati reaction
- SGOT (now AST)
- SGPT (now ALT)
- shake
- sheep cell agglutination (SCAT)
- Sia
- Sicard-Cantelouble
- sickle cell
- Sickledex
- Sicklequik
- sickling
- Siebold and Bradbury
- silver
- Sims
- skin
- skin puncture (for Behçet syndrome)
- skin window
- slide
- slide clumping factor
- slide coagulase
- SMAC
- SMA-6
- SMA-12
- SMA-20
- small increment sensitivity index (SISI)
- smear
- Smith
- sodium
- Soldaini
- Solera
- solubility screening (for sickle cell hemoglobin)
- somatomedin C
- Sonnenschein
- Southern blot
- soybean

test *(continued)*
- specific gravity
- spectrophotometric
- sperm penetration assay
- Spiegler
- Spiro
- spironolactone
- split renal function
- spot (for infectious mononucleosis)
- standard acid reflux (SART)
- standard serologic (for syphilis) (STS for syphilis)
- standing plasma
- starch
- starch-iodine
- stat
- Sterneedle tuberculin
- stimulated gastric secretion
- Stock
- Stokvis
- Stoll
- stool cytotoxin
- stool electrolyte
- stool osmolality
- stool osmotic gap
- Strassburg
- Struve
- Stypven time
- sucrose
- sucrose hemolysis
- sucrose lysis
- SUDS (Single Use Diagnostic System)
- sulfosalicylic acid turbidity
- sulfur
- Sullivan
- susceptibility
- sweat
- swordfish
- syphilis
- Szabo
- Tanret

test *(continued)*
- taurine
- Taylor
- TCPI Rapid (for HIV)
- Teichmann
- Tensilon
- Test-Tape urine glucose
- testosterone
  - free
  - total
- TestPackChlamydia
- tetrahydrocortisol (THF)
- tetrahydrodeoxycortisol
- thalleioquin
- thermostable opsonin
- thiocyanate
- Thompson
- Thormählen
- Thorn
- thromboplastin generation
- Thudichum
- thymol turbidity
- thyroglobulin (Tg)
- thyroid antibodies
- thyroid function (TFT)
- thyroid hemagglutination
- thyroid microsomal antibodies
- thyroid-stimulating hormone (TSH)
- thyroid suppression
- thyroid uptake of radioactive iodine
- thyrotropin-releasing hormone (TRH) stimulation
- thyroxine
  - free (FT_4)
  - free (index)
  - total
- thyroxine-binding globulin (TBG)
- thyroxine ratio, effective (ETR)
- thyroxine/TBG ratio
- TIBC (total iron-binding capacity)
- Tidy

test *(continued)*
- tilt
- tine
- tine tuberculin
- titratable acidity
- Tizzoni
- tolbutamide
- Tollens, Neuberg, and Schwket
- Torquay
- total catecholamine
- total fecal weight
- total iron-binding capacity (TIBC)
- toxigenicity
- TPHA (*Treponema pallidum* hemagglutination)
- TPI (*Treponema pallidum* immobilization)
- transcortin
- transferrin
- transketolase
- *Treponema pallidum* complement fixation
- Tretop
- trichophytin
- triglycerides (TG)
- triiodothyronine (T_3) resin uptake
- triiodothyronine (T_3) uptake
- triketohydrindene hydrate
- triolein-^{131}I absorption
- Trommer
- Trousseau
- tryptophan load
- TSH (thyroid stimulating hormone)
- tube coagulase
- tuberculin
- tuberculosis
- tubular reabsorption of phosphate (TRP)
- T_3 uptake
- two-stage prothrombin
- two-stage triolein
- typhoid fever

test *(continued)*
- tyramine
- tyrosine
- Tyson
- Tzanck
- Udranszky
- Uffelmann
- Ulrich
- Ultzmann
- Umber
- unheated serum reagin (USR)
- urea
- urea clearance
- urea concentration
- urea nitrogen
- urea nitrogen/creatinine ratio
- urease
- Urecholine supersensitivity
- uric acid
- Uricult dipslide
- urine (see Table, pp. 561-563)
- urine concentration
- urine sediment
- urine volume
- urobilin
- urobilinogen
- uroporphyrin
- urorosein
- USR (unheated serum reagin)
- vaginal cornification
- vaginal mucification
- Vagitest
- valine
- van Deen (for blood)
- van den Bergh
- van der Velden
- vanillylmandelic acid
- Van Slyke
- vasoactive intestinal polypeptide (VIP)
- VDRL (for syphilis)
- ViraPap

test *(continued)*
- Vironostika Mixt ELISA HIV antibody
- viscosity
- Vitali
- vitamin A
- vitamin A tolerance
- vitamin B_2
- vitamin B_6
- vitamin B_{12} absorption
- vitamin B_{12} intrinsic factor
- vitamin C
- vitamin C saturation
- vitamin D
- Vitamin D assay
- vitamin E
- Voelcker and Joseph
- Vogel and Lee
- Voges-Proskauer
- Volhard (for renal function)
- Vollmer tuberculin patch
- von Aldor
- von Jaksch
- von Kossa calcium
- von Maschke
- von Pirquet
- von Zeynek and Mencki
- Waaler-Rose
- Wagner
- Waldenström (for porphyrin in urine)
- Wang
- Warburg
- Wassermann
- water
- water-gurgle
- water-sipping
- water-soluble contrast esophageal swallow
- Watson-Schwartz
- Webster
- Weichbrodt

test *(continued)*
- Weidel
- Weil-Felix
- Weisz
- Welcozyme HIV 1+2 ELISA antibody
- Wender
- Wenzell
- Weppen
- Werner thyroid suppression
- Westergren sedimentation rate
- Western immunoblot
- Wetzel
- Weyl
- Wheeler–Johnson
- whiff
- Widal
- Widal agglutination
- Widal serum
- Wideroe
- Widmark
- Wijs
- Wilcoxon
- Williamson blood
- Winckler
- Wishart
- Witz
- Woldman
- Woodbury
- Wood's light
- Worm-Mueller
- Wormley (for alkaloids)
- Wurster (for tyrosine)
- xylose
- xylose absorption
- Yvon (for alkaloids)
- Zaleski
- Zimmermann
- zona-free hamster egg penetration
- Zsigmondy

Tes-Tape urine glucose test

test meal

test on venous blood for:
- bile pigments
- carbohydrates
- electrolytes
- hormones
- lipids
- nitrogenous wastes
- prescribed drugs
- proteins (including enzymes)
- toxic substances
- vitamins

Tes-Tape

test panel

test profile

test result
- abnormal
- high normal
- low normal
- normal

testicles, undescended

testicular artery

testicular atrophy

testicular cyst

testicular degeneration

testicular feminization syndrome

testicular hormone

testicular nerve

testicular tumor

testicular vein

testing
- antibiotic sensitivity
- compatibility (cross-match)

testing antibody

testing antigen

testing electrolyte

testis (pl. testes)
- appendix
- ectopic
- efferent ductules of
- rete
- undescended

testis-determining factor (TDF)

testis teratocarcinoma
testis teratoma
testosterone hormone
testosterone test
  free
  total
TestPackChlamydia (no spaces)
Testut, ligament of
tetanus
tetanus bacillus
tetany
tetrachrome stain
tetrahydrocortisol (THF) test
tetrahydrodeoxycortisol test
tetraiodothyronine (thyroxine, T_4)
tetralogy of Fallot
tetroxide, osmium
Teutleben ligament
Texas fever
texture
  beefy
  bumpy
  buttery
  fleshy
  grainy
  granular
  greasy
  meaty
  nodular
  rough
  rubbery
  smooth
T_4 (thyroxine)
T_4/TBG ratio (thyroxine/thyroxine-binding globulin)
TFT (thyroid function test)
T4/T8 ratio
T-4 helper/inducer cell
T-4 lymphocyte
T-4 lymphocyte count
T-8 suppressor/cytotoxic cell
Thai hemorrhagic fever
thalassemia
thalassemia major
thalassemia minor
thalleioquin test for quinine
thallium poisoning
Thayer-Martin culture medium
Thayer-Martin medium
theca (pl. thecae)
  externa
  interna
theca cell of stomach
theca-lutein cell
theca-lutein cyst
thecal abscess
thecal sac
Theile canal
Theile gland
Theiler virus
thelarche
T helper cell
thenar eminence
Theobald Smith phenomenon
therapeutic abortion
therapeutic level of drug
therapeutic malaria
therapeutic range of a drug
therapy
  radiation
  steroid
thermal capacity
thermal energy
Thermoactinomyces sacchari
thermocoagulation change
Thermomax microplate reader
thermostable opsonin test
thiamine
thiazide diabetes
thickened material
thickened plaque
thickening of skin
thick-walled gallbladder
thigh

thigh muscle
thin bone cortex
thin-layer chromatography
thin skin
thin-walled cyst
thin-walled gallbladder
thin-walled hemangiomatous nodule
thin-walled venous sinuses
thiocyanate test
thioflavine T stain
thionin
third-trimester placenta
thixotropy
Thoma fixative
Thoma-Zeiss counting chamber
Thompson ligament
Thompson test
thoracentesis fluid
thoracic aorta
thoracic aorta artery
thoracic aperture
thoracic artery
thoracic bones
thoracic cage
    bony
    osseocartilaginous
thoracic cavity
thoracic duct
thoracic inlet
thoracic kidney
thoracic outlet
thoracic stomach
thoracic vertebra
thoracic wall
thoracic wall bone
thoracoabdominal diaphragm
thoracoabdominal incision
thoracoabdominal nerve
thoracocentesis
thoracolumbar fascia
thorax (pl. thoraces)
thorax, floor of
Thormählen test for melanin in urine
Thorn test
thornlike intercellular bridges
thornlike projections
threadlike
threatened abortion
three-cornered bone
three-vessel umbilical cord
threshold
    convulsant
    galvanic
threshold sugar
throat culture
throat swab
thrombasthenia
thrombin-antithrombin III complex (TAT)
thrombin time
thromboangiitis obliterans
thrombocyte
thrombocytopenia
thromboembolic disease
thromboembolism
thrombomodulin
thrombophlebitis
thromboplastin
thromboplastin generation test
thrombosed hemorrhoid
thrombosis
    arterial stenosis without
    intravascular
    recurrent intravascular
    widespread intravascular
thrombosis in arteriosclerotic vessel
thrombosis of a venous sinus
Thrombosphere synthetic platelets
thrombotic infarct
thrombotic thrombocytopenic purpura (TTP)
thrombus
    antemortem
    fibrin

thrombus *(continued)*
- lamellated
- laminated
- mural
- organization of
- organized
- postmortem
- traumatic

thrombus embolus
thrush of oral cavity
Thudichum test for creatinine
thumb, principal artery of
thymic abscess
thymic atrophy
thymic dysplasia
thymic lymphopoietic
thymidine, uptake of isotopically tagged
thymol turbidity test
thymoma
thymus-dependent lymphocyte
thymus-derived lymphocyte
thymus gland
thymus hyperplasia of
thymus, medulla of
Thy-1 antigen
thyrocervical trunk
thyrocyte
thyroepiglottic ligament
thyroglobulin antibody
thyroglobulin (Tg) test
thyroglossal duct cyst
thyrohyoid ligament
thyroid, accessory
thyroidal clearance
thyroid antibodies test
thyroid artery
thyroid atrophy
thyroid capsule
thyroid carcinoma
thyroid crisis
thyroidectomy
thyroid degeneration
thyroid eminence
thyroid follicle
thyroid function test (TFT)
thyroid gland
- accessory
- enlarged
- hyperplasia of
- indurated
- tender
- woody hard

thyroid goiter
thyroid hemagglutination test
thyroid hormone
- T_3 (triiodothyronine)
- T_4 (tetraiodothyronine, thyroxine)

thyroiditis
- acute
- autoimmune
- chronic fibrous
- de Quervain
- fibrous
- Hashimoto
- invasive fibrous
- ligneous
- lymphocytic
- Riedel
- subacute
- subacute granulomatous

thyroid microsomal antibody
thyroid panel
thyroid profile
thyroid scan (fluorescent scan)
thyroid-stimulating hormone (TSH)
thyroid-stimulating hormone-releasing factor (TSH-RF)
thyroid suppression test for hyperthyroidism
thyroid tumor
thyroid uptake tests
- perchlorate discharge test
- RAI (radioactive iodine) uptake test

thyroid *(continued)*
  radioimmunoassay for TSH
  ^{99m}Tc-pertechnetate uptake test
  thyroxine ^{125}I uptake test
  thyroxine ^{131}I uptake test
  TSH stimulation test
  TRH stimulation test
  T_3 suppression test
thyroid uptake of radioactive iodine test
thyrotoxic complement-fixation factor
thyrotoxicosis
thyrotropic hormone
thyrotropin
thyrotropin receptor antibody
thyrotropin-releasing factor (TRF)
thyrotropin-releasing hormone (TRH)
thyrotropin-releasing hormone stimulation test
thyroxine (T_4, tetraiodothyronine)
  free
  total
thyroxine assays
  free thyroxine (FT_4)
  free thyroxine index (FT_4 index)
  protein bound iodine (PBI)
  serum thyroxine by column chromatography: T_4(C)
  total serum T_4
thyroxine-binding albumin
thyroxine-binding globulin (TBG)
thyroxine-binding globulin assays
thyroxine-binding prealbumin (TBPA)
thyroxine-binding protein (TBP)
thyroxine hormone
thyroxine I 125 (^{125}I) radioactive agent
thyroxine I 131 (^{131}I) radioactive agent
thyroxine index, free (FT_4 index)
  total T_4
  T_3 resin uptake test
thyroxine ratio, effective (ETR)
thyroxine/TBG ratio
thyroxine test, free (FT_4)

TIBC (total iron-binding capacity)
tibia bone, nutrient artery of
tibial artery, posterior
tibial collateral ligament
tibial nerve, anterior
tibiocalcaneal ligament
tibiofibular articulation
tibiofibular joint
tibiofibular ligament, anterior inferior
tibionavicular ligament
tibiotarsal articulation
tibiotarsal joint
tick bite
tickborne (or tick-borne)
tickborne encephalitis
tickborne fever
tickborne illness
tickborne viruses
Tidy test for albumin in urine
Tiedemann gland
tigering
tightly packed round cell
"tigroid" appearance from fat deposit
tigroid mass
tigroid retina
Tilden stain
tilted sacrum
time
  activated coagulation
  activated thromboplastin
  bleeding
  clotting
  coagulation
  dextrinizing
  euglobulin clot lysis (ECLT)
  fixed interval of
  Mielke bleeding
  one-stage prothrombin
  partial thromboplastin (PTT)
  prothrombin (PT)
  reptilase
  turnaround

time-of-flight measurement
timothy bacillus
T-independent antigen
tinea barbae
tinea capitis
tinea circinata
tinea corporis (ringworm)
tinea cruris (jock itch)
tinea faciei
tinea favosa
tinea glabrosa
tinea imbricata
tinea manuum
tinea nigra palmaris
tinea pedis (athlete's foot)
tinea unguium (dermatophytic onychomycosis)
tinea versicolor
tine test
tine tuberculin test
tip of coccyx
tip of spleen
Tiselius apparatus
Tiselius electrophoresis cell
tissue
  aberrant
  abnormal formation of connective
  absence of germinal centers in lymphoid
  acinar
  adenoid
  adipose
  aerated lung
  archival
  areolar
  areolar connective
  basement
  blood-forming
  bony
  brain
  breakdown of muscle
  brown adipose

tissue *(continued)*
  cancellous
  cardiac muscle
  cartilaginous
  cavernous
  cellular
  cerebral
  chondroid
  chorionic
  chromaffin
  cicatricial
  clear
  collagenous
  connective
  cortical
  crushed
  damaged
  dartoic
  dead
  debridement
  degenerated
  dense connective
  dermal
  destruction of
  devitalized
  disorganization of connective
  ectopic
  elastic
  endothelial
  epidermal
  epithelial
  erectile
  exocervical
  extracellular
  extraperitoneal
  exuberant granulation
  exuberant hypertrophic granulation
  fatty
  fatty connective
  fibroadipose
  fibroareolar
  fibrocartilaginous

tissue *(continued)*
fibrofatty
fibrofatty connective
fibrohyaline
fibromuscular
fibrosing granulation
fibrous
fibrous connective
fibrous scar
fibrovascular
flabby
gelatiginous
gelatinous
glandular
glial
granulation
gross examination of
grumous
gut-associated lymphoid (GALT)
healing
hematopoietic
hemolymphatic
hepatic
heterotopic
hyperplastic
infected
inflamed
intercellular
interlobular
interstitial
intertrabecular
joint
lacerated
lipomatous-like
living
loose connective
lymphatic
lymph node
lymphoid
lymphoreticular
mature scar
mesenchymal

tissue *(continued)*
mesenteric
mesocolonic fat
microscopic examination
muscle
muscular
myeloid
necrosis
necrotic
neoplastic
nerve
nervous
nidus of inflamed
nidus of necrotic
nodal
nonfunctioning
nongerminal
nonviable
normal bone
osseous
osteoid
parafollicular lymphoid
parenchymal
periappendiceal adipose
periarticular
peribronchial connective
pericolic adipose
periorbital
perisplenic soft
pliable
preparation of
proliferation of fibrous
regeneration of
regular connective
repair of damaged
representative
reticular connective
reticulated
scar
septal
soft
somatic

tissue *(continued)*
    spinal cord
    splenic
    subcutaneous
    subcutaneous connective
    subperitoneal fatty areolar
    synovial
    taenia
    tendon
    underlying
tissue antigen
tissue block
tissue change
tissue culture
tissue death due to
    abnormal antibodies
    circulatory impairment
    malignant tumor
tissue differentiation
tissue equivalent material
tissue factor
tissue fluid
tissue hormone
tissue lymph
tissue metamorphosis
tissue polypeptide antigen (TPA)
tissue section
    mounting of
    staining of
tissue space
tissue specimen
tissue typing
titer
    agglutination
    anti-deoxyribonuclease-B
    antibody
    antihyaluronidase
    ASO (antistreptolysin O)
    heterophile
    serologic
titratable acidity test
titration
Tizzoni stain
Tizzoni test for iron in tissues
T lymphocyte
Tm cell
T method of staining
TNM (tumor size, nodal involvement, metastatic progress) classification
TNM classification
TNM node
TNTC (too numerous to count)
tobacco nodule
Todaro tendon
Todd cirrhosis
Todd units
toe tag
toe, webbed
togavirus
Toison solution
Toison stain
tolbutamide test
Toldt, line of
Tollens, Neuberg, and Schwket test
toluene
toluidine blue
toluidine blue stain
toluol
tones, bowel
T1–T12 (thoracic vertebrae)
tongue
tongue bone
tongue gland
tongue, strawberry
tonofibril
tonofilament
tonsil
    eustachian
    faucial
    lingual
    Luschka
    palatine
    pharyngeal
tonsillar artery

tonsillar crypt
tonsillitis, follicular
tonsil of auditory tube
too numerous to count (TNTC)
tooth (pl. teeth)
Tooth atrophy
tophus (pl. tophi)
TORCH infections (toxoplasmosis, rubella, cytomegalovirus, herpes simplex)
Tornwaldt abscess
Torquay test for bile
torr (1 millimeter of mercury, mm Hg)
Torrance and Bothwell method
torsional deformity
torsion of spermatic cord
torso crease
tortuous aorta
tortuous tubule
Torulopsis candida
Torulopsis glabrata
torulopsosis
torulosis
torulus
torus
torus tubarius auditory tube
Toscana virus
total catecholamine test
total hematuria
total iron-binding capacity (TIBC)
total knee replacement
total lesion
total lung capacity (TLC)
total necrosis
total protein
total protein concentration of spinal fluid
totipotent cell
totipotential cell
toto, in
touch cell
touch prep
tough capsule
tourniquet test for capillary fragility
Tourtual canal
Touton giant cell
Towbin method of immunoblotting
toxemia, bacterial
toxemia of pregnancy
toxemic pneumonia
toxic atrophy
toxic cirrhosis
toxic goiter
toxic granulation
toxic granule
toxic hepatitis
toxic inflammation
toxic insult
toxic level
toxic myocarditis
toxic nephrosis
toxic neuritis
toxic pneumonia
toxic shock syndrome
toxic substances test on venous blood
toxic vacuolization
toxicologic
toxicology screen
toxicosis, Frank capillary
toxigenic
toxigenicity test
toxin
Toxocara canis
Toxoplasma body
Toxoplasma gondii
toxoplasmosis, congenital
toxoplasmotic myocarditis
TPA (tissue plasminogen activator)
TPA (tissue polypeptide antigen)
TP53 tumor suppressor gene
TPHA (*Treponema pallidum* hemagglutination) test
TPI (*Treponema pallidum* immobilization) test

trabecula (pl. trabeculae)
trabecular adenocarcinoma
trabecular bone
trabecular degeneration in bronchial walls
trabecular endoplasmic reticulum
trabecula, septomarginal
trabeculated
trachea
  annular ligament of
  carina of
  scabbard
tracheal artery
tracheal gland
tracheitis
tracheobronchial lavage
tracheobronchial lymph node
tracheobronchial mucosal inflammation
tracheobronchial mucosal necrosis
tracheobronchial tree
tracheoesophageal (TE)
tracheoesophageal junction
tracheoesophageal fistula
trachoma
trachoma gland
tract
  alimentary
  ascending nerve
  auditory
  biliary
  central tegmental
  cerebellorubral
  cerebellothalamic
  comma
  corticobulbar
  corticopontine
  corticospinal
  crossed pyramidal
  cuneocerebellar
  dead
  deiterospinal
  dentatothalamic
tract *(continued)*
  descending
  digestive
  direct pyramidal
  dorsolateral
  fastigiobulbar
  fistulous
  frontopontine
  frontotemporal
  gastrointestinal (GI)
  geniculocalcarine
  genital
  hepatic outflow
  ileal inflow
  Maissiat
  pancreaticobiliary
  pyramidal
  spinothalamic
  upper gastrointestinal (UGI)
  uveal
traction alopecia
traction artifact
traction diverticulum
traction epiphysis
trait
  dominant
  sickle cell
transaminase
  glutamic oxaloacetic (GOT)
  glutamic pyruvic (GPT)
  serum glutamic-oxaloacetic (SGOT)
  serum glutamic-pyruvic (SGPT)
transbronchial
transcobalamin 2 deficiency
transcortin test
transdermal patch for glucose monitoring
transducer cell
transect
transepithelial migration
transepithelial migration of chronic inflammatory cells

transferase
- gamma-glutamyl (GGT)
- glucuronyl
- terminal deoxynucleotidyl (TdT)

transfer factor
transferrin test
transformation zone
transforming factor
transforming gene
transforming growth factor
transfusion
- arterial
- autologous
- blood
- direct
- exchange
- exsanguination
- fetomaterial
- immediate
- indirect
- intraperitoneal
- intrauterine
- mediate
- mismatched blood
- packed red blood cell
- placental
- reciprocal
- twin-to-twin

transfusion hepatitis
transfusion malaria
transfusion nephritis
transfusion of incompatible blood
transfusion reaction
transfusion recipient
transient acantholytic dermatosis
transient hyperphenylalaninemia
transient neonatal systemic lupus erythematosus
transient phenylketonuria
transient proteinuria
transilluminate
transillumination
transitional cell
transitional cell carcinoma
transitional cell papilloma
transitional epithelial cell
transitional epithelium
transitional meningioma
transition zone
transitory gastroenteritis
transitory loss of consciousness
transitory papule
transketolase test
translocation
- chromosomal abnormality of
- reciprocal
- robertsonian

transmission electron microscope
transmural myocardial infarction
transneuronal atrophy
transneuronal degeneration
transparency
transparent
transpeptidase
- gamma-glutamyl (GGTP)
- serum gamma-glutamyl (SGGT)

transplant (or transplantation)
- allogeneic
- bone marrow
- cadaveric
- corneal
- heart
- heart-lung
- hematopoietic stem cell (HSC)
- heterotopic
- homotopic
- kidney
- liver
- living related donor
- living unrelated donor
- orthotopic
- pancreas
- renal
- syngeneic

transplant *(continued)*
  syngenesioplastic
  tendon
  tooth
transport medium
transport protein
transport vesicle
transposition of great vessels
transpyloric plane (TPP)
transseptal needle
transtubercular plane (TTP)
transudate
transudative
transumbilical plane (TUP)
transurethral resection of prostate (TURP)
transverse aorta
transverse artery of neck
transverse atlantal ligament
transverse band
transverse carpal ligament
transverse cerebral fissure
transverse cervical artery
transverse colon
transverse colon loop
transverse crural ligament
transverse facial artery
transverse genicular ligament
transverse humeral ligament
transverse ligament
transverse mesocolon
transverse metacarpal ligament
transverse metatarsal ligament
transverse muscle of tongue
transverse myelitis
transverse oval pelvis
transverse palatine folds
transverse pericardial sinus
transverse perineal artery
transverse perineal muscle
transverse process
transverse rectal fold
transverse scapular artery
transverse section
transverse sinus
transverse tarsal articulation
transverse tarsal joint
transverse tibiofibular ligament
transversus abdominis muscle
trapezium bone
trapezoid bone
trapezoid ligament
Traube semilunar space
trauma
  acoustic
  birth
  blunt
  multiple
  penetrating
  physical
traumatic alopecia
traumatic aneurysm
traumatic degeneration
traumatic herpes
traumatic inflammation
traumatic meningocele
traumatic neuritis
traumatic orchitis
traumatic pneumonia
traumatic scar
traumatic thrombus
traumatopneic wound
trauma to spinal cord
Trautmann triangular space
TRC (tanned red cell)
Treacher Collins syndrome
treatment, acid-wash
tree
  biliary
  hepatobiliary
  tracheobronchial
trefoil dermatitis
trefoil tendon
Treitz arch

Treitz, ligament of
trematode (fluke)
trench mouth
Treponema
Treponema buccale
Treponema carateum
Treponema pallidum
Treponema pallidum complement fixation test
Treponema pallidum immobilization (TPI) test
Treponema pallidum pertenue
Treponema pertenue
Treponema vincentii
treponematosis
Tretop test
triad
  acute compression
  Charcot
  Dieulafoy
  hepatic
  portal
  Saint
  Whipple
triangle
  anal
  auricular
  axillary
  Calot
  cardiohepatic
  carotid
  cephalic
  cervical
  clavipectoral
  crural
  cystohepatic
  deltoideopectoral
  digastric
  facial
  femoral
  Grynfeltt
  Henke
triangle *(continued)*
  Hesselbach
  inguinal
  Labbe
  Lesgaft
  Livingston
  lumbocostoabdominal
  mesenteric
  Pawlik
  Scarpa
  urogenital
  vertebrocostal
triangular bone
triangular fibrocartilage
triangular fibrocartilage complex
triangular fontanelle
triangular ligaments of liver
triangular muscle
triangular suprarenal gland
tributary
trichilemmoma
Trichinella myocarditis
Trichinella spiralis
trichinosis
trichinous embolism
trichinous myositis
trichocyst
trichoma
trichomonal vaginitis
Trichomonas tenax
Trichomonas vaginalis
trichomoniasis, vaginal
trichophytic granuloma
trichophytin test
Trichophyton
Trichophyton ajelloi
Trichophyton concentricum
Trichophyton equinum
Trichophyton fisheri
Trichophyton flavescens
Trichophyton floccosum
Trichophyton georgiae

Trichophyton gloriae
Trichophyton gourvilii
Trichophyton longifusum
Trichophyton mariatii
Trichophyton megninii
Trichophyton mentagrophytes
Trichophyton phaseoliforme
Trichophyton rubrum
Trichophyton schoenleinii
Trichophyton simii
Trichophyton soudanense
Trichophyton terrestre
Trichophyton tonsurans
Trichophyton vanbreuseghemii
Trichophyton verrucosum
Trichophyton violaceum
Trichosporon beigelii
trichosporosis
trichrome stain
trichuriasis (whipworm)
Trichuris trichiura
trick knee
tricuspid orifice
tricuspid valve
tricuspid valvular leaflet
trifid stomach
trigeminal cave
trigeminal impression
trigeminal nerve
trigger finger
triglyceride enzyme deficiency
triglyceride level, normal fasting
triglycerides (TG)
  long chain (LCT)
  medium chain (MCT)
  serum
trigone
  angles of
  collateral
  deltoideopectoral
  Henke
  hypoglossal
trigone *(continued)*
  Lieutaud
  Müller
  Pawlik
  vertebrocostal
trigone of bladder
trihexosidase, ceramide
triiodothyronine (T_3) hormone
triiodothyronine resin uptake test
triiodothyronine uptake test
triketohydrindene hydrate test
trimellitic anhydritic pneumonitis
triolein–^{131}I absorption test
triple phosphate
triquetral bone
triquetrohamate joint
triquetrum
Tris-HCl
trisomy
Triton X-100 buffer solution
trocar, aspiration
trocar plug
trochanter
  greater
  lesser
trochanteric bursitis
trochlea
trochlear
trochoid joint
trochoidal articulation
Trommer test for glucose in urine
trophic lesion
trophoblast
trophoblastic
trophozoite
tropical abscess
tropical ear
tropical eczema
tropical stomatitis
tropical swelling
tropic hormone
troponin T protein in cardiac muscle

trough, gingival
trough level
Trousseau test for bile in urine
Truant auramine–rhodamine stain
Trucut cutting biopsy needle
true aneurysm
true back muscles
true mole
true pelvis
true plasma
true proteinuria
true rib
truncus arteriosus
  embryonic
  persistent
trunk
  articulations of
  atrioventricular (AV)
  bifurcation of pulmonary
  brachiocephalic
  bronchomediastinal
  bronchomediastinal lymph
  celiac
  cordlike
  costocervical
  joints of
  lumbosacral
  lymph
  nerve
  posterior vagal
  thyrocervial
  vagal
trunk artery
trypan blue
Trypanosoma cruzi
Trypanosoma gambiense
Trypanosoma rhodesiense
trypanosome
trypticase soy agar
trypticase soy broth
tryptic soy agar with sRBC
trypsin G-banding stain
tryptophan load test
T_3 (triiodothyroninc)
T_3 resin uptake (triiodothyronine uptake)
TSH (thyroid stimulating hormone)
TTP (thrombotic thrombocytopenic purpura)
tubal abortion
tubal air cell
tubal canal
tubal ligation
tubal mole
tubal nephritis
tubal pregnancy
tube
  auditory
  bronchial
  calices (calyces)
  capillary
  corneal
  digestive
  endotracheal (ET)
  Eppendorf
  eustachian
  fallopian
  muscular
  nasogastric (NG)
  neural
  separator
  solid-phase extraction
  uterine
tube coagulase test
tubercle
  accessory
  acoustic
  adductor
  amygdaloid
  articular
  ashen
  auricular
  calcaneal
  carotid

tubercle *(continued)*
  conoid
  corniculate
  crown
  cuneiform
  darwinian
  dental
  dissection
  epiglottic
  fibrous
  genital
  Ghon
  greater
  iliac
  lesser
  Lister
  postmortem
  prominent scalene
  pubic
  scalene
  sella turcica
tubercle bacillus
tubercle of Darwin, auricular
tubercle of rib, facet for
tubercle of temporal bone, articular
tuberculin test
tuberculoid leprosy
tuberculoid lesion
tuberculoid myocarditis
tuberculosis
  avian
  bone
  disseminated
  exudative
  fulminant
  genitourinary
  hematogenous
  inhalation
  meningeal
  miliary
  postprimary
  primary
tuberculosis *(continued)*
  pulmonary
  renal
tuberculosis of bone
tuberculosis test
tuberculous abscess
tuberculous arthritis
tuberculous gumma
tuberculous infiltration
tuberculous meningitis
tuberculous myocarditis
tuberculous nephritis
tuberculous nodule
tuberculous pericarditis
tuberculous pneumonia
tuberculous salpingitis
tuberculous spondylitis
tuberculum
tuberosity (pl. tuberosities)
  bicipital
  calcaneal
  coracoid
  costal
  deltoid
  ischial
  omental
tuberous sclerosis
tuboabdominal pregnancy
tuboligamentary pregnancy
tubo-ovarian abscess
tubo-ovarian pregnancy
tubotympanic canal
tubouterine pregnancy
tubular aneurysm
tubular gland
tubular reabsorption of phosphate (TRP) test
tubule
  collecting
  connecting
  convoluted
  convoluted seminiferous

tubule *(continued)*
  dcntal
  dentinal
  discharging
  distal convoluted
  proximal convoluted
  renal
  seminiferous
  straight
  tortuous
tubulitis
tubuloacinar gland
tubuloalveolar gland
Tuffier inferior ligament
tufted cell
tuft, vascular
tularemia
tularemic pneumonia
tumor
  adrenal
  anaplastic
  Askin
  benign epidermal
  bladder
  bone
  breast
  Brenner
  brown
  carcinoid
  CNS (central nervous system)
  cutaneous
  dental
  discrete
  embryonal
  endocardial
  Ewing
  focal
  gastrin-secreting non-beta islet cell
  gastrointestinal
  giant cell
  globular
  grading

tumor *(continued)*
  granular cell
  granulosa cell
  gray
  gritty
  gross
  highly vascular
  intracranial
  invasive
  islet cell
  kidney
  Krukenberg
  liver
  lobulated
  locally invasive
  lung
  lymphoid
  main
  malignant
  malignant mesenchymal
  metastatic
  myxomatous
  ovarian
  pancreatic
  pancreatic islet cell
  paraffin
  parathyroid
  periampullary
  pituitary
  reddish
  retinal
  salivary gland
  scirrhous
  small cell
  submucosal
  subserosal
  testicular
  thyroid
  urinary
  uterine
  vascular cutaneous and hepatic
  virilizing adrenal

tumor *(continued)*
  Warthin (adenolymphoma)
  Wharton (cystadenoma)
  white
  Wilms
tumoral calcinosis
tumor angiogenic factor (TAF)
tumor antigen
tumor capsule
tumor embolism
tumor erosion
tumor marker
  AFP (alpha-fetoprotein)
  CA 15-2 RIA
  CA 15-3 antigen
  CA 15-3 breast cancer
  CA 19-9 antigenic
  CA 19-9 carbohydrate antigen
  CA 27.29
  CA 50
  CA 72-4 antigen
  CA 125 antigen
  CA 125 cross-reactivity
  CA 125 ovarian
  CA 125-11
  CA 195
  CA 549 breast cancer
  CA M26
  CA M29
  CEA (carcinoembryonic antigen)
  PSA (prostate-specific antigen)
tumor mass
tumor necrosis factor (TNF)
tumor registry
tumor-specific antigen
tumor staging
tumor suppressor gene
  APC (adenomatous polyposis coli)
  DCC (deleted in colon carcinoma)
  mutant
  NF (neurofibromatosis)
  NF1

tumor suppressor gene *(continued)*
  NF2
  p53
  RB1
  TP53
  VHL
  WT1
tumor virus
tunica adventitia
tunica albuginea
tunica fibrosa
tunica intima
tunica media
tunica mucosa
tunica muscularis
tunica propria
tunica serosa
tunica vaginalis
tunnel
  carpal
  cubital
  retropancreatic
  tarsal
tunnel cell
turbid fluid
turbidity
turbinate(d) bones
Turbo TMB colorimetric reader
turcica, sella
Türck degeneration
Türk cell
Türk irritation leukocyte
turnaround time
Turnbull blue
Turner biopsy needle
Turner syndrome
TURP (transurethral resection of prostate)
Tween-albumin broth culture
Tween-20
20-channel chemistry profile
24-hour urine specimen

twig
  cutaneous
  muscular
twigs to pelvic diaphragm
twigs to piriformis muscle
twin pregnancy
twin-to-twin transfusion
twisted
2060 virus
two-hour postprandial blood-sugar level
two-hour postprandial sugar
Twort-d'Herelle bacteriophagia phenomenon
two-stage prothrombin test
two-step indirect immunoperoxidase method
two-vessel umbilical cord
tympanic air cell
tympanic artery
tympanic bone
tympanic canal
tympanic cell
tympanic gland
tympanic membrane, perforated
tympanitic abscess
tympanocervical abscess
tympanohyal bone
tympanomastoid abscess
tympanostapedial junction
Tyndall light
type and crossmatch (T&C)
type, blood (blood group)
type I cell
type I diabetes mellitus
type 1 hereditary orotic aciduria
type I insulin-dependent diabetes
type II cell
type II diabetes mellitus
type II non-insulin-dependent diabetes
typhoid bacillus
typhoid fever
typhoid fever test
typhoid nodule
typhoid osteomyelitis
typhoid pleurisy
typhoid pneumonia
typhus
  endemic
  epidemic
  flea-borne
  louse-borne
  scrub
typhus nodule
typical rib
typing
  blood
  column
  tissue
typing and crossmatching of blood for transfusion
tyramine test
tyrosine test
Tyson gland
Tyson test for bile acids in urine
Tzanck cell
Tzanck smear of vagina
Tzanck test

U, u

ubiquinone
ubiquitin
U-cell lymphoma
UCHL1 monoclonal antibody
Udranszky test for bile acids
U echovirus
Uffelmann test
Uganda S virus
ulcer
- acute peptic
- anastomotic
- aphthous
- buccal
- cervical
- chiclero
- chronic
- chronic peptic
- corneal
- Curling
- Cushing
- cutaneous
- decubitus
- duodenal
- flask-shaped
- gastric
- genital
- granulomatous

ulcer *(continued)*
- healing
- herpes
- Hunner
- incised
- intestinal
- mucosal
- oral
- painless indurated
- penetrating
- peptic
- puncture
- rodent
- shallow mucosal
- urinary
- venereal

ulceration
- corneal
- gastrointestinal

ulcerative colitis
ulcerative dermatosis
ulcerative inflammation
ulcerative stomatitis
Ulex europaeus agglutinin 1
ulnar artery
ulnar bone
ulnar carpal artery

ulnar collateral artery
ulnar collateral ligament of elbow
ulnar collateral ligament of wrist
ulnar head
ulnocarpal ligament
ulnolunate ligament
ulnotriquetral ligament
Ulrich test for albumin
ultimobranchial gland
ultimobranchial pouch
ultracentrifugation
ultracentrifuge
ultramicrotome
ultrasound diagnosis
ultrathin section
ultraviolet light
ultraviolet radiation
ultravirus
Ultzmann test for bile pigments
Umber test for scarlet fever
umbilical artery in fetus
umbilical canal
umbilical cord
    three-vessel
    two-vessel
umbilical fold
umbilical hernia
umbilical ligament
umbilical region
umbilical vein
umbilicated
umbilicus
umbilicus granuloma
umbrella cell
unattended death
unciform bone
uncinarial dermatitis
uncinate process of pancreas
uncircumcised
unconjugated bilirubin, deposition of
uncontrolled diabetes
uncontused
unconventional virus
uncoupling protein
uncovertebral joint
uncus
undegenerated nerve cell
underlying tissue
undersurface of liver
undescended testicle
undescended testis
undifferentiated adenocarcinoma
undifferentiated carcinoma
undifferentiated carcinoma of thyroid
undifferentiated cell
undifferentiated columnar epithelial cell
undifferentiated leukemia
undifferentiated lymphoma
undigested food in stool
undilated
undulant fever
unencapsulated
unequivocal
unesterified free fatty acid
unformed stool
unheated serum reagin (USR) test
uniaxial joint
unicellular gland
unicellular microorganism
unicellular organism
unicornis, uterus
unilateral facial atrophy
unilobular cirrhosis
unilocular cyst
unilocular joint
unilocular pustule
un-ionized acid
unipennate muscle
unipolar cell
unit
    arbitrary
    Bessey-Lowry
    Bodansky

unit *(continued)*
  IU (international)
  King-Armstrong
  mIU (milli-international)
  motor
  pilosebaceous
  SI (Système International)
  Todd
uniting canal
units per volume
unmyelinated postganglionic fibers
Unna disease
Unna mark
Unna nevus
Unna-Pappenheim stain
Unna stain
Unna-Taenzer stain
unobstructed
unpaired visceral branches
unremarkable
unresolved pneumonia
unruptured follicles
unsaturated fatty acid
unsegmented neutrophils
unstable hemoglobin
unsuspected cause of death
unwinding protein
upper esophageal sphincter (UES)
upper extremity
upper gastrointestinal tract (UGI)
upper jaw bone
upper limb
upper lip
upper motor neuron lesion
Uppsala virus
uptake of isotopically tagged thymidine
urachal adenocarcinoma
urachal ligament
urachus
uranium nitrate
uranoschisis
uranyl acetate
uranyl acetate stain
urate, amorphous
urate calculus
urate crystals
urate crystals stain
urea (urea nitrogen)
urea clearance test
urea concentration test for renal efficiency
urea nitrogen (BUN, blood urea nitrogen)
urea nitrogen/creatinine ratio
urea nitrogen test
urea, urinary
Ureaplasma urealyticum
urease-producing organism
urease test
Urecholine supersensitivity test
uremia
uremic acidosis
uremic coma
uremic pneumonitis
uremic pruritus
uremic stomatitis
ureter
  circumcaval
  ectopic
  kinked
  postcaval
  retrocaval
  retroiliac
ureteral colic
ureteral meatus
ureteral opening
ureteral orifice
ureteric artery
ureteric calculus
ureteric pelvis
ureteric stone
ureteropelvic junction (UPJ)
ureterovesical junction (UVJ)
ureterovesical obstruction

urethra
  bulb of
  membranous
  prostatic
  spongy
urethral abscess
urethral artery
urethral bulb artery
urethral calculus
urethral crest
urethral discharge
urethral diverticulum
urethral gland
urethral groove
urethral hematuria
urethral orifice, external
urethral pressure profile
urethritis
  gonococcal
  gonorrheal
  gouty
  granular casts in
  nongonococcal
  nonspecific
  prophylactic
  simple
  specific
urethrovaginal fistula
uric acid
uric acid crystals in gout
uric acid infarct
uric acid test
Uricult dipslide test
urinalysis
urinary (see *urine*)
urinary abscess
urinary aldosterone
urinary amylase
urinary arsenic
urinary bladder
urinary bladder fundus
urinary calculus
urinary catecholamines
urinary creatinine
urinary excretion of coproporphyrin
urinary excretion of 5-hydroxyindoleacetic acid (5-HIAA)
urinary excretion of 17-ketosteroid
urinary hemoglobin
urinary 17-ketosteroid excretion
urinary lead level
urinary leukocyte esterase test (LET)
urinary metanephrines
urinary mucosa
urinary obstruction
urinary osmolality
urinary oxalate
urinary protein
urinary protein electrophoresis
urinary red blood cell (RBC)
urinary sediment
urinary smear
urinary specific gravity
urinary stone
urinary tract infection (UTI)
urinary tumor
urinary ulcer
urinary urea
urinary urobilinogen
urinary urobilinogen excretion
urine
  abnormal casts in
  acetone in
  albumin in
  amber color
  amorphous sediment in
  Bence Jones protein in
  bilirubin in
  black
  calcareous material in
  cells in sediment of
  chorionic gonadotropin in
  chylous
  clarity of

urine *(continued)*
  clean-catch
  clear
  cloudiness of
  cloudy
  Coca-Cola
  color of
  crude
  crystals in
  dark concentrated
  diabetic
  dried smears of
  dyspeptic
  febrile
  fragments of tissue in
  freshly voided
  gouty
  granular casts in
  high-colored
  homogeneous casts in
  honey
  hyaline casts in
  ketones in
  leakage of
  light-colored
  maple syrup odor in
  milky
  mucus shreds in
  myoglobin in
  nebulous
  odorous
  pink
  pregnancy
  protein in
  residual
  scanty
  smoky brown
  specific gravity of
  straw-colored
  turbidity of
  watery
  yellow

urine, abnormalities in
  bile
  bilirubin
  blood
  color changes due to
    abnormal waste products
    drugs
    pigments from foods
  crystals of sulfanilamide derivatives
  cystine
  epithelial cells
  fat
  glucose
  granular casts
  hemoglobin
  hyaline casts
  ketone bodies
  mucous casts
  occult blood
  proteins
  proteoses
  pus
  spermatozoa
  waxy casts

urine androgen level
urine bacilli
urine chloride
urine colony count
urine concentration test
urine culture
urine cytology
urine dip slide
urine electrolyte
urine estrogen level
urine glucose
urine leakage
urine osmolality
urine pH
urine/plasma ratio (U/P)
urine reaction
urine sediment test
urine smear

urine specimen
  catheterized
  clean catch
  clean-voided
  first-voided
  freshly voided
  midstream
  twenty-four hour
urine sediment test
urine specific gravity
urine stagnation
urine sugar
urine tests (see Table, pp. 561-563)
urine volume
uriniparous
urinocryoscopy
urinogenital
urinogenous
urinoglucosometer
urinoma
urinometer
urinophilous
urinosexual
urinous infiltration
uriposia
Uristix
uroacidimeter
uroammoniac
uroazotometer
urobilin
urobilinemia
urobilinogen
  fecal
  stool
  urinary
urobilinogen excretion
urobilinogen test
urobilin test
urobilinuria
urocanase deficiency
urocele
urochezia
urocystitis
Urocyte diagnostic cytometry system
uroerythrin
urofuscin
urofuscohematin
urogenital canal
urogenital diaphragm
urogenital region
urogenital triangle
urolithiasis
uropathy, obstructive
uroporphyrinogen-1-synthetase enzyme
uroporphyrin test
uropygial gland
urorosein test
urothelial cell
urothelium
urticaria
urticarial eruption
urticaria pigmentosa with systemic
  mastocytosis
urushiol (skin-sensitizing agent)
USR (unheated serum reagin) test
uta (leishmaniasis)
uteri, fundus
uterine artery
uterine calculus
uterine canal
uterine cavity
uterine cervical ganglion
uterine cervix
uterine didelphia
uterine dysfunctional bleeding
uterine fibroid
uterine fibromyoma
uterine fundus
uterine gland
uterine horn
uterine leiomyoma (leiomyomata)
uterine myometrium
uterine ostium
uterine polyp

uterine relaxing factor (URF)
uterine tube, ampulla of
uterine tumor
uteroabdominal pregnancy
uterocervical canal
uterosacral ligament
uterotubal junction
uterotubal pregnancy
uterovaginal canal
uterovaginal plexus
uterovesical junction
uterovesical ligament
uterovesical pouch
uterus
  adhesions of
  anteflexed
  anteverted
  aplastic
  bicameral
  bicornuate
  bilocular
  bipartite
  bleeding, dysfunctional
  boggy
  broad ligament of
  cervix of
  cochleate
  cornu of
  Couvelaire
  didelphic
  double
  double-mouthed
  duplex
  fetal
  fibroid
  gravid
  heart-shaped
  horn of
  hypoplastic
  infantile
  isthmus of
  pear-shaped

uterus *(continued)*
  pregnant
  pubescent
  retroflexed
  retroverted
  ribbon
  round ligament of
  saddle-shaped
  septate
uterus arcuatus
uterus bicameratus vetularum
uterus bicornis
uterus bicornis bicollis
uterus bicornis unicollis
uterus biforis
uterus bilocularis
uterus bipartitus
uterus cordiformis
uterus didelphys
uterus incudiformis
uterus masculinus
uterus parvicollis
uterus planifundalis
uterus rudimentarius
uterus septus
uterus simplex
uterus subseptus
uterus triangularis
uterus unicornis
UTI (urinary tract infection)
utricle
  prostatic
  urethral
utricular gland
utriculosaccular canal
uveal melanoma
uveal nevus
uveal tract
uveitis (pl. uveitides)
  anterior
  Förster
  granulomatous

uveitis *(continued)*
  lens-induced
  nongranulomatous
  phacoantigenic
  phacotoxic
  posterior

uveoparotid fever
U virus
UVJ (ureterovesical junction)
uvula of bladder

V, v

Vabra aspiration
vaccinia virus
vacuolar degeneration of adrenal and thyroid glands
vacuolar degeneration of sarcoplasm
vacuolar nephrosis
vacuolated cells
vacuolating virus
vacuolation of cells
vacuole
  autophagic
  contractile
  cytoplasmic
  fatty
vacuoles in stratum granulosum
vacuolization, toxic
Vacutainer
vagal trunk
vagina
  anterior fornix of
  azygos artery of
  Candida albicans infection of
  double
  fornix of
  genital warts of
  gonorrheal infection of
  herpes simplex lesions of
vagina *(continued)*
  Neisseria gonorrhoeae infection of
  squamous cell carcinoma of
  syphilitic chancres of
  Trichomonas vaginalis infection of
  vestibule of
vagina, ectocervix, endocervix (VCE) smear
vagina fundus
vaginal adenocarcinoma
vaginal adenosis
vaginal artery
vaginal atrophy
vaginal bands, transverse
vaginal canal
vaginal candidiasis
vaginal carcinoma
vaginal clear cell adenocarcinoma
vaginal cornification
vaginal cyst
vaginal cytology
vaginal epithelial abnormality
vaginal flora
vaginal fornix
vaginal gland
vaginal hypertrophy
vaginal intraepithelial neoplasia (VIN)

vaginal introitus, complete closure of
vaginal irrigation smear
vaginalis
- *Candida*
- *Gardnerella*
- *Neisseria*
- *Trichomonas*

vaginal microflora
vaginal mucification test
vaginal mucosa
vaginal opening
vaginal orifice
vaginal pH
vaginal plexus
vaginal secretion
vaginal smear
vaginal trichomoniasis
vaginal wall
vaginitis
- adhesive
- atrophic
- chlamydial
- desquamative inflammatory
- diphtheritic
- emphysematous
- *Gardnerella*
- monilial
- nonspecific
- senile
- trichomonal
- yeast

vaginomycosis
vaginosis, bacterial
Vagitest
vagus, auricular nerve of
vagus nerve
vagus pneumonia
valgus, cubitus
valine test
vallate papillae
vallecula (pl. valleculae)
vallecular pooling
valley fever
valproic acid
Valsalva antrum
Valsalva ligaments
valve
- anal
- aortic
- aortic semilunar
- atrioventricular
- ball
- bicuspid
- capillary
- cardiac
- caval
- coronary
- eustachian
- frenulum of
- globular
- ileocecal
- incompetent
- leaky mitral
- mitral
- pulmonary
- pulmonic
- rectal
- semilunar
- tricuspid
- venous

valve cusp
valve leaflet
valve of Bauhin
valve of coronary sinus
valve of Houston
valve of Kerckring
valve of navicular fossa
valvula (pl. valvulae)
valvular leaflet
valvular ring
valvular sclerosis
van Deen test for blood
van den Bergh test
van der Velden test

van Ermengen stain
van Gieson stain
van Heuven anatomic classification of
   diabetic retinopathy
van Horne canal
vanillylmandelic acid (VMA)
Vanox fluorescence microscope
Vanox-T microscope
Van Slyke apparatus
Van Slyke test
variant, clear cell
variation, alpha-beta
variceal column
variceal wall
varicella (chickenpox)
varicella pneumonia
Varicellavirus
varicella-zoster virus
varices (pl. of varix), esophageal
varicocele
varicose aneurysm
varicose eczema
varicose vein
varicosity (pl. varicosities)
variegated
variegate porphyria (VP)
variola (smallpox)
variola virus (now extinct)
varix (pl. varices)
   cirsoid
   conjunctival
   esophageal
vascular apron
vascular atrophy
vascular birthmark
vascular cirrhosis
vascular collapse
vascular congestion
vascular cutaneous and hepatic tumors
vascular disease of retina
vascular engorgement
vascular gland
vascular goiter
vascular hemophilia
vascular hypertension
vascularization in cornea
vascularization, patches of
vascular myxoma
vascular nephritis
vascular nevus
vascular osteitis
vascular plexus
vascular polyp
vascular sclerosis
vascular tuft
vascular wall
vasculitic rejection
vasculitis
   granulomatous
   obliterative
   systemic necrotizing
vas deferens, artery of
vasoactive cell
vasoactive intestinal peptide (VIP)
vasoactive intestinal polypeptide (VIP)
vasoconstriction
vasodilation
vasoformative cell
vasomotor nerve
vasopressin hormone
vasopressin-resistant diabetes
vasorum, vasa
Vater
   ampulla of
   papilla of
vaterian segment
vault
   cranial
   rectal
VCE (vagina, ectocervix, endocervix)
   smear
VDRL (Venereal Disease Research
   Laboratory)
VDRL antigen

VDRL test for syphilis
veal infusion
vector
  arthropod
  biological
  mechanical
vector-borne infection
vegetation, destructive
vegetations of cardiac valve
vegetative form
veil (or veiled) cell
Veillonella
Veillonella parvula
vein (see Table of Veins)
  accessory cephalic
  accessory hemiazygos
  accessory saphenous
  accessory vertebral
  accompanying
  anal
  anastomosing
  anastomotic
  angular
  anonymous
  antebrachial
  anterior cardiac
  anterior jugular
  appendicular
  aqueous
  arciform
  arcuate
  arterial
  ascending lumbar
  auditory
  auricular
  axillary
  azygos
  basal
  basilic
  basivertebral
  brachial
  brachiocephalic

vein *(continued)*
  bronchial
  capillary
  cardiac
  cardinal
  cavernous
  central
  cephalic
  cerebral
  cervical
  choroid
  ciliary
  circumflex
  colic
  common basal
  common cardinal
  common facial
  companion
  condylar emissary
  conjunctival
  coronary
  costoaxillary
  cutaneous
  cystic
  digital
  diploic
  dorsispinal
  duodenal
  embryonic umbilical
  emissary
  epigastric
  episcleral
  esophageal
  ethmoidal
  external pudendal
  facial
  femoral
  fibular
  frontal
  gastric
  gastroepiploic
  great cardiac

vein *(continued)*
- great saphenous
- hemiazygos
- hepatic
- ileocolic
- inferior pulmonary
- inferior rectal
- intercostal
- jugular
- labial
- left hepatic
- median antebrachial
- mesenteric
- middle cardiac
- middle rectal
- oblique
- pancreatic
- paraumbilical
- pericardial
- portal
- posterior auricular
- prepyloric
- pudendal
- pulmonary
- renal
- Retzius
- saphenous
- scrotal
- small cardiac
- splenic
- subclavian
- superior mesenteric
- superior pulmonary
- superior rectal
- systemic
- testicular
- varicose

vein stripper
velamentous insertion
velamentous placenta
vellus hair
Velpeau canal
velvetlike
velvety
vena cava
- inferior
- infrahepatic
- superior
- suprahepatic

Venereal Disease Research Laboratory (VDRL)
venereal ulcer
venereal warts
venereum, lymphogranuloma
venipuncture
venosum, ligamentum
venosus, sinus
venous angioma
venous blood
venous capillary
venous congestion
venous dorsal arch
venous embolism
venous groove
venous lake
venous ligament
venous network
venous obstruction
venous plexus
- prostatic
- vertebral
- vesical

venous sinus of brain
venous stasis
venous system, portal
venous valves
venous web
ventilation pneumonitis
ventral aorta
ventral hernia
ventral horn
ventral mesentery
ventral pancreatic bud
ventral primary ramus

ventral root
ventral sacrococcygeal ligament
ventral sacroiliac ligament
ventricle
  Arantius
  auxiliary
  cephalic
  cerebral
  double-inlet left
  double-inlet right
    associated with pulmonary stenosis
    doubly committed
    subaortic
    subpulmonic
    uncommitted
  double-outlet left
  double-outlet right
  Duncan (fifth)
  fifth
  fourth
  Galen
  laryngeal
  lateral
  left
  Morgagni
  pineal
  right (of heart)
  single
  sixth (Verga)
  Sylvius
  terminal
  third
  Verga
ventricles of brain
  fourth
  lateral (two)
  third
ventricular aneurysm
ventricular canal
ventricular free wall
ventricular ligament
ventricular loop
ventricular papillary muscle
ventricular septal defect
venule
vera, polycythemia
Verga lacrimal groove
Verga ventricle
verge, anal
Verhoeff elastic stain
vermian fossa
vermiform appendix
vermiform body
vermiform granule
vermilion border
verminous abscess
verminous dermatitis
vermis
vernal conjunctivitis
Verneuil canal
Vero cell culture
verruca vulgaris
verrucous carcinoma
verrucous hemangioma
verrucous nevus
verruga peruana
versicolor, tinea
vertebra (pl. vertebrae)
  articular process of
  basilar
  caudal
  cervical (C1 through C7)
  coccygeal
  codfish
  cranial
  dorsal (D)
  false
  lumbar (L1 through L5)
  sacral (S1 through S5)
  thoracic (T1 through T12)
  true
vertebral arch
vertebral artery

vertebral body
vertebral canal
vertebral column
vertebral foramen
vertebral fracture
vertebral groove
vertebral part of medial surface
vertebral pleural reflection
vertebral spinous process
vertebral venous plexus
vertebra prominens
vertebrocostal rib
vertebrocostal triangle
vertebrocostal trigone
vertebropelvic ligament
vertebrosternal rib
vertical cleft
vertical heart
vertical muscle of tongue
verumontanum
very low density lipoprotein (VLDL)
Vesalius bone
vesical artery
vesical calculus
vesical fistula
vesical hematuria
vesical plexus
vesical scrapings
vesical venous plexus
vesication
vesicle
  acoustic
  acrosomal
  air
  allantoic
  auditory
  blastodermic
  cerebral
  cervical
  cutaneous
  encephalic
  germinal

vesicle *(continued)*
  seminal
  transport
vesicle of endoplasmic reticulum
vesicoprostatic calculus
vesicoumbilical ligament
vesicourethral canal
vesicouterine fistula
vesicouterine ligament
vesicouterine pouch
vesicovaginal space
vesicular dermatitis
vesicular eruption
vesicular mole
vesicular nuclei
vesicular pharyngitis
vesicular stomatitis virus
vesiculation
Vesiculovirus
vessel
  afferent
  afferent lymph
  arcuate
  blood
  capillary
  chyle
  collateral
  collecting
  deep lymph
  efferent
  efferent lymph
  gastroepiploic
  intercostal
  internal pudendal
  kidney
  lymph
  musculophrenic
  pole of
  renal
  splenic
  superficial lymph
  superior gluteal

vessel leak
vestibular canal
vestibular ganglion
vestibular gland
vestibular hair cells
vestibular labyrinth
vestibular ligament
vestibular neuritis
vestibular schwannoma
vestibule
  aortic
  bulb of
  esophagogastric
  gastroesophageal
vestibule of vagina
vestigial fold
vestigial organ
Vetastain Elite kit
veto cell
V gene
VHDL (very high density lipoprotein)
VHL tumor suppressor gene
viable fetus
Vibrio alginolyticus
Vibrio cholerae
Vibrio damsela
Vibrio fetus
Vibrio fluvialis
Vibrio hollisae
Vibrio jejuni
Vibrio metschnikovii
Vibrio mimicus
vibrissae
Vidas image analyzer
vidian artery
vidian canal
Vieussens ansa
Vieussens loop
villi (pl. of villus)
villonodular synovitis
villous adenoma
villous atrophy
villous carcinoma
villous hypertrophy of synovial
  membrane
villous papilloma
villous placenta
villus (pl. villi)
  anchoring
  chorionic
  duodenal
  floating
  gallbladder
  intestinal
  placental
vimentin
Vim-Silverman needle
VIN (vaginal intraepithelial neoplasia)
Vincent infection
Vincent stomatitis
vinegar stain
violaceous
violet
  crystal
  gentian
  methyl
violet rash
violin-string adhesions
VIP (vasoactive intestinal polypeptide)
viral culture
viral encephalitis
viral exanthem
viral gastroenteritis
viral hemorrhagic fever
viral hepatitis
viral infection
viral inflammatory conditions
viral meningitis
viral myelitis
viral myocarditis
viral pericarditis
viral pneumonia
viral respiratory infection
viral septicemia

ViraPap test
ViraType
Virchow bone-splitting chisel
Virchow cells
Virchow gland
Virchow hydatid
Virchow-Robin space
viremia
Viridans streptococci
virilization
virilization of genitalia
virilizing adrenal tumor
virion
Virocult
virocyte
virology
Vironostika Mixt ELISA HIV
  antibody test
virulence
virus (pl. viruses) (see *pathogen* for
  names of viruses)
  adeno-associated
  animal
  arthropod-borne
  avian leukosis
  bacterial
  BK (BKV)
  bluetongue
  border disease
  cancer-inducing
  chikungunya
  common cold
  croup-associated (CA v.)
  cytomegalic inclusion disease
  defective
  dengue
  dermotropic
  DNA
  DNA tumor
  encephalomyocarditis
  enteric
  enteric orphan

virus *(continued)*
  enveloped
  epidemic keratoconjunctivitis
  helper
  hemadsorption
  herpangina
  infectious pancreatic necrosis
  infectious wart
  influenza
  iridescent
  latent
  lymphocyte-associated
  lytic
  masked
  measles
  milker's node
  molluscum contagiosum
  mosquito-borne
  mucosal disease
  mumps
  naked
  negative strand
  neurotropic
  newborn pneumonitis
  nonenveloped
  nonoccluded
  nononcogenic
  oncogenic
  orphan
  papilloma
  poliomyelitis
  polyoma
  rabies
  respiratory
  rubella
  satellite
  slow
  temperate
  tickborne or tick-borne
  unconventional
  vacuolating
  vesicular stomatitis

virusemia
virustatic
virus-transformed cell
viscera (pl. of viscus)
  abdominal
  abdominopelvic
  hollow
  intraperitoneal
  pelvic
visceral arch
visceral artery
visceral branches
visceral cleft, first
visceral edema
visceral embolism
visceral larva migrans
visceral layer
visceral leishmaniasis
visceral lymph node
visceral pelvic fascia
visceral pericardium
visceral peritoneum
visceral pleura
visceral skeleton
visceral surface of liver
viscerocranium, cartilaginous
viscid bile
viscosity
viscous (adj.)
viscous bile
viscous fluid
viscous greenish exudate
viscous lubricant
viscous metamorphosis
viscus (pl. viscera)
visual cell
visual field
visual impairment, progressive
visual pigment
visual receptor cells
visual zone
vital capacity (VC)
Vitali test for alkaloids
vital stain
vitamin
  antineuritic
  test on venous blood for
vitamin A (retinol, dehydroretinol)
vitamin A tolerance test
vitamin B_1 (thiamine)
vitamin B_6 (pyridoxine)
vitamin B_{12} (cobalamin)
vitamin B_{12} intrinsic factor test
vitamin B_{12} tagged with radioactive cobalt, oral administration of
vitamin C (ascorbic acid)
vitamin C saturation test
vitamin D (calciferol)
vitamin D_3 (calciferol, cholecalciferol)
vitamin D-binding protein (DBP)
vitamin D intoxication
vitamin deficiencies due to inherited metabolic disorders
  malabsorption
  malnutrition
vitamin D test
vitamin E (tocopherol)
vitamin E test
vitamin K (phytonadione, menaquinone, menadione)
Vitek
vitelline duct
vitelline fistula
vitelline gland
vitiligo
vitreous abscess
vitreous body
vitreous cell
vitreous chamber
vitreous humor
vitreous membrane
vitro, in
vivax fever
vivax malaria

vivo, in
VLDL (very low density lipoprotein)
VMA (vanillylmandelic acid)
vocal cord
  pachyderma of
  papilloma of
vocal ligament
Voelcker and Joseph test
Vogel and Lee test for mercury
Voges-Proskauer test
volar arch artery, superficial
volar artery, superficial
volar capitate
volar carpal artery
volar carpal ligament
volar interosseous artery
volar ligament
volar sling
volar ulnar sling
vole bacillus
Volhard test for renal function
Volkmann canal
Volkmann contracture
Vollmer tuberculin patch
volume
  blood
  plasma
  mean corpuscular (MCV)
  mean platelet (MPV)
  red cell
  vertebral
volume-corrected mitotic index
volume of packed cells
volumetric analysis
voluntary muscle
volvulus, cecal
vomer, alae of
vomer bone
vomerine canal
vomerobasilar canal
vomerorostral canal
vomerovaginal canal
vomiting
vomiting blood
vomitus
von Aldor test
von Bezold abscess
von Gierke disease
von Jaksch test
von Kossa calcium stain
von Kossa stain
von Kupffer cell
von Maschke test for creatinine
von Meyenburg complex
von Pirquet test
von Recklinghausen disease of bone
von Recklinghausen disease of skin
von Willebrand disease
von Willebrand factor (vWF)
von Willebrand factor antigen
von Zeynek and Mencki test
voodoo death
vortex mixed
VP (variegate porphyria)
vulgaris, pemphigus verruca
Vulpian atrophy
vulva, labial artery of
vulvar canal
vulvar dystrophy
vulvitis
vulvouterine canal
vulvovaginal gland
vulvovaginitis
vWF (von Willebrand factor) antigen
VZV (varicella-zoster virus)

W, w

Waaler-Rose test
Wagner test for occult blood
waist of scaphoid
Waldenström macroglobulinemia
Waldenström purpura
Waldenström test for urine porphyrin
Waldeyer fascia
Waldeyer gland
Waldeyer ring
Waldeyer space
wall
  abdominal
  anterior abdominal
  axial
  body
  bowel
  carotid
  cavity
  cell
  chest
  gallbladder
  midabdominal
  nasal cavity
  posterior abdominal
  thoracic
  vaginal
  variceal
wall akinesis
wallerian degeneration
Walther canal
Walther oblique ligament
wandering abscess
wandering cell
wandering gallbladder
wandering goiter
wandering histiocyte
wandering kidney
wandering pneumonia
Wangiella dermatitidis
Wang test
Warburg apparatus
wart (verruca vulgaris)
  dermal
  epidermal
  flat genital
  genital
  Hassall-Henle
  keratotic
  mosaic
  pitch
  plantar
  postmortem
  precancerous
  venereal

Warthin cell
Warthin-Finkeldey cell
Warthin-Finkeldey giant cell
Warthin-Finkeldey giant cell in
  lymphoid tissue and skin
Warthin sign
Warthin-Starry silver stain
Warthin-Starry tissue-staining method
Warthin tumor (adenolymphoma)
wartlike
wart virus, infectious
warty
warty papilloma
washed clot
washed sperm
washerman's mark dermatitis
washing
  bladder
  bronchial
  gastric
  sperm
washings and brushings
Wasmann gland
wasserhelle (water-clear) cells
Wassermann test
wastes
  creatinine
  urea
  nitrogen
wasting, muscle
water balance
water-borne gastroenteritis
water-borne infection
water-buffalo leprosy
water-clear cell of parathyroid
watered-silk retina
water-filled pouch
Waterhouse-Friderichsen syndrome
water itch
Waters Nova-Pak C18 reversed-phase
  column
water-soluble
water-soluble proteins
water test
watery diarrhea
watery stool
watery urine
Watson-Schwartz test
wave
  A
  B
  brain
  C
  cannon
  delta
  dicrotic
  fluid
  peristaltic
wax
  bone
  paraffin
  tubercle bacillus
wax block
waxy casts in urine
waxy degeneration of skeletal muscle
waxy kidney
Wayson stain
WB (Western blot)
WBC (white blood cell) count
    consisting of:
  bands
  basos (basophils)
  blasts
  differential
  eos (eosinophils)
  immature forms
  leukocytes
  lymphs (lymphocytes)
  monos (monocytes)
  neutrophils
  polys or PMNs (polymorpho-
    nuclear leukocytes)
  segs (segmented neutrophils)
  stabs

WBC/hpf (white blood cells per high-power field)
weakness of peripheral pulses
weal (wheal)
wear and tear pigments
web
 digital
 duodenal
 esophageal
 fibrous
 hepatic
 intestinal
 laryngeal
 postcricoid
 terminal
 venous
webbed digit
webbed finger
webbed neck
webbed penis
webbed toe
Weber-Christian panniculitis
Weber gland
Weber-Rendu-Osler disease
Weber staining method
weblike fold
wedge-and-groove joint
wedge bone
wedge-shaped
Weeks bacillus
weeping eczema
Wegener granulomatosis
Weibel-Palade body
Weibel-Palade granule
Weichbrodt test for globulin
Weidel test for uric acid
Weigert-Gram stain
Weigert iron hematoxylin
Weigert-Pal method
Weigert stain
weightbearing bone
weightbearing joints
weight-per-volume concentration
Weil disease
Weil-Felix agglutinins
Weil-Felix test
Weil myelin sheath stain
Weil stain
Weiss-Mallory syndrome
Weisz test
Weitbrecht ligament
Welch abscess
Welch bacillus
Welcozyme HIV 1+2 ELISA antibody test
well-differentiated adenocarcinoma
well-differentiated carcinoma
well-healed surgical incision
Wender test for glucose
Wenzell test for strychnine
Wepfer gland
Weppen test for morphine
Werdnig-Hoffmann spinal muscular atrophy
Werner thyroid suppression test
Wernicke encephalopathy
Wernicke field
Wesselsbron virus
Westberg space
Westcott cutting biopsy needle
Westergren method
Westergren sedimentation rate
Western blot (WB) analysis
Western blot procedure
Western blotting
western equine encephalitis antibody
Western immunoblot test
West Nile virus
Westphal zone
wet brain
wet gangrene
wet pleurisy with effusion
wet preparation
wet smear

Wetzel test
Weyl test for creatinine
Wharton jelly
Wharton tumor (cystadenoma)
wheal (also weal)
Wheeler and Johnson test
whettle bones
whiff test
whiplike cilia
whiplike process
Whipple triad
whipworm (trichuriasis)
whistling deformity
white atrophy
white bile
white blood cell (WBC)
white blood cell count
white blood cells per high-power field (WBC/hpf)
"white cell" (slang for white blood cell)
white cell casts
white corpuscle
"white count" (slang for white blood cell count)
white fatty stool
white gangrene
Whitehead deformity
white light
white line
white matter
white piedra
white plague
white pulp
white pulp of spleen
white ramus communicans
white sponge nevus
white thrombus
white tissue
white tumor
whitlow, herpetic
Whitmore bacillus
whole blood
whole protein
whooping cough (pertussis)
whorl
  coccygeal
  digital
  fingerprint
  keratin
whorled cell formation
whorled mass
WI-38 cells (Wistar Institute)
Wiberg classification of patellar types
Widal agglutination test
Widal serum test
wide-angle glaucoma
wide-mouth sac
Wideroe test
widespread bleeding
widespread intravascular thrombosis
widespread metastasis
Widmark test
width
  platelet distribution (PDW)
  red cell distribution
Wijsman method of end-labeling
Wijs test
Wilcoxon test
Wilder reticulum stain
wild-type DNA
Wilkie artery
Williams factor
Williamson blood test
Williams stain
Willis
  antrum of
  artery of
  circle of
Willis pancreas
Wilms tumor
Wilson disease
Wilson-Kimmelstiel disease
Winckler test for alkaloids
winding

windows of jejunum
windpipe
wing, ashen
wing cell
Winslow, foramen of
Winslow pancreas
Winslow ligament
Winterbottom sign
winter eczema
winter itch
wire-loop appearance
wire-loop lesion
wire, pacemaker
Wirsung canal
Wirsung duct
Wirtz-Conklin spore stain
wisdom teeth
Wishart test for acetonemia
Wiskott-Aldrich syndrome
within normal limits (WNL)
without irreversible injury
Witz test
WNL (within normal limits)
Woldman test
Wolfe breast carcinoma classification
Wolfer gland
wolffian cyst
Wolfring gland
Wolinella
Woodbury test
Wood's light test
woodworker's lung disease
woody
woolly-hair nevus
woolsorter's disease
woolsorter's pneumonia
work, blood
working diagnosis
worm (pl. worms) (see also *pathogen*)
  appendiceal
  bladder
  cecal

worm *(continued)*
  fluke
  guinea
  mucosal
  parasitic
  rectal
worm abscess
Wormley test for alkaloids
Worm-Mueller test
worms in appendix
worms in cecum
worms in mucosa of cecum and appendix
worms in rectum
wound
  abraded
  aseptic
  avulsed
  ballistic
  blowing
  clean
  closed
  contaminated
  contused
  craniocerebral penetrating
  crease
  cross-irrigation of
  cutaneous
  depths of
  exit
  gaping
  glancing
  gunshot (GSW)
  gutter
  high-energy gunshot
  high-velocity gunshot
  incised
  lacerated
  nonpenetrating
  open
  penetrating
  perforating

wound *(continued)*
- plantar puncture
- puncture
- septic
- seton
- stab
- subcutaneous
- sucking
- tangential
- tetanus-prone
- traumatopneic

wound hematoma
wound infection
wound repair
woven bone
wrenched knee
Wright stain
wrinkle
Wrisberg ligament
wrist
wrist joint
wrist tag
wrongful death suit
wry neck (torticollis)
WT1 tumor suppressor gene
Wucheraria bancrofti
Wu method
Wurster test
Wyeomyia melanocephala mosquito
Wyeomyia virus

X, x

xanthelasma
xanthemia
xanthochromia of cerebrospinal fluid
xanthochromic spinal fluid
xanthogranuloma, juvenile
xanthogranulomatous pyelonephritis
xanthoma
  disseminated
  eruptive
  malignant fibrous
  planar
  tendinous
  tuberoeruptive
  verruciform
xanthoma cell
xanthomatosis, cerebrotendinous
xanthomatous granuloma
xanthoma tuberosum
Xanthomonas
xanthosarcoma
xanthosis
xenobiotics
xenogenous
xenon skin clearance test
xenon washout technique measurement
xeroderma
xerosis
xerotic eczema
Xg blood group
xiphicostal ligaments of Macalister
xiphisternal articulation
xiphisternal joint
xiphoid appendix
xiphoid bone
xiphoid ligament
xiphoid process
X-linked gene
X-linked infantile agammaglobulinemia
x-ray dermatitis
xylene
xylose absorption test
xylose test
Xylohypha bantiana

Y, y

Yale SK virus
Yatapoxvirus
yaws (frambesia)
Y body
yeast
yeast fungus
yeast infection
yeastlike fungus
yellow
    acid
    fast
    alizarin
    brilliant
    butter
    corallin
    imperial
    Manchester
    metanil
    methyl
    naphthol
    Philadelphia
yellow atrophy
yellow cartilage
yellow crusted patches
yellow elastic fiber
yellow fever
yellow fever virus
yellowish-gray plaques
yellow jaundice
yellow marrow
yellow plaque, fibrofatty
yellow tissue
yellow urine
Yersinia
Yersinia enterocolitica (formerly *Pasteurella enterocolitica*)
Yersinia frederiksenii
Yersinia intermedia
Yersinia kristensenii
Yersinia pestis (formerly *Pasteurella pestis*)
Yersinia pseudotuberculosis (formerly *Pasteurella pseudotuberculosis*)
Y-linked gene
yoke, alveolar
yoke bone
yolk cell
Young diabetes
Y-shaped incision
Y-shaped ligament
Yvon test for alkaloids

Z, z

Zaleski test
Zenker fixative
Zenker fluid
Zenker solution
Ziemann dots
Zika fever
Zimmermann test
zona-free hamster egg penetration
zone
  abdominal
  apical
  border
  cervical
  cervical transformation
  ciliary
  contact area
  coronal
  cutaneous
  dentofacial
  dolorogenic
  entry
  ependymal
  epileptogenic
  erogenous
  fetal
  Flechsig primordial
  gingival

zone *(continued)*
  Golgi
  grenz
  His
  keratogenous
  medullary
  nephrogenic
  neutral
  occlusal
  peripheral
  periventricular
  placental
  portal
  pupillary
  Rolando
  segmental
  T
  thymus-dependent
  thymus-independent
  transition
  transitional
  transformation
  visual
  Westphal
zone of antibody excess
zone of antigen excess
zone of discontinuity

zonula adherens
zonula occludens
zonular space
zonule, ciliary
zoo blot analysis
zoster, herpes
Zsigmondy test
Zubrod scale
zuckergussleber
Zuckerkandl gland
zygapophyseal articulation
zygapophyseal joint
zygogenic cell
zygoma
zygomatic arch
zygomatic artery
zygomatic bone
zygomatic nerve
zygomaticofacial canal
zygomatico-orbital artery
zygomaticotemporal canal
zygomaticotemporal nerve
zygomatic process
zygomycetous fungus
zygomycosis
zygote
zymogen cell
zymogen granule
zymogenic cell
zymoid

Appendix

Table of Arteries

artery	arteria (pl. arteriae)
Abbott's artery	
abdominal aorta artery	arteria aorta abdominalis
aberrant artery	
aberrant obturator artery	
accessory meningeal artery	arteria meningea accessoria
accessory obturator artery	arteria obturatoria accessoria
accessory pudendal artery	arteria pudenda accessoria
accompanying artery of ischiadic nerve	arteria comitans nervi ischiadici
accompanying artery of median nerve	arteria comitans nervi mediani
acetabular artery	ramus acetabularis arteriae circumflexae femoris medialis
acromial artery	
acromiothoracic artery	
Adamkiewicz, artery of	arteria radicularis magna
adipose arteries of kidney	rami capsulares arteriae renis
adrenal artery, middle	arteria suprarenalis media
afferent artery of glomerulus	vas afferens glomeruli
alar artery of nose	
alveolar artery, inferior	arteria alveolaris inferior
alveolar arteries, superior, anterior	arteriae alveolares superiores anteriores
alveolar artery, superior, posterior	arteria alveolaris superior posterior
anastomotic atrial artery	ramus atrialis anastomoticus arteriae coronariae sinistrae
angular artery	arteria angularis
angular gyrus artery	arteria gyri angularis
anonymous artery	
anterior auricular artery	arteria auricularis anterior
anterior cecal artery	arteria cecalis anterior
anterior cerebellar artery	arteria cerebelli anterior
anterior cerebral artery	arteria cerebri anterior
anterior choroidal artery	arteria choroidea anterior
anterior ciliary artery	arteria ciliaris anterior

artery	arteria (pl. arteriae)
anterior circumflex humeral artery	arteria circumflexa humeri anterior
anterior communicating artery	arteria communicans anterior
anterior conjunctival artery	arteria conjunctivalis anterior
anterior descending artery	
anterior ethmoidal artery	arteria ethmoidalis anterior
anterior humeral circumflex artery	
anterior inferior cerebellar artery	arteria cerebelli inferior anterior
anterior inferior segmental artery of kidney	arteria segmenti anterioris inferioris renis
anterior intercostal arteries	rami intercostales anteriores
anterior interosseous artery	arteria interossea anterior
anterior interventricular artery	ramus interventricularis anterior arteriae coronariae sinistrae
anterior labial arteries	arteriae labiales anteriores
anterior lateral malleolar artery	arteria malleolaris anterior lateralis
anterior medial malleolar artery	arteria malleolaris anterior medialis
anterior mediastinal arteries	rami mediastinales arteriae thoracicae internae
anterior meningeal artery	arteria meningea anterior
anterior parietal artery	arteria parietales anterior
anterior peroneal artery	ramus arteriae fibularis anterior
anterior radial carpal artery	arteria radialis carpalis
anterior spinal artery	arteria spinalis anterior
anterior superior alveolar arteries	arteriae alveolares superiores anteriores
anterior superior dental artery	arteria alveolaris anterior superior
anterior superior segmental artery of kidney	arteria segmenti anterioris superioris renis
anterior temporal artery	arteria temporalis anterior
anterior tibial artery	arteria tibialis anterior
anterior tibial recurrent artery	arteria recurrens tibialis anterior
anterior tympanic artery	arteria tympanica anterior
anterolateral central arteries	arteriae centrales anterolaterales
anterolateral striate arteries	arteriae centrales anterolaterales
anterolateral thalamostriate arteries	arteriae centrales anterolaterales
apicoposterior artery	
appendicular artery	arteria appendicularis
arch of aorta	arteria arcus aortae

artery	arteria (pl. arteriae)
arciform artcries	arteriae arcuatae renis
arcuate artery of foot	arteria arcuata pedis
arcuate arteries of kidney	arteriae arcuatae renis
articular artery, proper, of little head of fibula	ramus circumflexus fibulae arteriae tibialis posterioris
ascending artery	arteria ascendens
ascending aorta	arteria aorta ascendens
ascending cervical artery	arteria cervicalis ascendens
ascending palatine artery	arteria palatina ascendens
ascending pharyngeal artery	arteria pharyngea ascendens
atrial anastomotic artery	ramus atrialis anastomoticus arteriae coronariae sinistrae
atrial arteries	arteriae atriales
atrioventricular node, artery to	ramus nodi atrioventricularis
atrioventricular nodal artery	ramus nodi atrioventricularis arteriae coronariae dextrae
auditory artery, internal	arteria labyrinthina
auricular arteries, anterior	rami auriculares anteriores arteriae temporalis superficialis
auricular artery	arteria auricularis
axillary artery	arteria axillaris
axis thoracic artery	arteria thoracica axillaris
azygos arteries of vagina	vaginales arteriae uterinae
basilar artery	arteria basilaris
brachial artery	arteria brachialis
brachiocephalic artery	truncus brachiocephalicus
bronchial arteries	rami bronchiales
buccal artery, buccinator artery	arteria buccalis
bulbourethral artery	arteria bulbi urethrae
bulb of penis, artery of	arteria bulbi penis
bulb of vestibule of vagina, artery of	arteria bulbi vestibuli vaginae
calcaneal arteries	rami calcanei
calcarine artery	
calf, artery of	arteria sural
callosomarginal artery	arteria callosomarginalis
capsular artery	arteria suprarenalis
caroticotympanic arteries	arteriae caroticotympanicae
carotid artery	
caudal artery	arteria sacralis mediana

artery	arteria (pl. arteriae)
caudate lobe, artery of	arteria lobi caudati
cavernous artery	
cecal artery	arteria caecalis
celiac artery	
central arteries	arteriae centrales
central artery of retina, Zinn's artery	arteria centralis retinae
central sulcus artery	arteria sulci centralis
cephalic artery	arteria carotis communis
cerebellar artery	arteria cerebelli
cerebral artery, cerebral arteries	arteria cerebri, arteriae cerebrales
cervical artery	arteria cervicalis
cervicovaginal artery	arteria cervicovaginalis
Charcot's artery	
chief artery of thumb	arteria princeps pollicis
choroid artery, anterior	arteria choroidea anterior
ciliary arteries	arteriae cilliares
circle of Willis	
circumflex artery	ramus circumflexus arteriae coronariae sinistrae
circumflex artery, deep, internal	ramus profundus arteriae circumflexae femoris medialis
circumflex femoral artery, lateral	arteria circumflexa femoris lateralis
circumflex femoral artery, medial	arteria circumflexa femoris medialis
circumflex humeral artery, anterior	arteria circumflexa anterior humeri
circumflex humeral artery, posterior	arteria circumflexa posterior humeri
circumflex iliac artery, deep	arteria circumflexa iliaca profunda
circumflex iliac artery, superficial	arteria circumflexa iliaca superficialis
circumflex scapular artery	arteria circumflexa scapulae
clavicular artery	
clitoris, artery of, deep	arteria profunda clitoridis
clitoris, artery of, dorsal	arteria dorsalis clitoridis
coccygeal artery	arteria sacralis mediana
cochlear artery	ramus cochlearis arteriae labyrinthi
Cohnheim's artery	arteria terminalis
coiled artery	
colic artery	arteria colica
collateral artery	arteria collateralis
common carotid artery	arteria carotis communis
common hepatic artery	arteria hepatica communis

artery	arteria (pl. arteriae)
common iliac artery	arteria iliaca communis
common interosseous artery	arteria interossea communis
common palmar digital artery	arteria digitalis palmaris communis
common plantar digital artery	arteria digitalis plantaris communis
communicating artery of cerebrum	arteria communicans cerebri
companion artery	
conducting artery	
conjunctival artery	arteria conjunctivalis
conus artery	ramus coni arteriosi arteriae coronariae
copper-wire artery	
corkscrew artery	
coronary artery of heart	arteria coronaria
coronary artery of stomach	arteria gastrica
corpus cavernosum	
cortical artery	
costocervical trunk artery	
cremasteric artery	arteria cremasterica
cricothyroid artery	ramus cricothyroideus
crural artery	
cystic artery	arteria cystica
deep artery of clitoris	arteria profunda clitoridis
deep artery of penis	arteria profunda penis
deep artery of thigh	arteria profunda femoris
deep auricular artery	arteria auricularis profunda
deep brachial artery	arteria profunda brachii
deep cervical artery	arteria cervicalis profunda
deep circumflex iliac artery	arteria circumflexa iliaca profunda
deep epigastric artery	arteria epigastrica profunda
deep external pudendal artery	arteria pudenda profunda externa
deep femoral artery	arteria femoralis profunda
deep iliac circumflex artery	arteria circumflexa iliaca superficialis
deep lingual artery	arteria profunda linguae
deep palmar arch	arcus palmaris profundus
deep penis artery	arteria profunda penis
deep plantar artery	ramus plantaris profundus
deep temporal artery	arteria temporalis profunda
deep volar branch of ulnar artery	arteria ulnaris
deferential artery	arteria ductus deferentis
deltoid artery	ramus deltoideus arteriae profundae brachii

artery	arteria (pl. arteriae)
dental artery	arteria alveolaris
descending branch of occipital artery	arteria occipitalis descendens
descending genicular artery	arteria anastomotica magna
descending palatine artery	arteria palatina descendens
descending scapular artery	arteria scapularis descendens
diaphragmatic arteries	arteriae phrenicae inferiores
digital arteries	arteriae digitales
digital collateral artery	arteria digitalis palmaris propria
distributing artery	
dorsal artery of clitoris	arteria dorsalis clitoridis
dorsal artery of foot	arteria dorsalis pedis
dorsal artery of great toe	arteria dorsalis hallucis
dorsal artery of nose	arteria dorsalis nasi
dorsal artery of penis	arteria dorsalis penis
dorsal carpal artery	arteria dorsalis carpal
dorsal digital artery	arteria digitalis dorsalis
dorsal interosseous artery	arteria interossea dorsalis
dorsal metacarpal artery	arteria metacarpalis dorsalis
dorsal nasal artery	arteria dorsalis nasi
dorsalis pedis artery	arteria dorsalis pedis
dorsalis penis artery	arteria dorsalis penis
dorsal metacarpal artery	arteria metacarpea dorsalis
dorsal metatarsal artery	arteria metatarsea dorsalis
dorsal nasal artery	arteria nasi externa
dorsal pancreatic artery	arteria pancreatica dorsalis
dorsal scapular artery	arteria dorsalis scapulae
Drummond, artery of (marginal artery of colon)	
ductus deferens, artery of	arteria ductus deferentis
duodenal arteries	arteriae pancreaticoduodenales inferiores
efferent artery of glomerulus	vas efferens glomeruli
elastic artery	
emulgent artery	arteria renalis
end artery (terminal artery)	
epigastric artery	arteria circumflexa iliaca
epiphyseal artery	
episcleral arteries	arteriae episclerales
esophageal arteries	rami esophagei arteriae gastricae

artery	arteria (pl. arteriae)
ethmoidal artery	arteria ethmoidalis
external carotid artery	arteria carotis externa
external iliac artery	arteria iliaca externa
external mammary artery (lateral thoracic artery)	arteria thoracica lateralis
external maxillary artery (facial artery)	arteria maxillaris externa
external pudendal arteries	arteriae pudendae externae
external spermatic artery (cremasteric artery)	
facial artery	arteria facialis
fallopian artery	areria uterina
femoral artery	arteria femoralis
fibular artery (peroneal artery)	arteria fibularis
foot, artery of, dorsal	arteria dorsalis pedis
frontal artery (supratrochlear artery)	arteria supratrochlearis
frontobasal artery, lateral	arteria frontobasalis lateralis
funicular artery	arteria testicularis
gastric artery	arteria gastrica
gastroduodenal artery	arteria gastroduodenalis
gastroepiploic artery	arteria gastro-omentalis
gastro-omental artery	arteria gastro-omentalis
genicular artery	arteria genicularis
glaserian artery (anterior tympanic)	arteria tympanica anterior
glomerular artery	
gluteal artery	arteria glutealis
great anastomotic artery	arteria radicularis magna
greater palatine artery	arteria palatina major
great pancreatic artery	arteria pancreatica magna
great radicular artery	arteria radicularis magna
great superior pancreatic artery (dorsal)	arteria pancreatica magna superior
helicine arteries of penis	arteriae helicinae penis
hemorrhoidal artery	arteria rectalis
hepatic artery	arteria hepatica
Heubner, artery of (medial striate artery)	
highest intercostal artery (superior)	rami intercostales superiores
highest thoracic artery (superor)	arteria thoracica superior
humeral artery (brachial artery)	arteria humeri
hyaloid artery	arteria hyaloidea
hyoid artery	ramus suprahyoideus arteriae lingualis

artery	arteria (pl. arteriae)
hypogastric artery (internal iliac artery)	arteria iliaca interna
hypophysial artery	arteria hypophysialis
ileal arteries	arteriae ileales
ileocolic artery	arteria ileocolica
iliac artery	arteria iliaca
iliolumbar artery	arteria iliolumbalis
inferior alveolar artery	arteria alveolaris inferior
inferior cerebellar artery	arteria cerebelli inferior
inferior dental artery	arteria alveolaris inferior
inferior epigastric artery	arteria epigastrica inferior
inferior gastroduodenal artery	arteria gastroduodenalis inferior
inferior genicular artery	arteria genicularis inferior
inferior gluteal artery	arteria glutea inferior
inferior hemorrhoidal artery	arteria rectalis inferior
inferior hypophysial artery	arteria hypophysialis inferior
inferior labial artery	arteria labialis inferior
inferior laryngeal artery	arteria laryngea inferior
inferior lateral genicular artery	arteria genus inferior lateralis
inferior medial genicular artery	arteria genus inferior medialis
inferior mesenteric artery	arteria mesenterica inferior
inferior pancreatic artery	arteria pancreatica inferior
inferior pancreaticoduodenal artery	arteria pancreaticoduodenalis inferior
inferior phrenic artery	arteria phrenica inferior
inferior profunda artery	arteria profunda inferior
inferior rectal artery	arteria rectalis inferior
inferior segmental artery of kidney	arteria segmenti inferioris renis
inferior suprarenal artery	arteria suprarenalis inferior
inferior thyroid artery	arteria thyroidea inferior
inferior tympanic artery	arteria tympanica inferior
inferior ulnar collateral artery	arteria collateralis ulnaris inferior
inferior vesical artery	arteria vesicalis inferior
infracostal artery	ramus costalis lateralis arteriae thoracicae internae
infrahyoid artery	arteria infrahyoideus
infraorbital artery	arteria infraorbitalis
infrascapular artery	arteria infrascapularis
innominate artery	truncus brachiocephalicus
inguinal arteries	rami inguinales arteriae femoralis
innominate artery	truncus brachiocephalicus

artery	arteria (pl. arteriae)
insular arteries	arteriae insulares
intercostal arteries	rami intercostales arteriae thoracicae
interlobar arteries of kidney	arteriae interlobares renis
interlobular arteries of kidney	arteriae interlobulares renis
interlobular arteries of liver	arteriae interlobulares hepatis
intermediate atrial artery	ramus atrialis intermedius
intermediate temporal artery	arteria temporalis intermedia
intermetacarpal arteries	arteriae metacarpales palmares
internal auditory artery (labyrinthine)	arteria labyrinthi
internal carotid artery	arteria carotis interna
internal iliac artery	arteria iliaca interna
internal malleolar artery	arteria malleolaris interna
internal mammary artery (thoracic)	arteria thoracica interna
internal maxillary artery	arteria maxillaris interna
internal palpebral artery	arteria palpebralis interna
internal plantar artery	arteria plantaris interna
internal pubic artery	arteria pubicus interna
internal pudendal artery	arteria pudenda interna
internal spermatic artery (testicular)	arteria testicularis interna
internal thoracic artery	arteria thoracica interna
interosseous artery	arteria interossea
interosseous palmar artery	arteria palmaris interossea
intersegmental artery	
interventricular artery	ramus interventricularis
intestinal arteries (ileal or jejunal)	arteriae intestinales
jejunal arteries	arteriae jejunales
kidney, arteries of (segmental arteries of kidney)	arteriae renis
Kugel's anastomotic artery	arteria anastomotica auricularis magna
labial arteries of vulva	rami labiales arteriae femoralis
labyrinthine artery	arteria labyrinthi
lacrimal artery	arteria lacrimalis
laryngeal artery	arteria laryngea
lateral calcaneal artery	arteria calcanei lateralis
lateral circumflex femoral artery	arteria circumflexa femoris lateralis
lateral circumflex artery of thigh	arteria circumflexa femoris lateralis
lateral costal artery	
lateral frontobasal artery	arteria frontobasalis lateralis
lateral inferior genicular artery	arteria genicularis lateralis inferior

artery	arteria (pl. arteriae)
lateral malleolar arteries	rami malleolares laterales
lateral nasal artery	arteria nasi lateralis
lateral occipital artery	arteria occipitalis lateralis
lateral palpebral artery	arteria palpebralis lateralis
lateral plantar artery	arteria plantaris lateralis
lateral sacral artery	arteria sacralis lateralis
lateral striate arteries	arteriae centrales anterolaterales
lateral tarsal artery	arteria tarsea lateralis
lateral thoracic artery	arteria thoracica lateralis
left anterior descending coronary artery	ramus interventricularis anterior arteriae coronariae sinistrae
left colic artery	arteria colica sinistra
left coronary artery	arteria coronaria sinistra
left gastric artery	arteria gastrica sinistra
left gastroepiploic artery	arteria gastro-omentalis sinistra
left gastro-omental artery (left gastroepiploic artery)	
left hepatic artery	ramus sinister arteriae hepaticae propriae
left pulmonary artery	arteria pulmonalis sinistra
lenticulostriate arteries (Charcot's artery) (lateral striate arteries)	
lesser palatine artery	arteria palatina minor
lienal artery (splenic artery)	
lingual artery	arteria lingualis
lingual artery, dorsal	arteria lingualis dorsalis
lobar artery	
long central artery (medial striate artery)	
long ciliary artery	arteria ciliaris longa
long posterior ciliary artery	arteria ciliaris posterior longa
long thoracic artery (lateral)	arteria thoracica lateralis
lowest lumbar arteries	arteriae lumbales imae
lowest thyroid artery	arteria thyroidea ima
lumbar artery	arteria lumbalis
macular arteries	
malleolar artery	arteria malleolaris
mammary artery	arteria thoracica
mandibular artery	arteria alveolaris inferior
marginal artery	ramus marginalis

artery	arteria (pl. arteriae)
marginal artery of colon (artery of Drummond, Riolan's arc)	arteria marginalis coli
masseteric artery	arteria masseterica
mastoid artery	rami mastoidei arteriae auricularis posterioris
maxillary artery	arteria maxillaris
medial artery of foot, superficial	ramus superior arteriae plantaris medialis
medial circumflex femoral artery	arteria circumflexa femoris medialis
medial frontobasal artery	arteria frontobasalis medialis
medial malleolar arteries	arteriae malleolares posteriores mediales
medial palpebral artery	
medial striate artery	
medial tarsal artery	
median artery	arteria comitans nervi mediani
median sacral artery	arteria sacralis mediana
mediastinal arteries, anterior	rami mediastinales arteriae thoracicae internae
mediastinal arteries, posterior	rami mediastinales aortae thoracicae
medullary artery	arteria nutriens
meningeal artery, accessory	ramus meningeus accessorius arteriae meningeae mediae
meningeal artery, anterior	ramus meningeus anterior arteriae ethmoidalis anterioris
meningeal artery, middle	arteria meningea media
meningeal artery, posterior	arteria meningea posterior
mental artery	arteria mentalis
mesencephalic arteries	arteriae mesencephalicae
mesenteric artery	arteria mesenterica
metacarpal arteries	arteriae metacarpales
metaphyseal artery	
metatarsal artery	arteria metatarsae
middle capsular artery	arteria suprarenalis media
middle cerebral artery	arteria cerebri media
middle colic artery	arteria colica media
middle collateral artery	arteria collateralis media
middle genicular artry	arteria articularis azygos
middle hemorrhoidal artery	

artery	arteria (pl. arteriae)
middle meningeal artery	arteria meningea media
middle rectal artery	arteria rectalis media
middle sacral artery	arteria sacralis media
middle suprarenal artery	arteria suprarenalis media
middle temporal artery	arteria temporalis media
middle vesical artery	arteria vesicalis media
Mueller, arteries of	arteriae helicinae penis
musculophrenic artery	arteria musculophrenica
mylohyoid artery	ramus mylohyoideus arteriae alveolaris inferioris
myomastoid artery	ramus occipitalis arteriae auricularis posterioris
nasal artery, dorsal	arteria dorsalis nasi
nasopalatine artery	arteria sphenopalatina
Neubauer's artery	arteria thyroidea ima
nodal artery	
nose, dorsal artery of	arteria dorsalis nasi
nutrient artery	arteria nutricia
obliterated hypogastric artery	
obliterated umbilical artery	
obturator artery	arteria obturatoria
occipital artery	arteria occipitalis
omental artery	
omphalomesenteric artery	
ophthalmic artery	arteria ophthalmica
orbital artery	
orbitofrontal artery (lateral frontobasal)	
ovarian artery	arteria ovarica
palatine artery	arteria palatina
palmar metacarpal artery	arteria metacarpea palmaris
palpebral arteries	arteriae palpebrales
pancreatic artery	arteria pancreatica
pancreaticoduodenal artery	arteria pancreaticoduodenalis
paracentral artery	arteria paracentralis
parietal arteries, anterior and posterior	arteriae parietales anterior et posterior
parieto-occipital artery	arteria parieto-occipitalis
parieto-temporal artery	
pectoral artery	
pelvic artery, posterior	arteria iliaca interna

artery	arteria (pl. arteriae)
penis, deep artery of	arteria profunda penis
penis, dorsal artery of	arteria dorsalis penis
perforating arteries	arteriae perforantes
pericallosal artery	arteria pericallosa
pericardiac arteries, posterior	rami pericardiaci aortae thoracicae
pericardiacophrenic artery	arteria pericardiacophrenica
perineal artery	arteria perinealis
periosteal artery	
peroneal artery, fibular artery	arteria peronea, arteria fibularis
pharyngeal artery, ascending	arteria pharyngea ascendens
phrenic arteries	arteriae phrenicae
plantar artery	arteria plantaris
plantar metatarsal artery	arteria metatarsea plantaris
pontine arteries	arteriae pontis
popliteal artery	arteria poplitea
postcentral sulcal artery	arteria sulci postcentralis
posterior alveolar artery	arteria alveolaris posterior
posterior auricular artery	arteria auricularis posterior
posterior cecal artery	arteria cecalis posterior
posterior cerebral artery	arteria cerebri posterior
posterior choroidal artery	arteria choroidea posterior
posterior circumflex humeral artery	arteria circumflexa humeri posterior
posterior communicating artery	
posterior descending coronary artery	ramus interventricularis posterior arteriae coronariae dextrae
posterior humeral circumflex	artria circumflexa humeri posterior
posterior inferior cerebellar artery	arteria cerebelli posterior inferior
posterior intercostal artery	
posterior interosseous artery	arteria interossea posterior
posterior pancreaticoduodenal artery	arteria pancreaticoduodenalis posterior
posterior scapular artery	arteria scapulae posterior
posterior scrotal artery	arteria scrotalis posterior
posterior septal artery of nose	arteria nasalis posterior septi
posterior spinal artery	arteria spinalis posterior
posterior superior alveolar artery	arteria alveolaris superior posterior
posterior temporal artery	arteria temporalis posterior
posterior tibial artery	arteria tibialis posterior
posterior tibial recurrent artery	arteria recurrens tibialis posterior
posterior tympanic artery	arteria tympanica posterior

artery	arteria (pl. arteriae)
posterolateral central artery	arteriae centrales posterolaterales
posteromedial central arteries	arteriae centrales posteromediales
precentral sulcal artery	arteria sulci precentralis
princeps pollicis artery	arteria princeps pollicis
precuneal artery	arteria precunealis
prepancreatic artery	arteria prepancreatica
presegmental artery	arteria presegmenti
prevertebral artery	arteria prevertebralis
principal artery of thumb	arteria princeps pollicis
profunda brachii artery	arteria profunda brachii
profunda femoris artery	arteria profunda femoris
proper hepatic artery	arteria hepatica propria
proper palmar digital artery	arteria digitalis palmaris propria
proper plantar digital artery	arteria digitalis plantaris propria
pterygoid arteries	rami pterygoidei
pterygoid canal, artery of	arteria canalis pterygoidei
pubic artery	ramus pubicus arteriae epigastricae inferioris
pudendal arteries	arteriae pudendae externae
pulmonary artery	truncus pulmonalis
pyloric artery	arteria gastrica dextra
quadriceps artery of femur	ramus descendens arteriae circumflexae femoris lateralis
radial artery	arteria radialis
radial artery of index finger	arteria volaris radialis indicis
radial carpal artery	
radial collateral artery	arteria collateralis radialis
radial recurrent artery	arteria recurrens radialis
radiate arteries of kidney	arteriae interlobulares renis
radicular arteries	rami spinales arteriae vertebralis
ranine artery	arteria profunda linguae
rectal artery	arteria rectalis
recurrent artery	arteria centralis longa
recurrent artery, radial	arteria recurrens radialis
recurrent artery, tibial, anterior	arteria recurrens tibialis anterior
recurrent artery, tibial, posterior	arteria recurrens tibialis posterior
recurrent artery, ulnar	arteria recurrens ulnaris
recurrent interosseous artery	arteria interossea recurrens
recurrent radial artery	arteria recurrens radialis

artery	arteria (pl. arteriae)
recurrent ulnar artery	arteria recurrens ulnaris
renal artery, renal arteries	arteria renalis, arteriae renales
retinal artery	
retrocostal artery	ramus costalis lateralis arteriae thoracicae internae
retroduodenal artery	arteria retroduodenalis
retroesophageal subclavian artery	artery subclavia rctroesophagei
revehent artery	vas efferens glomeruli
right colic artery	arteria colica dextra
right coronary artery	arteria coronaria dextra
right gastric artery	arteria gastrica dextra
right gastroepiploic artery	arteria gastro-omentalis dextra
right hepatic artery	ramus dexter arteriae hepaticae propriae
right pulmonary artery	arteria pulmonalis dextra
round ligament of uterus, artery of	arteria ligamenti teretis uteri
sacral arteries	arteriae sacrales
sacrococcygeal artery	arteria sacralis mediana
saphenous artery	
scapular artery	arteria scapulare
sciatic artery	arteria comitans nervi ischiadici
scrotal arteries, anterior	rami scrotales anteriores arteriae femoralis
scrotal arteries, posterior	rami scrotales posteriores arteriae pudendae internae
segmental artery	arteria segmenti
semilunar ganglion artery	
septal arteries, anterior	rami interventriculares septales
septal arteries, posterior	rami interventricularis posterioris
short central artery	arteria centralis brevis
short ciliary artery	arteria ciliaris brevis
short gastric artery	arteriae gastricae breves
short posterior ciliary artery	arteria ciliaris posterior brevis
sigmoid arteries	arteriae sigmoideae
sinoatrial nodal artery, sinuatrial (S-A) node artery	ramus nodi sinuatrialis arteriae coronaria dextra
somatic artery	
spermatic artery, external	arteria cremasterica
spermatic artery, internal	arteria testicularis
sphenopalatine artery	arteria sphenopalatina

artery	arteria (pl. arteriae)
spinal arteries	rami spinales arteriae vertebralis
spiral artery	
splanchnic artery	
splenic artery	arteria splenica
stapedial artery	
sternal arteries, posterior	rami sternales arteriae thoracicae internae
sternocleidomastoid artery, superior	ramus sternocleidomastoideus arteriae thyroideae superioris
straight arteries of kidney	arteriolae rectae renis
striate arteries	arteriae centrales anterolaterales
stylomastoid artery	arteria stylomastoidea
subclavian artery	arteria subclavia
subcostal artery	arteria subcostalis
sublingual artery	arteria sublingualis
submaxillary glandular artery	
submental artery	arteria submentalis
subscapular artery	arteria subscapularis
sulcal artery	
superficial brachial artery	arteria brachialis superficialis
superficial cervical artery	arteria cervicalis superficialis
superficial circumflex iliac artery	arteria circumflexa iliaca superficialis
superficial epigastric artery	arteria epigastrica superficialis
superficial external pudendal artery	arteria pudenda superficialis externa
superficial iliac circumflex artery	arteria circumflexa iliaca superficialis
superficial palmar arch artery	arteria arcus palmaris superficialis
superficial perineal artery	arteria perinealis superficialis
superficial petrosal artery	
superficial temporal artery	arteria temporalis superficialis
superficial volar artery	
superficial volar arch artery	
superior cerebellar artery	arteria cerebelli superior
superior epigastric artery	arteria epigastrica superior
superior gluteal artery	arteria glutea superior
superior hemorrhoidal artery	arteria rectalis superior
superior hypophysial artery	arteria hypophysialis superior
superior intercostal artery	arteria intercostalis suprema
superior labial artery	arteria labialis superior
superior laryngeal artery	arteria laryngea superior
superior lateral genicular artery	arteria genus superior lateralis

artery	arteria (pl. arteriae)
superior medial genicular artery	arteria genus superior medialis
superior mesenteric artery	arteria mesenterica superior
superior pancreaticoduodenal artery	arteria pancreaticoduodenalis superior
superior phrenic artery	arteria phrenica superior
superior profunda artery	arteria profunda superior
superior rectal artery	arteria rectalis superior
superior segmental artery of kidney	arteria segmenti superioris renis
superior suprarenal arteries	arteriae suprarenales superiores
superior thoracic artery	arteria thoracica superior
superior thyroid artery	arteria thyroidea superior
superior tympanic artery	arteria tympanica superior
superior ulnar collateral artery	arteria collateralis ulnaris superior
superior vesical artery	arteria vesicalis superior
supraduodenal artery	arteria supraduodenalis
suprahyoid artery	arteria superhyoideus
supraorbital artery	arteria supraorbitalis
suprarenal artery, aortic	arteria suprarenalis media
suprascapular artery	arteria suprascapularis
supratrochlear artery	arteria supratrochlearis
sural artery	arteria suralis
sylvian artery	arteria cerebri media
tarsal artery	arteria tarsalis
temporal artery	arteria temporalis
terminal artery (Cohnheim's artery)	
testicular artery	arteria testicularis
thalamostriate arteries, anterolateral	arteriae centrales anterolaterales
thoracic artery	arteria thoracica
thoracicoacromial artery	arteria thoracoacromialis
thoracodorsal artery	arteria thoracodorsalis
thymic arteries	rami thymici arteriae thoracicae internae
thyroid artery	arteria thyroidea
thyroid artery, inferior, of Cruveilhier	ramus cricothyroideus arteriae thyroideae superioris
thyroid ima artery	arteria thyroidea ima
tibial artery	arteria tibialis
tonsillar artery	ramus tonsillaris arteriae facialis
tracheal artery	
transverse artery of neck	arteria transversa cervicis
transverse cervical artery	arteria transversa cervicis

artery	arteria (pl. arteriae)
transverse facial artery	arteria transversa faciei
transverse perineal artery	arteria transversa perinealis
transverse scapular artery	arteria transversa scapulae
trunk artery	
tubo-ovarian artery	arteria ovarica
tympanic artery	arteria tympanica
ulnar artery	arteria ulnaris
ulnar carpal artery	
ulnar collateral artery, inferior	arteria collateralis ulnaris inferior
ulnar collateral artery, superior	arteria collateralis ulnaris superior
umbilical artery	arteria umbilicalis
upper limb, arteries of	arteriae membri superioris
ureteric artery	
urethral artery	arteria urethralis
urethral bulb artery	
uterine artery	arteria uterina
uterine artery, aortic	arteria ovarica
vaginal artery	arteria vaginalis
venous arteries	venae pulmonales
ventricular arteries	arteriae ventriculares
vermiform artery	arteria appendicularis
vertebral artery	arteria vertebralis
vesical artery, inferior	arteria vesicalis inferior
vesical arteries, superior	arteriae vesicales superiores
vestibular arteries	rami vestibulares arteriae labyrinthi
vidian artery	arteria canalis pterygoidei
visceral artery	
vitelline artery	arteria vitellina
volar carpal artery	
volar interosseous artery	arteria interossea volaris
Zinn, artery of	arteria centralis retinae
zygomatic artery	
zygomatico-orbital artery	arteria zygomatico-orbitalis

Table of Bones

bone (region)	os (pl. ossa)
acetabulum	os acetabuli
acromial bone	os acromiale
	os acromiale secondarium
ankle bone	talus
atlas (neck)	atlas
axis (neck)	axis
basilar bone	os basilare
Bertin's bone	
blade bone	scapula
breast bone	sternum
Breschet's bone	os suprasternale
calcaneus (foot)	calcaneus; os calcis; os tarsi fibulare
capitate bone (wrist)	os capitatum; os carpale distale tertium
carpal bones (wrist)	ossa carpi; ossa carpalia
central bone (wrist)	os centrale
clavicle (shoulder)	clavicula
coccyx (lower back)	os coccygis
compact bone	substantia compacta
concha, inferior nasal (skull)	concha nasalis inferior
cortical bone	substantia corticalis
cranial bones	ossa cranii; ossa cranialia
cuboid bone (foot)	os cuboideum
cuneiform bone, intermediate (foot)	os cuneiforme intermedium
cuneiform bone, lateral (foot)	os cuneiforme laterale
cuneiform bone, medial (foot)	os cuneiforme mediale
digits, bones of	ossa digitorum
elbow bone (olecranon process of ulna)	cubitus
epipteric bone (Flower's bone)	
ethmoid bone	os ethmoidale
fabella (knee)	
facial bones	ossa facialia; ossa faciei
femur (thigh)	femur

bone (region)	os (pl. ossa)
fibula (leg)	fibula
flat bone	os planum
Flower's bone (epipteric bone)	
foot, bones of	ossa pedis
frontal bone (skull)	os frontale
digits of hand	ossa digitorum manus
digits of foot	ossa digitorum pedis
Goethe's bone (preinterparietal bone)	
greater multangular bone	trapezium
hamate bone (wrist)	os hamatum; os carpale distale quartum
hand, bones of (carpals, metacarpals, phalanges)	ossa manus
heel bone	calcaneus
hip bone (pelvis and hip)	os coxae
hollow bone (pneumatic bone)	
hooked bone (hamate bone)	
humerus (arm)	humerus
hyoid bone (neck)	os hyoideum
iliac bone; ilium (pelvis)	os ilii; os ilium
incisive bone	os incisivum
incus (ear)	incus
inferior limb, bones of (os coxae, pelvis, patella, tibia, fibula, tarsus metatarsus, digits of foot)	ossa membri inferioris
innominate bone (hip bone)	os coxae
intermaxillary bone	os incisivum
interparietal bone	os interparietale
irregular bone	os irregulare
ischial bone; ischium (pelvis)	os ischii
jaw bone (mandible)	mandibula
jugal bone (zygomatic bone)	os zygomaticum
Krause's bone (small bone)	
lacrimal bone (skull)	os lacrimale
lamellar bone	
lesser multangular bone (trapezoid)	os trapezoideum
lingual bone (hyoid bone)	
long bone (pipe bone)	os longum
lunate bone (wrist)	os lunatum
malar bone	os zygomaticum

bone (region)	**os** (pl. **ossa**)
malleus (ear)	malleus
mandible (lower jaw)	mandibula
mastoid bone of occipital bone	margo mastoideus squamae occipitalis
maxilla (skull, upper jaw)	maxilla
metacarpal bones (hand)	ossa metacarpalia
metacarpal bone, third or middle	os metacarpale tertium
metatarsal bones (foot)	ossa metatarsalia
nasal bone (nose)	os nasale
navicular bone of foot	os naviculare; os centrale tarsi
navicular bone of hand	os scaphoideum
nonlamellar bone (woven bone)	
occipital bone (skull)	os occipitale
palatine bone (skull)	os palatinum
parietal bone (skull)	os parietale
patella (knee)	patella
pelvis	os pelvicum
penis bone	os penis
perichondral bone (periosteal bone)	
periosteal bone (perichondral bone)	
peroneal bone (fibula)	
petrosal bone	
phalanges (pl. of phalanx) (fingers, toes)	ossa digitorum
phalanx, proximal	os phalanx proximalis
phalanx, middle	os phalanx media
phalanx, distal	os phalanx distalis
ping-pong bone	
pipe bone (long bone)	
Pirie's bone (dorsal talonavicular bone)	
pisiform bone (wrist)	os pisiforme
pneumatic bone	os pneumaticum
postsphenoid bone	
preinterparietal bone (Goethe's bone)	
premaxillary bone	os incisivum
presphenoid bone	
pubic bone (pelvis)	os pubis; mons pubis
pyramidal bone (triquetral bone)	os triquetrum
radius (forearm)	radius
replacement bone (endochondral bone)	
reticulated bone (woven bone)	

bone (region)	os (pl. ossa)
rib, ribs	os costae, os costale; ossa costalis
rider's bone (cavalry bone, exercise bone)	
Riolan's bone	
sacrum (lower back)	os sacrum
scaphoid bone (wrist)	os scaphoideum
scapula (shoulder)	scapula
scroll bones	
septal bone (interalveolar septum)	
sesamoid bones of hand	ossa sesamoidea manus
sesamoid bones of foot	ossa sesamoidea pedis
shank bone (cannon bone; tibia)	
shin bone (tibia)	
short bone	os breve
sieve bone	
skull, bones of	ossa cranii
sphenoid bone (base of skull)	os sphenoidale
splint bone (fibula)	
spongy bone	
stapes (ear)	stapes
sternum (chest)	sternum
superior limb, bones of (humerus, radius, ulna, carpus, metacarpus, digits of hand)	ossa membri superioris
suprainterparietal bone	
suprasternal bones	ossa suprasternalia
sutural bones	ossa suturalia; ossa fonticulorum
tail bone (coccyx)	os coccygis
talus (ankle)	talus; os tarsi tibiale
tarsal bones (ankle and foot)	ossa tarsi
temporal bone (skull)	os temporale
thigh bone (femur)	
thoracic bones	ossa thoracis
three-cornered bone (triquetral bone)	os triquetrum
tibia (leg)	tibia
tongue bone (hyoid bone)	
trabecular bone	
trapezium bone (wrist)	os trapezium; os carpale distale primum
trapezoid bone (wrist)	os trapezoideum; os carpale distale secundum

bone (region)	**os** (pl. **ossa**)
triangular bone	os trigonum
triquetral bone (wrist)	os triquetrum
turbinate bone, inferior (inferior nasal concha)	
tympanic bone	
ulna (forearm)	ulna
unciform bone (hamate bone)	
upper jaw bone (maxilla)	
vertebrae (back)	
vertebrae, cervical	vertebrae cervicales
vertebrae, thoracic (dorsal)	vertebrae thoracicae
vertebrae, lumbar	vertebrae lumbales
vertebrae, sacral	vertebrae sacrales
vertebrae, coccygeal	vertebrae coccygeae
Vesalius' bone; vesalian bone	os vesalianum pedis
vomer (skull)	vomer
wedge bone (intermediate cuneiform)	
woven bone (nonlamellar; reticulated)	
yoke bone (zygomatic bone)	
zygomatic bone (skull)	os zygomaticum

Table of Normal Laboratory Values

All are adult values, unless otherwise specified.

Abbreviations and symbols used in these tables:

±	plus or minus
≤	less than or equal to
≥	greater than or equal to
/	per
%	percent
<	less than
>	greater than
μ	micron
μ^3	cubic micron
μg	microgram
μmol	micromole
μU	microunit
d	day
dL	deciliter
EU	Ehrlich units
g	gram
Hb	hemoglobin
hr.	hour
IU	international unit
kg	kilogram
L	liter
mEq	milliequivalent
mg	milligram
mIU	international milliunit
mL	milliliter
mmol	millimole
mOsm	milliosmole
mU	milliunit
ng	nanogram
pg	picogram
s	seconds
U	unit

Blood	
acetaldehyde	<0.2 mg/L
acetoacetate	negative
acid hemolysis test (Ham's test)	<5% lysis
acetone	negative
acid phosphatase	0 to 7 mU/mL, or less than 3 ng/mL
acidified serum test (Ham's test)	<5% lysis
ACT (activated coagulation time)	107 ± 13 s
ACTH (adrenocorticotropic hormone)	25 to 100 pg/mL
activated coagulation time (ACT)	107 ± 13 s
activated partial thromboplastin time (APTT)	25 to 35 s
adrenocorticotropic hormone (ACTH)	25 to 100 pg/mL
AFP (alpha-fetoprotein) tumor marker	0 to 10 ng/mL
A/G (albumin/globulin) ratio	1.1 to 2.3
alanine aminotransferase—see *ALT*.	
albumin	3 to 5 g/dL
albumin/globulin (A/G) ratio	1.1 to 2.3
aldolase	1 to 8 U/L
aldosterone	supine, 3 to 10 ng/dL upright, 5 to 30 ng/dL
alkaline phosphatase	10 to 32 mU/mL, or 30 to 120 U/L
alpha$_1$-antitrypsin	105 to 200 mg/dL
alpha-1-fetoprotein, serum (AFP)	<40 ng/mL
ALT (alanine aminotransferase) (formerly SGPT)	0 to 17 mU/mL
aminotransferase—see *ALT* and *AST*.	
ammonia	0 to 50 μmol/L
ammonia nitrogen	15 to 45 μg N/dL
amylase	0-88 U/L
ANA (antinuclear antibody)	negative
angiotensin I	11 to 88 pg/mL
angiotensin II	arterial, 2.4 ± 1.2 ng/dL venous, 50% to 75% of arterial
anion gap	7 to 16 mmol/L
anti-centromere screen and titer	negative
alpha$_1$-antichymotrypsin	30 to 60 mg/dL
antideoxyribonuclease B titer (anti-DNAse titer)	$\leq$170 units

Blood

antidiuretic hormone (ADH) (vasopressin) mOsmol/kg	
270-280:	<1.5 pg/mL
280-285:	<2.5 pg/mL
285-290:	1 to 5 pg/mL
290-295:	2 to 7 pg/mL
295-300:	4 to 12 pg/mL
anti-DNA antibodies	
indirect fluorescence	negative in 1:10 dilution
Farr method	<20% of DNA bound
Ginsberg/Keiser	≤1μg/mL
antihyaluronidase (AH) titer	≤128 units
antinuclear antibody (ANA)	negative
antistreptolysin-O (ASO) titer	≤166 Todd units
alpha$_1$-antitrypsin	105 to 200 mg/dL
antithrombin III (AT-III)	
radioimmunodiffusion	plasma, 21 to 30 mg/dL serum, 17 to 25 mg/dL
amidolytic	plasma, 85 to 115% of standard serum, 55 to 80% of standard
APTT (activated partial thromboplastin time)	25 to 35 s
arterial blood gases—see *blood gases*.	
ascorbic acid	0.6 to 2.0 mg/dL
ASO (antistreptolysin-O) titer	≤166 Todd units
aspartate aminotransferase—see *AST*.	
AST (aspartate aminotransferase) (formerly SGOT)	0 to 19 mU/mL
bands (banded neutrophils) on WBC differential	3% to 5%
base excess	-3 to +3
basos (basophils) on WBC differential	0 to 0.75%
beta carotene	60 to 200 μg/dL
bicarbonate (CO_2), arterial	23 to 29 mEq/L
bile acids, total	
fasting	0.3 to 2.3 μg/mL
2-hr. postprandial	1.8 to 3.2 μg/mL

Blood

bilirubin	
direct (conjugated)	0.1 to 0.4 mg/dL
indirect (unconjugated)	0.2 to 0.7 mg/dL
total	0.3 to 1.2 mg/dL
bleeding time	
Duke	1 to 5 minutes
Ivy	2 to 7 minutes
Simplate	2.75 to 8 minutes
blood factors—see *factors*.	
blood gases, arterial	
calculated bicarbonate	18 to 23 mmol/L
PCO_2	35-45 mm Hg
pH	7.35-7.45
PO_2	75-100 mm Hg
oxygen (O_2) saturation	96-100%
blood volume	8.5 to 9.0% of body weight females, 50 to 75 mL/kg males, 52 to 83 mL/kg
bone marrow differential (%)	
myeloblasts	0.3 to 5.0
promyelocytes	1 to 8
myelocytes	
neutrophilic	5 to 19
eosinophilic	0.5 to 3.0
basophilic	0 to 0.5
metamyelocytes	13 to 32
polymorphonuclear neutrophils	7 to 30
polymorphonuclear eosinophils	0.5 to 4.0
polymorphonuclear basophils	0.0 to 0.7
lymphocytes	3 to 17
plasma cells	0 to 2
monocytes	0.5 to 5.0
reticulum cells	0.1 to 2.0
megakaryocytes	0.03 to 3.0
pronormoblasts	1 to 8
normoblasts	7 to 32
BUN (blood urea nitrogen)	10 to 26 mg/dL
calcitonin (hCT)	<100 pg/mL

Blood

calcium	
ionized	4.25 to 5.25 mg/dL or 1/13 to 1.32 mmol/L
total	9.2 to 11 mg/dL
cancer antigen (CA-125)	0 to 35 U/mL
capillary fragility test	<5 to 10 petechiae on forearm halfway between systolic and diastolic pressures
carbon dioxide	
partial pressure (PCO_2)	35 to 45 mm Hg
total	23 to 31 mmol/L
carbon monoxide	nonsmokers, <2% total Hb smokers, <10% total Hb
carcinoembryonic antigen (CEA)	nonsmokers, <3 ng/mL smokers, <5 ng/mL
cardiac isoenzymes (CK, creatine kinase)	
CK-BB	absent
CK-MB	absent
CK-MM	present
carotenoids	0.5 to 3.0 μg/mL
catecholamines, serum (random)	
norepinephrine	104 to 548 pg/mL
epinephrine	<88 pg/mL
dopamine	<136 pg/mL
CBC (complete blood count)	
hematocrit	females, 35 to 46% males, 41 to 53%
hemoglobin	females, 12 to 16 g/dL males, 13.5 to 17.5 g/dL
MCH (mean corpuscular hemoglobin)	25.4 to 34.6 pg/cell
MCHC (mean corpuscular hemoglobin concentration)	32 to 36 g/dL
MCV (mean corpuscular volume)	80 to 105 μ^3
RBC (red blood cell) count	3.5 to 6.0 million
WBC (white blood cell) count	4,500 to 10,000
(see also *white blood cell differential*)	
CD2 (T11) total T cells	70 to 94%
CD3 (T3) mature T cells	57 to 91%
CD4/CD3 lymphocyte ratio	CD4 = 32 to 68% CD3 = 57 to 91%

Blood	
CD4/CD8 lymphocyte ratio	CD4 = 32 to 68% CD3 = 57 to 91% CD8 = 10 to 36%
cell count—see *white count differential.*	
ceruloplasmin	14 to 40 mg/dL
C (complement components or inhibitor proteins, C1–C9, not subscripts)	
$C1_s$ esterase inhibitor immuno-differential	2.1 to 4.1 mg/dL
C1q, serum	5.1 to 7.9 mg/dL
C2, serum	1.9 to 2.5 mg/dL
C3, serum	83 to 177 mg/dL
C4, serum	12 to 36 mg/dL
C5, serum	3.8 to 9.0 mg/dL
C6, serum	4.0 to 7.2 mg/dL
C7, serum	4.9 to 7.0 mg/dL
C8, serum	4.3 to 6.3 mg/dL
C9, serum	4.7 to 6.9 mg/dL
chloride (Cl), serum	96 to 106 mEq/L
cholesterol	
HDL (high-density lipoprotein)	>35 mg/dL recommended
LDL (low-density lipoprotein)	<130 mg/dL recommended
total	<200 mg/dL recommended
cholic acid	0.20±0.17 μg/mL
cholinesterase II	
RID	0.5 to 1.5 mg/dL
DuPont ACA	7 to 19 U/mL
chorionic gonadotropin	nondetectable unless pregnant
7-10 days	>5.0 mIU/mL
30 days	>100 mIU/mL
40 days	>2000 mIU/mL
10 weeks	50,000 to 100,000 mIU/mL
14 weeks	10,000 to 20,000 mIU/mL
trophoblastic disease	>100,000 mIU/mL
citrulline, serum	12 to 55 μmol/L
CK (creatine kinase)	females, 0 to 150 IU/L males, 0 to 175 IU/L
CK (creatine kinase) isoenzymes—see *cardiac isoenzymes.*	
coagulation (clotting) time	5 to 15 minutes

Blood

coagulation factors—see *Factors*.	
cold hemolysin test (Donath-Landsteiner)	negative
Coombs test, direct and indirect	negative
copper	70 to 155 μg/dL
corticosterone	0.13 to 2.3 μg/dL
cortisol, serum	8:00 AM, 5 to 23 μg/dL 4:00 PM, 3 to 15 μg/dL 10:00 PM, ≤50% of 8:00 AM value
C-peptide	≤5.0 ng/mL
C-reactive protein (CRP)	68 to 820 ng/mL
creatine kinase—see *cardiac isoenzymes*.	
creatinine, serum	0.7 to 1.5 mg/dL
creatinine clearance	88 to 137 mL/minute
CRP (C-reactive protein)	68 to 820 ng/mL
cryoglobulin screen	negative
cyanide, serum	nonsmokers, 0.004 mg/L smokers, 0.006 mg/L
dehydroepiandrosterone (DHEA)	1.7 to 5.2 ng/mL
dehydroepiandrosterone sulfate ($DHEA\text{-}SO_4$)	females, 0.11 to 3.38 μg/mL males, 1.99 to 3.34 μg/mL
deoxycholic acid, total	0.22±0.13 μg/mL
dihydrotestosterone (DHT)	adult females, 10 to 40 ng/dL adult males, 60 to 300 ng/dL
2,3 diphosphoglycerate (2,3 DPG)	12.27 ±1.87 μmol/g Hb
electrolytes	
bicarbonate (CO_2)	23 to 29 mEq/L
chlorides (Cl)	96 to 106 mEq/L
potassium (K)	3.5 to 5.0 mEq/L
magnesium (Mg)	1.3 to 2.5 mEq/L
sodium (Na)	136 to 146 mEq/L
electrophoresis	
globulin	0.1 to 0.4 g/dL
alpha-1	0.4 to 1.1 g/dL
alpha-2	0.5 to 1.6 g/dL
beta	0.5 to 1.4 g/dL
gamma	0.7 to 1.2 g/dL
hemoglobin	HbA >95% HbA2 1.5% to 3.5% HbF <2%

Blood	
eosinophils (eos) on WBC differential	1% to 3%
eosinophil count	50 to 350 cells/mL
erythrocyte count (RBC)	3.5 million to 5.5 million/mL
erythrocyte sedimentation rate (ESR or sed rate)	Wintrobe: 0 to 15 mm/hr. Westergren: 0 to 20 mm/hr.
erythropoietin	
hemagglutination	25 to 125 mIU/mL
RIA	<5 to 20 mIU/mL
bioassay	5 to 18 mU/mL
ESR (erythrocyte sedimentation rate)	Wintrobe: 0 to 15 mm/hr. Westergren: 0 to 20 mm/hr.
estradiol, serum	females, 10 to 500 pg/mL (varies with menstrual cycle) males, 8 to 36 pg/mL
estriol	
free	positive with pregnancy, 3.5 to 34.0 μg/L
total serum	males and nonpregnant females, <2 mg/mL positive with pregnancy, 30 to 350 ng/mL
estrogens, total	menstruating, 61 to 437 pg/mL prepubertal/postmenopausal females, ≤40 pg/mL males, 40 to 115 pg/mL
estrogen receptor assay (ERA)	>10 fmol/mg protein
estrone (E1)	female pubertal, 0 to 80 pg/mL female adult, 20 to 150 pg/mL male pubertal, 11 to 21 pg/mL male adult, 30 to 170 pg/mL
factors, blood coagulation	
factor I (fibrinogen)	200 to 400 mg/dL
factor II (prothrombin)	0.5 to 1.5 U/mL
factor II antigen	75% to 125% of normal
factor V	0.5 to 2.0 U/mL
factor VII	65% to 135% of normal
factor VIII (antihemophiliac)	55% to 145% of normal
factor VIII antigen	50% to 200% of normal
factor IX	60% to 140% of normal
factor X	60% to 130% of normal

Blood

factors, blood coagulation *(continued)*	
factor XI	65% to 135% of normal
factor XII (Hageman)	65% to 150% of normal
factor XIII (fibrin stabilizing)	0.02 to 0.05 U/mL
fatty acid profile	
oleic	26 to 45%
palmitic	23 to 25%
stearic	10 to 14%
linoleic	8 to 16%
fatty acids, total	190 to 420 mg/dL
ferritin	females, 12 to 150 ng/mL males, 15 to 200 ng/mL
fibrin lysis time	>60 minutes
fibrinogen	200 to 400 mg/dL
5'-nucleotidase	1 to 12 U/L
fluoride	0.01 to 0.2 μg/mL
folate	
serum	3 to 12 ng/mL
red blood cell	153 to 605 ng/mL
follicle stimulating hormone (FSH)	menstruating females, 4 to 90 mIU/mL pregnant females, low to undetectable postmenopausal females, 40 to 250 mIU/mL males, 4 to 25 mIU/mL
free thyroxine index—see *thyroxine index*.	
fructose	1 to 6 mg/dL
FTA-IgM, serum (fluorescent treponemal antibody)	nonreactive
galactose	<5 mg/dL
gamma-glutamyl transpeptidase—older name for GGT (*gamma-glutamyl-transferase)*	
gastrin, serum	<60 years old, <100 pg/mL >60 years old, 100 to 800 pg/mL
GGT (gamma-glutamyltransferase) (formerly gamma-glutamyl transpeptidase or GGTP)	5 to 40 U/L
GGTP (gamma-glutamyl transpeptidase)—see *GGT.*	

Blood	
glucose	fasting, 70 to 110 mg/dL 2 hr. postprandial, <120 mg/dL
glucose tolerance test (GTT)	fasting, 70 to 110 mg/dL at 1 hr., 120 to 170 mg/dL at 1-1/2 hr., 100 to 140 mg/dL at 2 hr., 70 to 120 mg/dL
glycerol, free	0.29 to 1.72 mg/dL
glycosylated hemoglobin (Hgb Al_c)	5.6 to 7.5%
gold	<10 μg/dL (therapeutic, 38-50)
growth hormone (hGH or GH)	females, <10 ng/mL males, <2 ng/mL
Ham's acidified serum test	<5% lysis
haptoglobin	
RID	30 to 175 mg/dL
nephelometry	25 to 175 mg/dL
haptoglobin/hemopexin (under two years)	
haptoglobin	100 to 300 mg/dL
hemopexin	40 to 100 mg/dL
HCG, hCG (human chorionic gonadotropin) tumor marker	<2 mIU/mL
HDL (high density lipoprotein) cholesterol	>35 mg/dL recommended
hematocrit (HCT, Hct)	females, 35 to 46% males, 41 to 53%
hemoglobin (Hb)	females, 12 to 16 g/dL males, 13.5 to 17.5 g/dL
hemoglobin A	>95%
hemoglobin A2 (HbA2)	1.5% to 3.5%
hemoglobin A1C (HbA_{1C})	
electrophoresis	5.6 to 7.5%
column	6 to 9%
hemoglobin electrophoresis	HbA >95% HbA2 1.5% to 3.5% HbF <2%
hemoglobin F	<2.0
hemoglobin H (HbH)	No precipitation at 40 minutes
high-density liproprotein (HDL) cholesterol	>35 mg/dL recommended
human chorionic gonadotropin (HCG, hCG) tumor marker	<2 mIU/mL
hydroxyproline	females, 0 to 34 μmol/L males, 0 to 42 μmol/L

Blood	
immunoglobulins	
IgA	60 to 383 mg/dL
IgD	0 to 8 mg/dL
IgE	0 to 230 IU/mL
IgG	600 to 1900 mg/dL
IgM	40 to 345 mg/dL
insulin, 12-hr. fasting	<60 years old, 7 to 24 μU/mL >60 years old, 6 to 35 μU/mL
ionized calcium	4.25 to 5.25 mg/dL
iron	newborn, 100 to 250 μg/dL infant, 40 to 100 μg/dL child, 50 to 120 μg/dL adult females, 40 to 150 μg/dL adult males, 50 to 160 μg/dL
iron-binding capacity, total (TIBC)	250 to 410 μg/dL
iron saturation	20 to 55%
isocitrate dehydrogenase (ICD)	1.2 to 7.0 U/L
isoenzymes, serum by agarose gel electrophoresis	
Fraction 1	14 to 26% of total
Fraction 2	29 to 39% of total
Fraction 3	20 to 26% of total
Fraction 4	8 to 16% of total
Fraction 5	6 to 16% of total
ketone bodies	
qualitative	negative
quantitative	0.5 to 3.0 mg/dL
lactate	venous, 4.5 to 20 mg/dL arterial, 4.5 to 14.4 mg/dL
lactate dehydrogenase (LDH)	50 to 220 U/L
lactose	<0.5 mg/dL
LDH (lactate dehydrogenase)	50 to 220 U/L
LDL (low-density lipoprotein) cholesterol	<130 mg/dL recommended
lead	0 to 50 μ/dL
leucine	75 to 175 μmol/L
lipase	
Cherry-Crandall	0 to 1.5 units
Tietz	0.1 to 1.0 U/mL
lipase, BMD	<180 U/L
lipoprotein electrophoresis	distinct beta band

Blood	
liver functions	
acid phosphatase	0 to 7 mU/mL
alkaline phosphatase	10 to 32 mU/mL
ALT (formerly SGPT)	0 to 17 mU/mL
AST (formerly SGOT)	0 to 19 mU/mL
bilirubin	
direct (conjugated)	0.1 to 0.4 mg/dL
indirect (unconjugated)	0.2 to 0.7 mg/dL
total	0.3 to 1.1 mg/dL
low-density lipoprotein (LDL) cholesterol	<130 mg/dL recommended
luteinizing hormone (LH)	
females:	
follicular	follicular phase, 5-30 mIU/mL
midcycle	75 to 150 mIU/mL
luteal	3 to 40 mIU/mL
postmenopausal	30 to 200 mIU/mL
males	6 to 23 mIU/mL
lymphs (lymphocytes)	25% to 33%
lysozyme (muramidase)	5 to 15 μg/mL
magnesium (Mg)	1.3 to 2.5 mEq/L
MB isoenzyme, bands, or fraction	<5%
MCH (mean corpuscular hemoglobin)	25.4 to 34.6 pg/cell
MCHC (mean corpuscular hemoglobin concentration)	32 to 36 g/dL
MCV (mean corpuscular volume)	80 to 105 microns
mercury	<5 μg/dL
methanol	<0.15 mg/dL
methemalbumin	negative
methionine	6 to 40 μmol/L
methemoglobin (MetHb)	0.06 to 0.24 g/dL or 0 to 1.5% of total hemoglobin
monos (monocytes) on WBC differential	3% to 7%
myoglobin	6 to 85 ng/mL
5'-nucleotidase	1 to 12 U/L
orosomucoid	55 to 140 mg/dL
osmolality	
serum	275 to 295 mOsmol/kg
urine/serum ratio	1 to 3; >3 after 12 hr. fluid restriction
oxygen (O_2) saturation	96-100%
oxytocin	<3.2 μU/mL

Blood	
partial thromboplastin time (PTT)	35 to 40 s
PCO_2 (partial pressure of carbon dioxide)	35-45 mm Hg
pH (measures acidity)	7.35-7.45
phosphatase	
acid	0 to 7 mU/mL, or less than 3 ng/mL
alkaline	10 to 32 mU/mL, or 30 to 120 U/L
phosphate, serum	3.0 to 4.5 mEq/L
phospholipids, total	<65 years old, 125 to 275 mg/dL >65 years old, 196 to 366 mg/dL
phosphorus, inorganic	3 to 4.5 mg/dL (or 1 to 1.5 mEq/L)
plasma volume	females, 28 to 45 mL/kg males, 25 to 43 mL/kg
phenylalanine	0.8 to 1.8 mg/dL
platelets	150,000 to 400,000/mL
PMNs or polys (polymorphonuclear neutrophils) on WBC differential	54 to 62%
prealbumin, serum	8 to 31 mg/dL
potassium (K)	3.5 to 5.0 mEq/L
PO_2 (partial pressure of oxygen)	75-100 mm Hg
progesterone	
pubertal females	0 to 13 ng/mL
adult females	0.02 to 0.9 ng/mL follicular phase
adult females	6 to 30 ng/mL luteal phase
pubertal males	0.11 to 0.26 ng/mL
adult males	0.12 to 0.3 ng/mL
prolactin	
nonpregnant females	5 to 40 ng/mL
pregnant females	<80 to <400 ng/mL
adult males	up to 20 ng/mL
protein	
albumin	3 to 5 g/dL
globulin	1.5 to 3.7 g/dL
total	6 to 8 g/dL
prostaglandins	
E	25 to 200 pg/mL
F	25 to 150 pg/mL
prostate specific antigen (PSA)	
healthy men	0 to 2.8 ng/mL
post prostatectomy	<0.2 ng/mL
prothrombin time (PT, pro time)	12 to 14 s

Blood	
protoporphyrin	<50 μg/dL
PSA (prostate specific antigen)	
healthy men	0 to 2.8 ng/mL
post prostatectomy	<0.2 ng/mL
pseudocholinesterase	
RID	0.5 to 1.5 mg/dL
DuPont ACA	7 to 19 U/mL
PTH-intact (parathyroid hormone)	10 to 65 pg/mL
PT (pro time, prothrombin time)	12 to 14 s
PTT (partial thromboplastin time)	35 to 40 s
pyruvic acid	0.3 to 0.9 mg/dL
sulfhemoglobin (SHb)	≤1.0% of total hemoglobin
RA latex (rheumatoid arthritis)	negative
red blood cells	3.5-6.0 million
red blood cell indices—see *CBC*.	
red cell distribution width (RDW)	<15%
red cell volume	females, 19 to 31 mL/kg males, 20 to 36 mL/kg
renin	supine, 1.6±1.5; standing, 4.5±2.9
reticulocyte count	
range	0.5 to 1.5%
absolute count	25,000 to 75,000/mL
reverse triiodothyronine (rT_3)	30 to 80 ng/dL
riboflavin (vitamin B_2)	See *Urine* section below.
RPR (rapid plasma reagin)	negative
secretin	37±8 pg/mL
sedimentation rate	Wintrobe: 0 to 15 mm/hr. Westergren 0 to 20 mm/hr.
segs (segmented neutrophils) on WBC differential; also *polys* and *PMNs*	54 to 62%
selenium	10 to 34 μg/dL
serotonin	whole blood, 39 to 361 ng/mL
SGOT (serum glutamic oxalo-acetic transaminase)—see *AST*.	
SGPT (serum glutamic pyruvic transaminase)—see *ALT*.	
sodium (Na)	136 to 146 mEq/L
somatomedin C	0.4 to 2.0 U/mL
somatotropin (growth hormone)	females, <10 ng/mL males, <2 ng/mL

Blood	
stab (also "band," banded neutrophil)	3% to 5%
sucrose	mean, 0.06 mg/dL
sulfate	2.9 to 3.5 mg/dL
testosterone, free	
prepubertal females	0.04 ±0.01 ng/dL
adult females	0.31±0.07 ng/dL
prepubertal males	0.04±0.01 ng/dL
adult males	7.9±2.3 ng/dL
testosterone, total	
prepubertal females	6.6±2.5 ng/dL
adult females	37±10 ng/dL
prepubertal males	6.6±2.5 ng/dL
adult males	572±135 ng/dL
thrombin time	±2 s when control is 9 to 13 s, or 14.5 to 18.9 s
thyroid function tests	
T_3 (triiodothyronine) uptake	25% to 38%
T_4 (thyroxine)	4.4 to 9.9 μg/dL
TSH (thyroid stimulating hormone)	2 to 10 μU/mL
thyroid antibodies	≤1:10 dilution
thyroid microsomal antibodies	nondetectable
thyroid stimulating hormone (TSH)	2 to 10 μU/mL
thyroid uptake of radioactive iodine	2 hr.: <6% 6 hr.: 3 to 20% 24 hr.: 8 to 30%
thyrotropin-releasing hormone (TRH)	5 to 60 pg/mL
thyroxine (T_4)	
free	0.8 to 2.4 ng/dL
serum (total)	4.4 to 9.9 μg/dL pregnant females, 6.1 to 17.6 μg/dL
thyroxine-binding globulin (TBG)	15 to 34 μg/mL
thyroxine index, free (FT_4I)	5.5 to 10
TIBC (total iron-binding capacity)	250 to 410 μg/dL
tourniquet test	<5 to 10 petechiae on forearm halfway between systolic and diastolic pressures
transcortin	females, 1.6 to 2.5 mg/dL pregnant females, 4.7 to 7.0 mg/dL males, 1.5 to 2.0 mg/dL
transferrin	200 to 400 mg/dL
transketolase	9 to 12 μmol/hr./mL whole blood

Blood	
triglycerides	35 to 160 mg/dL
triiodothyronine	
T_3-RIA	115 to 190 ng/dL
free	230 to 660 pg/dL
total	150 to 250 ng/dL
reverse (rT_3)	30 to 80 ng/dL
2,3 diphosphoglycerate (2,3 DPG)	12.27 $\pm$1.87 μmol/g Hb
tyrosine	0.8 to 1.3 mg/dL
urea nitrogen	8 to 23 mg/dL
urea nitrogen/creatinine ratio	12:1 to 20:1
uric acid	2.2 to 7.7 mg/dL
valine	141 to 317 μmol/L
vasoactive intestinal polypeptide (VIP)	20 to 53 pg/mL
VDRL (Venereal Disease Research Lab)	nonreactive
viscosity, serum	1.10 to 1.22 Centipoise
vitamin	
A	30 to 65 μg/dL
B_2 (riboflavin)	See *Urine* section below.
B_6	3.6 to 18 ng/mL
B_{12}	110 to 800 pg/mL
C	0.6 to 2.0 mg/dL
D	1,25-dihydroxy: 20 to 45 pg/mL 25-hydroxy: 15 to 18 ng/mL
E	5.0 to 20 μg/mL
white blood cells	4,500 to 10,000
white blood cell differential	
polys or PMNs (polymorphonuclear neutrophils [or leukocytes], also known as segmented neutrophils)	54% to 62%
bands (banded [immature] neutrophils, also called "stabs")	3% to 5%
lymphs (lymphocytes)	25% to 33%
eos (eosinophils)	1% to 3%
monos (monocytes)	3% to 7%
basos (basophils)	0 to 0.75%
xylose absorption test	child, 1 hr.: >30 mg/dL adult, 2 hr.: >25 mg/dL
zinc	70 to 150 μg/dL

Urine	
acetoacetate	negative
acetone	negative
alanine (24-hr. urine)	8 to 48 mg/d
albumin	negative (less than 80 mg/d)
ammonia nitrogen	500 to 1200 mg/d
ammonium chloride loading test	pH should fall to ≤5.2 two to eight hours after dosing
amorphous	few
amylase	1 to 17 U/hr.
bacteria	few or moderate
bilirubin	negative
blood	negative
calcium, 24-hr.	<300 mg/d
casts	negative
catecholamines, 24-hr.	
epinephrine	<15 μg/d
norepinephrine	<100 μg/d
chloride, 24-hr.	110 to 250 mEq/d
citrulline, 24-hr.	0.4 to 8 mg/d
color	yellow, straw, or colorless
copper, 24-hr.	0 to 50 μg/d
coproporphyrin, 24-hr.	30 to 250 μg/d
cortisol, free, 24-hr.	10 to 100 μg/d
creatine	females, <100 mg/d males, <40 mg/d
creatinine, 24-hr.	14 to 26 mg/kg/d
crystals	few
cystine or cysteine	random, negative 24-hr., 10 to 100 mg/d
DHEA (dehydroepiandrosterone), 24-hr.	0 to 2.3 ng/mL
endothelial cells	few or moderate
estrogen, 24-hr.	menstruating females, 4 to 100 μg/d postmenopausal females, <10 μg/d pregnant females, <45,000 μg/d males, 5 to 25 μg/d
estradiol, 24-hr.	females, 0 to 14 μg/d males, 0 to 6 μg/d
estriol, total, 24-hr.	6 to 42 mg/d with pregnancy
FIGLU, 24 hr. after dose of histidine	<35 mg/d
5-HIAA (5-hydroxyindoleacetic acid)	random, negative; 24-hr., 2 to 8 mg/d

Urine	
fluoride	0.2 to 1.1 μg/mL
folate absorption test, 24-hr.	45±7% of dose
glucose	negative
glycine, 24-hr.	59 to 294 mg/d
glycolic acid, 24-hr.	15 to 60 mg/d
hemoglobin/myoglobin	negative
homocystine, random	negative
homovanillic acid (HVAA), 24-hr.	child, 3 to 16 μg/mg creatinine adult, <15 mg/d
17-hydroxycorticosteroids, 24-hr.	children, 1 to 5.6 mg/d females, 2 to 8 mg/d males, 3 to 10 mg/d
5-HIAA (5-hydroxyindoleacetic acid)	random, negative; 24-hr., 2 to 8 mg/d
ketones	negative
17-ketosteroids, 24-hr.	4 to 18 mg/d
lactose	12 to 40 mg/dL
lead	<80 μg/d
leucine, 24-hr.	3 to 70 mg/d
magnesium, 24-hr.	6 to 10 mEq/d
mercury, 24-hr.	<20 μg/L (toxic >150 μg/L)
metanephrine, total, 24-hr.	0.05 to 1.20 μg/mg creatinine
microscopic	
amorphous	few
bacteria	few or moderate
epithelial cells/hpf	few or moderate
hyaline casts/hpf	negative or occasional (0 to 1)
crystals	few
mucus	few
RBC/hpf (red blood cells per high-power field)	negative
WBC/hpf (white blood cells per high-power field)	negative
mucus	few or moderate
nitrite	negative
occult blood	negative
pH	4.5 to 8.0
phenylalanine, 24-hr.	trace to 17 mg/d
phosphorus, inorganic, 24-hr.	0.4 to 1.3 g/d
porphobilinogen	random, negative; 24-hr., 0 to 2 mg/d

Urine	
protein, 24-hr.	<150 mg/d
red blood cells	negative
riboflavin (vitamin B2)	80 to 269 μg/g creatinine
sediment	clear or cloudy
selenium, 24-hr.	10 to 100 μg/L
17-hydroxycorticosteroids, 24-hr.	children, 1 to 5.6 mg/d females, 2 to 8 mg/d males, 3 to 10 mg/d
17-ketosteroids, 24-hr.	4 to 18 mg/d
specific gravity	1.002 to 1.030 random; 24-hr., 1.015 to 1.025
sucrose	mean, 2.2 mg/dL
tetrahydrocortisol (THF), 24-hr.	0.5 to 1.5 mg/d
tetrahydrodeoxycortisol, 24-hr.	<1000 μg/d
urobilinogen, 24-hr.	0.5 to 4.0 EU/d
uroporphyrin, 24-hr.	<50 μg/d
vanillylmandelic acid (VMA), 24-hr.	1 to 9 mg/d
volume	females, 600 to 1600 mL/d males, 800 to 1800 mL/d
white blood cells	negative
xylose absorption test (5-hr.)	child, 16 to 33% of ingested dose adult, 5 g dose at 5 hr. >1.2 adult, 25 g dose at 5 hr., >4.0

Miscellaneous Body Fluids

cerebrospinal fluid (CSF)	
chloride	118 to 132 mEq/L
electrophoresis	mostly albumin
glutamine	6 to 16 mg/dL
myelin basic protein	<4 ng/mL
pressure	70 to 180 mm water
volume	child, 60 to 100 mL adult, 100 to 160 mL
feces	
coproporphyrin, 24-hr.	400 to 1200 μg/d
fat, 72-hr.	<7 g/d
nitrogen, total	≤2 g N/d
occult blood	negative
protoporphyrin, 24-hr.	<1500 μg/d
urobilinogen	40 to 280 mg/d
uroporphyrin, 24-hr.	10 to 40 μg/d
gastric acid	0 to 5 mEq/L fasting 10 to 60 mEq/L post stimulation
semen	
volume	2 to 4 mL
sperm count	>20 million/mL
motility	>60%
morphology	>60% normal forms
sweat	
sweat chloride	normal, 0 to 35 mEq/L marginal, 30 to 70 mEq/L cystic fibrosis, 60 to 200 mEq/L
synovial fluid differential (%)	
polymorphonuclear cells	0 to 25
monocytes	0 to 71
lymphocytes	0 to 78
clasmatocytes	0 to 26
unclassified	0 to 21
synovial cells	0 to 12

Table of Muscles

muscle	musculus (pl. musculi)
abdominal muscles	musculi abdominis
abdominal external oblique muscle	musculus obliquus externus abdominis
abdominal internal oblique muscle	musculus obliquus internus abdominis
abductor digiti minimi muscle of foot (abductor muscle of little toe)	musculus abductor digiti minimi pedis
abductor digiti minimi muscle of hand (abductor muscle of little finger)	musculus abductor digiti minimi manus
abductor hallucis muscle (great toe)	musculus abductor hallucis
abductor pollicis brevis muscle (abductor muscle of thumb, short)	musculus abductor pollicis brevis
abductor pollicis longus muscle (abductor muscle of thumb, long)	musculus abductor pollicis longus
accessory flexor muscle of foot (quadratus plantae muscle)	musculus flexor accessorius
adductor muscle, short	musculus adductor brevis
adductor muscle of great toe	musculus adductor hallucis
adductor muscle, long	musculus adductor longus
adductor muscle, great	musculus adductor magnus
adductor minimus muscle (adductor muscle, smallest)	musculus adductor minimus
adductor pollicis muscle (thumb)	musculus adductor pollicis
Aeby's cutaneomucous muscle	
agonistic muscles	
Albinus' muscle	
anconeus muscle	musculus anconeus
antagonistic muscles	
anterior auricular muscle	musculus auricularis anterior
anterior cervical intertransverse muscles	musculi intertransversarii anteriores cervicis
anterior rectus muscle of head	musculus rectus capitis anterior
anterior scalene muscle	musculus scalenus anterior

muscle	musculus (pl. musculi)
anterior serratus muscle	musculus serratus anterior
anterior tibial muscle	musculus tibialis anterior
antigravity muscles	
antitragus muscle	musculus antitragicus
arrector pili muscles (erector muscles of hairs)	musculi arrectores pilorum
articular muscle	musculus articularis
articular muscle of elbow	musculus articularis cubiti
articular muscle of knee	musculus articularis genus
articular muscle of knee	articularis genu musculus
aryepiglottic muscle	musculus aryepiglotticus
auditory ossicles, muscles of	musculi ossiculorum auditus
axillary arch muscle	pectorodorsalis musculus
back muscles	musculi dorsi
Bell's muscle (ureteric bridge)	
biceps brachii muscle (biceps muscle of arm)	musculus biceps brachii
biceps femoris muscle (biceps muscle of thigh)	musculus biceps femoris
bipennate muscle	musculus bipennatus
Bochdalek's muscle	musculus triticeoglossus
Bovero's muscle ("sucking muscle")	musculus cutaneomucosus
Bowman's muscle (ciliary muscle)	musculus ciliaris
brachial muscle (brachialis)	musculus brachialis
brachiocephalic muscle	musculus brachiocephalicus
brachioradial muscle (brachioradialis)	musculus brachioradialis
Braune's muscle	musculus puborectalis
broadest muscle of back	musculus latissimus dorsi
bronchoesophageal muscle	musculus bronchoesophageus
Brücke's muscle (Crampton's muscle)	
buccinator muscle	musculus buccinator
buccopharyngeal muscles (also, constrictor muscles of pharynx, superior)	musculi pars buccopharyngea
bulbocavernous muscle	musculus bulbospongiosus
canine muscle	musculus levator anguli oris
cardiac muscle	
Casser's perforated muscle (casserian muscle)	musculus coracobrachialis (ligamentum mallei anterius)

muscle	musculus (pl. musculi)
ceratocricoid muscle	musculus ceratocricoideus
cervical iliocostal muscle	musculus iliocostalis cervicis
cervical interspinal muscles	musculi interspinalis cervicis
cervical longissimus muscle (neck)	musculus longissimus cervicis
cervical muscles	musculi colli
cervical rotator muscles	musculi rotatores cervicis
Chassaignac's axillary muscle	
chin muscle	musculus mentalis
chondroglossus muscle	musculus chondroglossus
chondropharyngeal muscles (constrictor muscle of pharynx, middle)	musculi pars chondropharyngea (constrictor pharyngis medius)
ciliary muscle	muscularis ciliaris
coccygeal (coccygeus) muscle(s)	musculus coccygeus, musculi coccygei
Coiter's muscle	musculus corrugator supercilii
compressor muscle of naris	
congenerous muscles	
constrictor muscle of pharynx, inferior	musculus constrictor pharyngis inferior
constrictor muscle of pharynx, middle	musculus constrictor pharyngis medius
constrictor muscle of pharynx, superior	musculus constrictor pharyngis superior
coracobrachial muscle (coracobrachialis)	musculus coracobrachialis
corrugator muscle	corrugator supercilii musculus
corrugator cutis muscle of anus	musculus corrugator cutis ani
corrugator supercilii muscle	musculus corrugator supercilii
Crampton's muscle (Bruecke's muscle)	
cremaster muscle (Riolan's muscle)	musculus cremaster
cricoarytenoid muscle, lateral	musculus crico-arytenoideus lateralis
cricoarytenoid muscle, posterior	musculus crico-arytenoideus posterior
cricopharyngeal muscle	musculus cricopharyngeus
cricothyroid muscle	musculus cricothyroideus
cruciate muscle	musculus cruciatus
cutaneomucous muscle (the "sucking muscle," also called Aeby's muscle, Bovero's muscle, Klein's muscle, Krause's muscle, mucocutaneous muscle)	musculus cutaneomucosus
cutaneous muscle	musculus cutaneus
dartos muscle of scrotum	musculus tunica dartos
deep muscles of back (true back muscles)	musculi dorsi
deep flexor muscle of fingers	musculus flexor digitorum profundus

muscle	musculus (pl. musculi)
deep transverse perineal msucle	musculus transversus perinei profundus
deltoid muscle	musculus deltoideus
depressor muscle of angle of mouth	musculus depressor anguli oris
depressor muscle of epiglottis	musculus thyroepiglottic
depressor muscle of eyebrow	musculus depressor supercilii
depressor muscle of lower lip	musculus depressor labii inferioris
depressor muscle of septum of nose	musculus depressor septi
depressor superciliary muscle	musculus depressor supercilii
detrusor muscle of urinary bladder	musculus detrusor urinae (musculus detrusor vesicae)
diaphragm, diaphragmatic muscle	diaphragma
digastric muscle	musculus digastricus
dilator muscle	musculus dilatator
dilator muscle of ileocecal sphincter	musculus dilator pylori ilealis
dilator muscle of pupil	musculus dilator pupillae
dilator muscle of pylorus	musculus dilator pylori gastroduodenalis
dorsal interosseous muscles of foot	musculi interossei dorsalis pedis
dorsal interosseous muscles of hand	musculi interossei dorsalis manus
dorsal muscles (muscles of back)	musculi dorsi
dorsal sacrococcygeal muscle	musculus sacrococcygeus dorsalis
Dupré's muscle	musculus articularis genu
Duverney's muscle	musculus orbicularis oculi
elevator muscle of anus	musculus levator ani
elevator muscle of prostate	musculus levator prostatae
elevator muscles of rib	musculi levatores costarum
elevator muscle of scapula	musculus levator scapulae
elevator muscle of soft palate	musculus levator veli palatini
elevator muscle of upper eyelid	musculus levator palpebrae superioris
elevator muscle of upper lip	musculus levator labii superioris
elevator muscle of upper lip and wing of nose	musculus levator labii superioris alaeque nasi
emergency muscles	
epicranial muscle	musculus epicranius
epimeric muscle	
epitrochleoanconeus muscle	musculus epitrochleoanconaeus
erector muscles of hairs (arrector pili)	musculi arrectores pilorum
erector muscle of penis	musculus ischiocavernosus
erector muscle of spine	musculus erector spinae

muscle	musculus (pl. musculi)
eustachian muscle	musculus tensor tympani
expression, muscles of	musculi faciales
extensor muscle of fingers	musculus extensor digitorum
extensor muscle of great toe, long	musculus extensor hallucis longus
extensor muscle of great toe, short	musculus extensor hallucis brevis
extensor muscle of hand, short (Pozzi's muscle)	musculus extensor digitorum brevis manus
extensor muscle of index finger	musculus extensor indicis
extensor muscle of little finger	musculus extensor digiti minimi
extensor muscle of thumb, long	musculus extensor pollicis longus
extensor muscle of thumb, short	musculus extensor pollicis brevis
extensor muscle of toes, long	musculus extensor digitorum longus
extensor muscle of toes, short	musculus extensor digitorum brevis
extensor muscle of wrist, radial, long	musculus extensor carpi radialis longus
extensor muscle of wrist, radial, short	musculus extensor carpi radialis brevis
extensor muscle of wrist, ulnar	musculus extensor carpi ulnaris
external intercostal muscles	musculi intercostales externi
external oblique muscle	musculus obliquus externus abdominis
external obturator muscle	musculus obturator externus
external pterygoid muscle	lateral pterygoid musculus
external sphincter muscle of anus	
extraocular muscles	musculi bulbi
extrinsic muscles	
eyeball muscles (extraocular muscles)	
facial and masticatory muscles	musculi faciales et masticatores
facial expression, muscles of	musculi faciales
facial muscles	musculi faciales
fast muscle (white muscle)	
fauces (the throat), muscles of	musculi palati et faucium
femoral muscle	musculus vastus intermedius
fibular muscle, long	musculus peroneus longus
fibular muscle, short	musculus peroneus brevis
fibular muscle, third	musculus peroneus tertius
fixation muscles, fixator muscles	
fixator muscle of base of stapes	musculus fixator baseos stapedis
flexor muscle of fingers, deep	musculus flexor digitorum profundus
flexor muscle of fingers, superficial	musculus flexor digitorum superficialis
flexor muscle of great toe, long	musculus flexor hallucis longus
flexor muscle of great toe, short	musculus flexor hallucis brevis

muscle	musculus (pl. musculi)
flexor muscle of little finger, short	musculus flexor digiti minimi brevis manus
flexor muscle of little toe, short	musculus flexor digiti minimi brevis pedis
flexor muscle of thumb, short	musculus flexor pollicis brevis
flexor muscle of thumb, long	musculus flexor pollicis longus
flexor muscle of toes, short	musculus flexor digitorum brevis
flexor muscle of toes, long	musculus flexor digitorum longus
flexor muscle of wrist, radial	musculus flexor carpi radialis
flexor muscle of wrist, ulnar	musculus flexor carpi ulnaris
Folius' muscle	ligamentum mallei laterale
fusiform muscle (spindle-shaped muscle)	musculus fusiformis
Gantzer's muscle	
gastrocnemius muscle	musculus gastrocnemius
Gavard's muscle	
gemellus muscle, inferior	musculus gemellus inferior
gemellus muscle, superior	musculus gemellus superior
genioglossal muscle	musculus genioglossus
geniohyoid muscle	musculus geniohyoideus
glossopalatine muscle (palatoglossus)	musculus palatoglossus
glossopharyngeal muscle	pars glossopharyngea musculi constrictoris pharyngis superioris
gluteal muscle, greatest	musculus gluteus maximus
gluteal muscle, least	musculus gluteus minimus
gluteal muscle, middle	musculus gluteus medius
gracilis muscle	musculus gracilis
great adductor muscle	musculus adductor magnus
greater pectoral muscle	musculus pectoralis major
greater posterior rectus muscle of head	musculus rectus capitis posterior major
greater psoas muscle	musculus psoas major
greater rhomboid muscle	musculus rhomboideus major
greater zygomatic muscle	musculus zygomaticus major
Guthrie's muscle	sphincter urethrae
hamstring muscles	
head, muscles of	musculi capitis
Hilton's muscle	musculus aryepiglotticus
Horner's muscle	musculus orbicularis oculi
Houston's muscle	compressor venae dorsalis penis
hyoglossal (hyoglossus) muscle	musculus hyoglossus

muscle	musculus (pl. musculi)
iliac muscle	musculus iliacus
iliacus minor muscle	musculus iliacus minor
iliococcygeal muscle	musculus iliococcygeus
iliocostal muscle	musculus iliocostalis
iliocostal muscle of neck	musculus iliocostalis cervicis
iliocostal muscle of loins	musculus iliocostalis lumborum
iliocostal muscle of thorax	musculus iliocostalis thoracis
iliopsoas muscle	musculus iliopsoas
incisive muscles of inferior lip	musculi incisivi labii inferioris
incisive muscles of lower lip	musculi incisivi labii inferioris
incisive muscles of superior lip	musculi incisivi labii superioris
incisive muscles of upper lip	musculi incisivi labii superioris
index extensor muscle	musculus extensor indicis
inferior constrictor muscle of pharynx	musculus constrictor pharyngis inferior
inferior gemellus muscle	musculus gemellus inferior
inferior longitudinal muscle of tongue	musculus longitudinalis inferior
inferior oblique muscle	musculus obliquus inferior
inferior oblique muscle of head	musculus obliquus capitis inferior
inferior posterior serratus muscle	serratus posterior inferior musculus
inferior rectus muscle	musculus rectus inferior
inferior tarsal muscle	musculus tarsalis inferior
infrahyoid muscles	musculi infrahyoidei
infraspinous muscle	musculus infraspinatus
innermost intercostal muscle	musculus intercostalis intimus
inspiratory muscles	
intercostal muscles	musculi intercostales
interfoveolar muscle	ligamentum interfoveolare
intermediate great muscle	musculus vastus intermedius
internal intercostal muscle	musculus intercostalis internus
internal oblique muscle	musculus obliquus internus abdominis
internal obturator muscle	musculus obturator internus
internal pterygoid muscle	musculus pterygoideus medialis
interosseous muscles	musculi interossei
interspinal muscles	musculi interspinales
intertransverse muscles	musculi intertransversarii
intra-auricular muscles	
intraocular muscles	
intrinsic muscles	
intrinsic muscles of foot	

muscle	**musculus** (pl. **musculi**)
involuntary muscles	
iridic muscles	
ischiocavernous muscle	musculus ischiocavernosus
Jarjavay's muscle	
Jung's pyramidal auricular muscle	
Klein's cutaneomucous muscle	
Kohlrausch's muscle	
Koyter's muscle	musculus corrugator supercilii
Krause's cutaneomucous muscle	musculus cutaneomucosus
Landstrom's muscle (umlaut o)	
Langer's axillary arch muscle	
larynx, muscles of	musculi laryngis
lateral cricoarytenoid muscle	musculus cricoarytenoideus lateralis
lateral great muscle	musculus vastus lateralis
lateral lumbar intertransversarii muscles	musculi intertransversarii laterales lumborum
lateral pterygoid muscle	musculus pterygoideus lateralis
lateral rectus muscle	musculus rectus lateralis
lateral rectus muscle of the head	musculus rectus capitis lateralis
lateral vastus muscle	musculus vastus lateralis
latissimus dorsi muscle	musculus latissimus dorsi
lesser rhomboid muscle	musculus rhomboid minor
lesser zygomatic muscle	musculus zygomaticus minor
levator ani muscle	musculus levator ani
levator muscles (see *elevator muscles*)	
lingual muscles	musculi linguae
long abductor muscle of thumb	musculus abductor pollicis longus
long adductor muscle	musculus adductor longus
long extensor muscle of great toe	musculus extensor hallucis longus
long extensor muscle of thumb	musculus extensor pollicis longus
long extensor muscle of toes	musculus extensor digitorum longus
long fibular muscle	musculus peroneus longus
long flexor muscle of great toe	musculus flexor hallucis longus
long flexor muscle of thumb	musculus flexor pollicis longus
long flexor muscle of toes	musculus flexor digitorum longus
long muscle of head	musculus longus capitis
longissimus muscle	musculus longissimus
longissimus muscle of back (thorax)	musculus longissimus thoracis
longissimus muscle of head	musculus longissimus capitis

muscle	musculus (pl. musculi)
longissimus muscle of neck	musculus longissimus cervicis
longitudinal muscle of tongue, inferior	musculus longitudinalis inferior linguae
longitudinal muscle of tongue, superior	musculus longitudinalis superior linguae
long muscle of head	musculus longus capitis
long muscle of neck	musculus longus colli
long palmar muscle	musculus palmaris longus
long peroneal muscle	musculus peroneus longus
long radial extensor muscle of wrist	musculus extensor carpi radialis longus
lumbar iliocostal muscle	musculus interspinalis lumborum
lumbar interspinal muscles	musculus interspinalis lumborum
lumbar quadrate muscle	musculus quadratus lumborum
lumbar rotator muscles	musculi rotatores lumborum
lumbrical muscles of foot	musculi lumbricales pedis
lumbrical muscles of hand	musculi lumbricales manus
Marcacci's muscle	
masseter muscle	musculus masseter
medial great muscle	musculus vastus medialis
medial lumbar intertransverse muscles	musculi intertransversarii mediales lumborum
medial pterygoid muscle	musculus pterygoideus medialis
medial rectus muscle	musculus rectus medialis
medial vastus muscle	musculus vastus medialis
mentalis muscle	musculus mentalis
Merkel's muscle	musculus ceratocricoideus
mesothenar muscle	musculus adductor pollicis
middle constrictor muscle of pharynx	musculus constrictor pharyngis medius
middle scalene muscle	musculus scalenus medius
mucocutaneous muscle	
Mueller's muscle	musculus orbitalis
multifidus muscles (intermediate layer of transversospinalis muscles)	musculi multifidi
multipennate muscle	musculus multipennatus
mylohyoid muscle	musculus mylohyoideus
nasal muscle	musculus nasalis
neck, muscles of	musculi colli
nonstriated muscle (smooth muscle)	
notch of helix, muscles of	musculus incisurae helicis
oblique arytenoid muscle	musculus arytenoideus obliquus
oblique auricular muscle	musculus obliquus auriculae

muscle	musculus (pl. musculi)
oblique muscle of abdomen, external	musculus obliquus externus abdominis
oblique muscle of abdomen, internal	musculus obliquus internus abdominis
oblique muscle of head, inferior	musculus obliquus capitis inferior
oblique muscle of head, superior	musculus obliquus capitis superior
obturator muscle, external	musculus obturator externus
obturator muscle, internal	musculus obturator internus
occipitofrontal muscle	musculus occipitofrontalis
Ochsner's muscles	
ocular muscles	musculi bulbi
Oddi's muscle (sphincter)	
Oehl's muscles	
omohyoid muscle	musculus omohyoideus
opposing muscle of little finger	musculus opponens digiti minimi
opposing muscle of thumb	musculus opponens pollicis
orbicular muscle	musculus orbicularis
orbicular muscle of eye	musculus orbicularis oculi
orbicular muscle of mouth	musculus orbicularis oris
orbital muscle	musculus orbitalis
organic muscle (visceral musscle)	
palate and fauces, muscles	musculi palati et faucium
palatine muscles	musculi palati
palatoglossus muscle	musculus palatoglossus
palatopharyngeal muscle	musculus palatopharyngeus
palmar interosseous muscle	musculus interosseus palmaris
palmar muscle, short	musculus palmaris brevis
palmar muscle, long	musculus palmaris longus
papillary muscle	musculus papillaris
pectinate muscles	musculi pectinati
pectineal muscle	musculus pectineus
pectoral muscle, greater	musculus pectoralis major
pectoral muscle, smaller	musculus pectoralis minor
pectorodorsalis muscle (axillary arch)	
penniform muscle	musculus unipennatus
perineal muscles	musculi perinei
peroneal muscle, long	musculus fibularis longus
peroneal muscle, short	musculus fibularis brevis
peroneal muscle, third	musculus fibularis tertius
pharyngopalatine muscle	musculus palatopharyngeus
Phillips' muscle	

muscle	musculus (pl. musculi)
piriform muscle	musculus piriformis
plantar interosseous muscle	musculus interosseus plantaris
plantar muscle	musculus plantaris
plantar quadrate muscle	musculus quadratus plantae
platysma muscle	musculus platysma
pleuroesophageal muscle	musculus pleuroesophageus
popliteal muscle	musculus popliteus
posterior auricular muscle	musculus retrahens aurem
posterior cervical intertransverse muscles	musculi intertransversarii posteriores cervicis
posterior cricoarytenoid muscle	musculus cricoarytenoideus posterior
posterior scalene muscle	musculus scalenus posterior
posterior tibial muscle	musculus tibialis posterior
Pozzi's muscle (extensor digitorum brevis muscle of hand)	musculus extensor digitorum brevis manus
procerus muscle	musculus procerus
pronator muscle, quadrate	musculus pronator quadratus
pronator muscle, round	musculus pronator teres
psoas muscle, greater	musculus psoas major
psoas muscle, smaller	musculus psoas minor
pterygoid muscle	musculus pterygoideus
pubococcygeal muscle	musculus pubococcygeus
puboprostatic muscle	musculus puboprostaticus
puborectal muscle (Braune's muscle)	musculus puborectalis
pubovaginal muscle	musculus pubovaginalis
pubovesical muscle	musculus pubovesicalis
pyloric sphincter muscle	musculus sphincter pyloricus
pyramidal auricular muscle (Jung's m.)	musculus pyramidalis auriculae
quadrate (four-sided) muscle	musculus quadratus
quadrate muscle of loins	musculus quadratus lumborum
quadrate muscle of lower lip	musculus depressor labii inferioris
quadrate muscle of sole	musculus quadratus plantae
quadrate muscle of thigh	musculus quadratus femoris
quadrate muscle of upper lip	musculus quadratus labii superioris
radial flexor muscle of wrist	musculus flexor carpi radialis
rectococcygeus muscle	musculus rectococcygeus
rectourethral muscle	musculus recto-urethralis
rectouterine muscle	musculus recto-uterinus
rectovesical muscle	musculus rectovesicalis

muscle	musculus (pl. musculi)
rectus abdominis muscle (rectus muscle of abdomen)	musculus rectus abdominis
rectus muscle of head, anterior	musculus rectus capitis anterior
rectus muscle of head, lateral	musculus rectus capitis lateralis
rectus muscle of head, greater posterior	musculus rectus capitis posterior major
rectus muscle of head, smaller posterior	musculus rectus capitis posterior minor
rectus femoris muscle (rectus muscle of thigh)	musculus rectus femoris
red muscle (slow muscle)	
Reisseisen's muscles	
rhomboid muscle, greater	musculus rhomboideus major
rhomboid muscle, lesser	musculus rhomboideus minor
ribbon muscles	musculi infrahyoidei
rider's muscles (adductor muscles of thigh)	
Riolan's muscle (cremaster muscle)	musculus cremaster
risorius muscle (Albinus' muscle, Santorini's muscle)	musculus risorius
rotator muscles	musculi rotatores
rotator muscles of neck	musculi rotatores cervicis
rotator muscles of back	musculi rotatores lumborum
rotator muscles of thorax	musculi rotatores thoracis
Rouget's muscle	
round pronator muscle	musculus pronator teres
Ruysch's muscle	
sacrococcygeal muscle	musculus sacrococcygeus
salpingopharyngeal muscle	musculus salpingopharyngeus
Santorini's muscle	musculus risorius
sartorius muscle (tailor's muscle)	musculus sartorius
scalene muscle, anterior	musculus scalenus anterior
scalene muscle, middle	musculus scalenus medius
scalene muscle, posterior	musculus scalenus posterior
scalene muscle, smallest (Albinus' m., Sibson's m.)	musculus scalenus minimus
scalp muscle (epicranius muscle)	
Sebileau's muscle	
second tibial muscle	musculus tibialis secundus
semimembranous muscle	musculus semimembranosus
semispinal muscle	musculus semispinalis
semispinal muscle of head	musculus semispinalis capitis

muscle	musculus (pl. musculi)
semispinal muscle of neck	musculus semispinalis cervicis
semispinal muscle of thorax	musculus semispinalis thoracis
semitendinous muscle	musculus semitendinosus
serratus anterior muscle	musculus serratus anterior
serratus posterior inferior muscle	musculus serratus posterior inferior
serratus posterior superior muscle	musculus serratus posterior superior
shawl muscle (trapezius muscle)	
short adductor muscle	musculus adductor brevis
short extensor musscle of great toe	musculus extensor hallucis brevis
short extensor muscle of thumb	musculus extensor pollicis brevis
short extensor muscle of toes	musculus extensor digitorum brevis
short fibular muscle	musculus peroneus brevis
short flexor muscle of great toe	musculus flexor hallucis brevis
short flexor muscle of little finger	musculus flexor digiti minimi brevis
short flexor muscle of little toe	musculus flexor digiti minimi brevis
short flexor muscle of thumb	musculus flexor pollicis brevis
short flexor muscle of toes	musculus flexor digitorum brevis
short palmar muscle	musculus palmaris brevis
short peroneal muscle	musculus peroneus brevis
short radial extensor muscle of wrist	musculus extensor carpi radialis brevis
Sibson's muscle	musculus scalenus minimus
skeletal muscles	musculi skeleti
slow muscle (red muscle)	
smaller muscle of helix	musculus helicis minor
smaller pectoral muscle	musculus pectoralis minor
smaller posterior rectus muscle of head	musculus rectus capitis posterior minor
smaller psoas muscle	musculus psoas minor
smallest scalene muscle	musculus scalenus minimus
smooth muscle (unstriated, unstriped, visceral)	
Soemmerring's muscle (levator muscle of thyroid gland)	
soleus muscle	musculus soleus
somatic muscles	musculi skeleti
sphincter muscle of anus	musculus sphincter ani
sphincter muscle of bile duct	musculus sphincter ductus choledochi
sphincter muscle of hepatopancreatic ampulla	musculus sphincter ampullae hepatopancreaticae
sphincter muscle of pupil	musculus sphincter pupillae

muscle	musculus (pl. musculi)
sphincter muscle of pylorus	musculus sphincter pyloricus
sphincter muscle of urethra	musculus sphincter urethrae
sphincter muscle of urinary bladder	musculus sphincter vesicae urinariae
spinal muscle	musculus spinalis
spinal muscle of head	musculus spinalis capitis
spinal muscle of neck	musculus spinalis cervicis
spinal muscle of thorax	musculus spinalis thoracis
spindle-shaped muscle	musculus fisiform
splenius muscle of head	musculus splenius capitis
splenius muscle of neck	musculus splenius cervicis
stapedius muscle	musculus stapedius
sternal muscle	musculus sternalis
sternochondroscapular muscle	musculus sternochondroscapularis
sternoclavicular muscle	musculus sternoclavicularis
sternocleidomastoid muscle	musculus sternocleidomastoideus
sternocostal muscle	musculus transversus thoracis
sternohyoid muscle	musculus sternohyoideus
sternomastoid muscle (sternocleidomastoid)	
sternothyroid muscle	musculus sternothyroideus
strap muscles	
striated muscle	
styloauricular muscle	musculus styloauricularis
styloglossus muscle	musculus styloglossus
stylohyoid muscle	musculus stylohyoideus
stylopharyngeal muscle	musculus stylopharyngeus
subanconeus muscle	musculus articularis cubiti
subclavian muscle	musculus subclavius
subcostal muscle	musculus subcostalis
subcrural muscle	musculus articularis genu
suboccipital muscles	musculi suboccipitales
subquadricipital muscle	musculus articularis genu
subscapular muscle	musculus subscapularis
subvertebral muscles	musculi hypaxial
superficial back muscles	
superficial flexor muscle of fingers	musculus flexor digitorum superficialis
superficial lingual muscle (of tongue)	
superficial transverse perineal muscle (Theile's muscle)	musculus transversus perinei superficialis
superior auricular muscle	musculus auricularis superior

muscle	musculus (pl. musculi)
superior constrictor muscle of pharynx	musculus constrictor pharyngis superior
superior gemellus muscle	musculus gemellus superior
superior longitudinal muscle of tongue	musculus longitudinalis superior
superior oblique muscle	musculus obliquus superior
superior oblique muscle of head	musculus obliquus capitis superior
superior posterior serratus muscle	musculus serratus posterior superior
superior rectus muscle	musculus rectus superior
superior tarsal muscle (Mueller's muscle)	musculus tarsalis superior
supinator muscle	musculus supinator
supraclavicular muscle	musculus supraclavicularis
suprahyoid muscles	musculi suprahyoidei
supraspinalis muscle	musculus supraspinalis
supraspinous muscle	musculus supraspinatus
suspensory muscle of duodenum (Treitz' ligament)	musculus suspensorius duodeni
synergic or synergistic muscles	
tailor's muscle (sartorius muscle)	
temporal muscle	musculus temporalis
temporoparietal muscle	musculus temporoparietalis
tensor muscle of fascia lata	musculus tensor fasciae latae
tensor muscle of soft palate	musculus tensor veli palati
tensor tarsi muscle	musculus orbicularis oculi
tensor muscle of tympanic membrane (Toynbee's muscle)	musculus tensor tympani
teres major muscle	musculus teres major
teres minor muscle	musculus teres minor
Theile's muscle (superficial transverse perineal muscle)	
third peroneal muscle	musculus peroneus tertius
thoracic interspinal muscle	musculi thoracic interspinalis
thoracic intertransverse muscles	musculi intertransversarii thoracis
thoracic longissimus muscle	musculus longissimus thoracis
thoracic rotator muscles	musculi rotatores thoracis
thorax, muscles of	musculi thoracis
thyroarytenoid muscle	musculus thyroarytenoideus
thyroepiglottic muscle (depressor muscle of epiglottis)	musculus thyroepiglotticus
thyrohyoid muscle	musculus thyrohyoideus

muscle	musculus (pl. musculi)
tibial muscle, anterior	musculus tibialis anterior
tibial muscle, posterior	musculus tibialis posterior
Tod's muscle (oblique auricular muscle)	
tongue, muscles of	musculi linguae
Toynbee's muscle	musculus tensor tympani
tracheal muscle	musculus trachealis
tracheloclavicular muscle	musculus tracheloclavicularis
trachelomastoid muscle	musculus longissimus capitis
tragicus muscle	musculus tragicus
(Valsalva's muscle)	
transverse arytenoid muscle	musculus arytenoideus transversus
transverse muscle of abdomen	musculus transversus abdominis
transverse muscle of auricle	musculus transversus auriculae
transverse muscle of chin	musculus transversus menti
transverse muscle of nape	musculus transversus nuchae
transverse muscle of neck	musculus transversus nuchae
transverse muscle of thorax	musculus transversus thoracis
transverse muscle of tongue	musculus transversus linguae
transversospinal muscle	musculus transversospinalis
trapezius muscle	musculus trapezius
Treitz' muscle (suspensory muscle of duodenum)	
triangular muscle	musculus triangularis
triceps muscle of arm	musculus triceps brachii
triceps muscle of hip	musculus triceps coxae
triceps muscle of calf	musculus triceps surae
trigonal muscle	
true (deep) muscles of back	musculi dorsi
two-bellied muscle (digastric muscle)	musculus digastricus
ulnar extensor muscle of wrist	musculus extensor carpi ulnaris
ulnar flexor muscle of wrist	musculus flexor carpi ulnaris
unipennate muscle	musculus unipennatus
unstriated muscle, unstriped muscle (smooth muscle)	
urogenital diaphragm, muscles of	musculi diaphragmatis urogenitalis
uvula, muscle of	musculus uvulae
Valsalva's muscle	
vastus intermedius muscle (intermediate great muscle)	musculus vastus intermedius

muscle	musculus (pl. musculi)
vastus lateralis muscle (lateral great muscle)	musculus vastus lateralis
vastus medialis muscle (medial great muscle)	musculus vastus medialis
ventral sacrococcygeal muscle	musculus sacrococcygeus ventralis
vertical muscle of tongue	musculus verticalis linguae
visceral muscle (smooth)	
vocal muscle	musculus vocalis
voluntary muscle	
white muscle (fast muscle)	
Wilson's muscle (urethral sphincter)	musculus sphincter urethrae
wrinkler muscle of eyebrow	musculus corrugator supercilii
yoked muscles	
zygomatic muscle, greater	musculus zygomaticus major
zygomatic muscle, lesser	musculus zygomaticus minor

Table of Nerves

nerve	nervus (pl. nervi)
abdominopelvic splanchnic nerves	
abducent nerve	nervus abducens
accelerator nerves	
accessory nerve	nervus accessorius
accessory nerve, vagal	ramus internus nervi accessorii
accessory phrenic nerves	nervi phrenici accessorii
acoustic nerve	
afferent nerve (centripetal; esodic)	
alveolar nerve, inferior	nervus alveolaris inferior
alveolar nerves, superior	nervi alveolares superiores
ampullar nerve, anterior	nervus ampullaris anterior
ampullar nerve, inferior	nervus ampullaris inferior
ampullar nerve, lateral	nervus ampullaris lateralis
ampullar nerve, superior	nervus ampullaris superior
anal nerves, inferior	nervi rectales inferiores
Andersch's nerve (tympanic)	
anococcygeal nerves	nervi anococcygei
anterior ampullar nerve	nervus ampullaris anterior
anterior antebrachial nerve (anterior interosseous nerve)	
anterior auricular nerves	nervi auriculares anteriores
anterior crural nerve (femoral nerve)	
anterior cutaneous nerves of abdomen (thoracoabdominal nerves)	
anterior ethmoidal nerve	nervus ethmoidalis anterior
anterior femoral cutaneous nerves	rami cutanei anteriores nervi femoralis
anterior interosseous nerve	nervus interosseous anterior
anterior labial nerves	nervi labiales anteriores
anterior scrotal nerves	nervi scrotales anteriores
anterior supraclavicular nerve (medial supraclavicular nerve)	
anterior tibial nerve (deep peroneal nerve)	

nerve	nervus (pl. nervi)
aortic nerve (Cyon's nerve, depressor nerve of Ludwig, Ludwig's nerve)	
Arnold's nerve	ramus auricularis nervi vagi
articular nerve	nervus articularis
auditory nerve (cochlear)	nervus vestibulocochlearis
augmentor nerves (cervical splanchnic nerves)	
auricular nerves, anterior	nervi auriculares anteriores
auricular nerve, great	nervus auricularis magnus
auricular nerve, internal	ramus posterior nervi auricularis magni
auricular nerve, posterior	nervus auricularis posterior
auricular nerve of vagus nerve	ramus auricularis nervi vagi
auriculotemporal nerve	nervus auriculotemporalis
autonomic nerve	nervus autonomicus
axillary nerve	nervus axillaris
baroreceptor nerve (pressoreceptor nerve)	
Bell's long thoracic nerve	nervus thoracicus longus
Bock's nerve	ramus pharyngeus ganglii pterygopalatini
buccal nerve	nervus buccalis
buccinator nerve (buccal nerve)	
cardiac nerve, cervical, inferior	nervus cardiacus cervicalis inferior
cardiac nerve, cervical, middle	nervus cardiacus cervicalis medius
cardiac nerve, cervical, superior	nervus cardiacus cervicalis superior
cardiac nerve, inferior	nervus cardiacus cervicalis inferior
cardiac nerve, middle	nervus cardiacus cervicalis medius
cardiac nerve, superior	nervus cardiacus cervicalis superior
cardiac nerves, supreme	rami cardiaci cervicales superiores nervi vagi
cardiac nerves, thoracic	rami cardiaci thoracici
cardiopulmonary splanchnic nerves	
caroticotympanic nerve	nervus carotidotympanicus
carotid sinus nerve (Hering's sinus)	ramus sinus carotici
cavernous nerves of clitoris	nervi cavernosi clitoridis
cavernous nerves of penis	nervi cavernosi penis
celiac nerves	rami coeliaci nervi vagi
centrifugal nerve (efferent)	
centripetal nerve (afferent)	

nerve	nervus (pl. nervi)
cerebral nerves	nervi craniales
cervical nerves	nervi cervicales
cervical splanchnic nerves (augmentor nerves)	
chorda tympani nerve	chorda tympani
ciliary nerves	nervi ciliares
circumflex nerve (axillary)	nervus axillaris
cluneal nerves	rami clunium
coccygeal nerve	nervus coccygeus
cochlear nerve	nervus cochlearis
common fibular nerve (common peroneal)	
common palmar digital nerves	nervi digitales palmares communes
common peroneal nerve	nervus fibularis communis
common plantar digital nerves	nervi digitales plantares communes
cranial nerves	nervi craniales
cranial nerve, eighth (acoustic)	nervus vestibulocochlearis
cranial nerve, eleventh (accessory	nervus accessorius
cranial nerve, fifth (trigeminal)	nervus trigeminus
cranial nerves, first (olfactory)	nervi olfactorii
cranial nerve, fourth (trochlear)	nervus trochlearis
cranial nerve, ninth (glossopharyngeal)	nervus glossopharyngeus
cranial nerve, second (optic)	nervus opticus
cranial nerve, seventh (facial)	nervus facialis
cranial nerve, sixth (abducens)	nervus abducens
cranial nerve, tenth (vagal)	nervus vagus
cranial nerve, third (oculomotor)	nervus oculomotorius
cranial nerve, twelfth (hypoglossal)	nervus hypoglossus
crural interosseous nerve	nervus interosseus cruris
cubital nerve (ulnar nerve)	nervus ulnaris
cutaneous femoral nerve, lateral	nervus cutaneus femoris lateralis
cutaneous nerve	nervus cutaneus
cutaneous nerve, femoral	nervus cutaneus femoralis
cutaneous nerve of arm, lateral, inferior	nervus cutaneus brachii lateralis inferior
cutaneous nerve of calf, medial	nervus cutaneus surae medial
cutaneous nerve of foot, dorsal, lateral	nervus cutaneus dorsalis lateralis
cutaneous nerve of forearm, medial	nervus cutaneus antebrachii medialis
cutaneous nerve of neck, anterior	nervus transversus colli
cutaneous nerve of thigh, posterior	nervus cutaneus femoralis posterior
Cyon's nerve (aortic)	

nerve	nervus (pl. nervi)
dead nerve (nonvital dental pulp)	
deep fibular nerve (deep peroneal)	
deep peroneal nerve	nervus fibularis profundus
deep petrosal nerve	nervus petrosus profundus
deep temporal nerves	nervi temporales profundi
dental nerve, inferior	nervus alveolaris inferior
depressor nerve of Ludwig (aortic)	
diaphragmatic nerve	nervus phrenicus
digastric nerve	ramus digastricus nervi facialis
digital nerves, dorsal, radial	nervi digitales dorsales nervi radialis
dorsal nerve of clitoris	nervus dorsalis clitoridis
dorsal digital nerves	
dorsal digital nerves of foot	nervi digitales dorsales pedis
dorsal digital nerves of hand	
dorsal interosseous nerve (posterior interosseous)	
dorsal lateral cutaneous nerve (lateral dorsal cutaneous)	
dorsal medial cutaneous nerve (medial dorsal cutaneous n.)	
dorsal nerve of penis	nervus dorsalis penis
dorsal nerve of scapula (dorsal scapular)	
dorsal scapular nerve	nervus dorsalis scapulae
dorsal nerves of toes	
efferent nerve (centrifugal nerve)	
eighth cranial nerve (vestibulocochlear nerve)	nervus vestibulocochlearis
eleventh cranial nerve (accessory nerve)	nervus accessorius
encephalic nerves	nervi craniales
esodic nerve (afferent nerve)	
ethmoidal nerve, anterior	nervus ethmoidalis anterior
excitor nerve	
excitoreflex nerve	
exodic nerve	
external acoustic meatus, nerve of	nervus meatus acustici externi
external carotid nerves	nervi carotici externi
external respiratory nerve of Bell (long thoracis nerve)	
external saphenous nerve (sural nerve)	

nerve	nervus (pl. nervi)
external spermatic nerve (genital branch of genitofemoral nerve)	
facial nerve	nervus facialis
femoral cutaneous nerve, intermediate	
femoral nerve	nervus femoralis
fibular nerve, superficial	nervus fibularis superficialis
fifth cranial nerve (trigeminal nerve)	nervus trigeminus
first cranial nerve (olfactory nerve)	nervus olfactorius
fourth cranial nerve (trochlear nerve)	nervus trochlearis
fourth lumbar nerve	nervus furcalis
frontal nerve	nervus frontalis
furcal nerve (fourth lumbar nerve)	
fusimotor nerves	
Galen's nerve	
gangliated nerve	
gastric nerves	truncus vagalis anterior and truncus vagalis posterior
genitocrural nerve (genitofemoral nerve)	
genitofemoral nerve	nervus genitofemoralis
glossopharyngeal nerve (ninth cranial nerve)	nervus glossopharyngeus
gluteal nerve, inferior	nervus gluteus inferior
great auricular nerve	nervus auricularis magnus
greater occipital nerve	nervus occipitalis major
greater palatine nerve	nervus palatinus major
greater petrosal nerve	
greater splanchnic nerve	nervus splanchnicus major
greater superficial petrosal nerve	nervus petrosus major
great sciatic nerve	
gustatory nerves	
hemorrhoidal nerves, inferior	nervi rectales inferiores
Hering's sinus nerve (carotid sinus)	
hypogastric nerve	nervus hypogastricus
hypoglossal nerve (twelfth cranial)	nervus hypoglossus
iliohypogastric nerve	nervus iliohypogastricus
ilioinguinal nerve	nervus ilio-inguinalis
inferior alveolar nerve	nervus alveolaris inferior
inferior cervical cardiac nerve	nervus cardiacus cervicalis inferior
inferior cluneal nerves	nervi clunium inferiores

nerve	nervus (pl. nervi)
inferior dental nerve (inferior alveolar)	
inferior gluteal nerve	nervus gluteus inferior
inferior hemorrhoidal nerves	
inferior laryngeal nerve	nervus laryngeus inferior
inferior lateral brachial cutaneous nerve	nervus cutaneus brachii lateralis inferior
inferior maxillary nerve	
inferior rectal nerves	nervi rectales inferiores
inferior vesical nerves	
infraoccipital nerve	nervus suboccipitalis
infraorbital nerve	nervus infraorbitalis
infratrochlear nerve	nervus infratrochlearis
inhibitory nerve	
intercarotid nerve	
intercostal nerves	nervi intercostales
intercostobrachial nerves	nervi intercostobrachiales
intercostohumeral nerves	
intermediary nerve	nervus intermedius
intermediate nerve	nervus intermedius
intermediate dorsal cutaneous nerve	
Jacobson's nerve (tympanic)	nervus tympanicus
jugular nerve	nervus jugularis
lacrimal nerve	nervus lacrimalis
Lancisi, nerves of	
Langley's nerves (pilomotor nerves)	
Latarget's nerve (superior hypogastric plexus)	
laryngeal nerve, recurrent	nervus laryngealis recurrens
lateral ampullar nerve	nervus ampullaris lateralis
lateral antebrachial cutaneous nerve	nervus cutaneus antebrachii lateralis
lateral anterior thoracic nerve	
lateral cutaneous nerve of calf	
lateral cutaneous nerve of forearm	
lateral cutaneous nerve of thigh	
lateral dorsal cutaneous nerve	nervus cutaneus dorsalis lateralis
lateral femoral cutaneous nerve	nervus cutaneus femoris lateralis
lateral pectoral nerve	nervus pectoralis lateralis
lateral plantar nerve	nervus plantaris lateralis
lateral popliteal nerve	
lateral supraclavicular nerve	nervus supraclavicularis lateralis

nerve	nervus (pl. nervi)
lateral sural cutaneous nerve	nervus cutaneus surae lateralis
lesser internal cutaneous nerve	
lesser occipital nerve	nervus occipitalis minor
lesser palatine nerves	nervi palatini minores
lesser petrosal nerve	
lesser splanchnic nerve	nervus splanchnicus minor
lesser superficial petrosal nerve	nervus petrosus minor
levator ani, nerve to	
lingual nerve	nervus lingualis
long buccal nerve	
long ciliary nerve	nervus ciliaris longus
longitudinal nerves of Lancisi	
long saphenous nerve	
long subscapular nerve	
long thoracic nerve	nervus thoracicus longus
lower lateral cutaneous nerve of arm	
lowest splanchnic nerve	nervus splanchnicus imus
Ludwig's nerve (aortic nerve)	
lumbar nerves	nervi lumbales
lumbar splanchnic nerves	nervi splanchnici lumbales
lumboinguinal nerve	ramus femoralis nervi genitofemoralis
Luschka, nerve of	
mandibular nerve	nervus mandibularis
masseteric nerve	nervus massestericus
masticator nerve	
maxillary nerve	nervus maxillaris
medial antebrachial cutaneous nerve	nervus cutaneus antebrachii medialis
medial anterior thoracic nerve	
medial brachial cutaneous nerve	nervus cutaneus brachii medialis
medial cutaneous nerve of arm	
medial cutaneous nerve of forearm	
medial cutaneous nerve of leg	
medial dorsal cutaneous nerve	nervus cutaneus dorsalis medialis
medial pectoral nerve	nervus pectoralis medialis
medial plantar nerve	nervus plantaris medialis
medial popliteal nerve	
medial supraclavicular nerve	nervus supraclavicularis medialis
medial sural cutaneous nerve	nervus cutaneus surae medialis
median nerve	nervus medianus

nerve	nervus (pl. nervi)
meningeal nerve	ramus meningeus medius nervi maxillaris
mental nerve	nervus mentalis
middle cervical cardiac nerve	nervus cardiacus cervicalis medius
middle cluneal nerves	nervi clunium medii
middle meningeal nerve	
middle supraclavicular nerve	
mixed nerve	nervus mixtus
motor nerve	nervus motorius
motor nerve of tongue	nervus hypoglossus
musculocutaneous nerve	nervus musculocutaneus
musculocutaneous nerve of leg	nervus fibularis profundus
musculospiral nerve (radial)	nervus radialis
myelinated nerve	
mylohyoid nerve	nervus mylohyoideus
nasal nerve	
nasociliary nerve	nervus nasociliaris
nasopalatine nerve	nervus nasopalatinus
ninth cranial nerve (glossopharyngeal nerve)	nervus glossopharyngeus
obturator nerve	nervus obturatorius
oculomotor nerve	nervus oculomotorius
olfactory nerves	nervi olfactorii
ophthalmic nerve	nervus ophthalmicus
optic nerve (second cranial nerve)	nervus opticus
orbital nerve	
palatine nerve, anterior	nervus palatinus major
parasympathetic nerve	
parotid nerves	rami parotidei nervi auriculotemporalis
pathetic nerve	
pectoral nerve, lateral	nervus pectoralis lateralis
pelvic splanchnic nerves	nervi pelvici splanchnici
parasympathetic nerve	
perforating cutaneous nerve	
perineal nerves	nervi perineales
peroneal nerve, common	nervus fibularis communis
phrenic nerve	nervus phrenicus
pneumogastric nerve	nervus vagus
popliteal nerve, external	nervus fibularis communis

nerve	nervus (pl. nervi)
popliteal nerve, internal	nervus tibialis
popliteal nerve, lateral	nervus fibularis communis
popliteal nerve, medial	nervus tibialis
posterior ampullar nerve	nervus ampullaris posterior
posterior antebrachial nerve	
posterior antebrachial cutaneous nerve	nervus cutaneus antebrachii posterior
posterior auricular nerve	nervus auricularis posterior
posterior brachial cutaneous nerve	nervus cutaneus brachii posterior
posterior cutaneous nerve of arm	
posterior cutaneous nerve of forearm	
posterior cutaneous nerve of thigh	
posterior ethmoidal nerve	nervus ethmoidalis posterior
posterior femoral cutaneous nerve	nervus cutaneus femoris posterior
posterior interosseous nerve	nervus interosseus posterior
posterior labial nerves	nervi labiales posteriores
posterior scapular nerve	
posterior scrotal nerves	nervi scrotales posteriores
posterior supraclavicular nerve	
posterior thoracic nerve	
presacral nerve	plexus hypogastricus superior
pressor nerve	
pressoreceptor nerve	
proper palmar digital nerves	nervi digitales palmares proprii
proper plantar digital nerves	nervi digitales plantares proprii
pterygoid nerve	nervus pterygoideus
pterygoid canal, nerve of	nervus canalis pterygoidei
pterygopalatine nerves	nervi pterygopalatini
pudendal nerve	nervus pudendus
pudic nerve (pudendal)	nervus pudendus
quadrate muscle of thigh, nerve of	nervus musculi quadrati femoris
radial nerve	nervus radialis
recurrent nerve	nervus laryngealis recurrens
recurrent laryngeal nerve	nervus laryngeus recurrens
recurrent meningeal nerve	nervus meningeus recurrens
recurrent ophthalmic nerve	ramus tentorii nervi ophthalmici
saccular nerve	nervus saccularis
sacral nerves	nervi sacrales
sacral splanchnic nerves	nervi splanchnici sacrales
saphenous nerve	nervus saphenus

nerve	nervus (pl. nervi)
sartorius, nerve to	
Scarpa's nerve	nervus nasopalatinus
sciatic nerve	nervus ischiadicus
second cranial nerve (optic nerve)	nervus opticus
secretomotor nerve	
secretory nerve	
sensory nerve	nervus sensorius
seventh cranial nerve (facial nerve)	nervus facialis
short ciliary nerve	nervus ciliaris brevis
short saphenous nerve	nervus saphenus brevis
sinus nerve	ramus sinus carotici nervi glossopharyngei
sinus nerve of Hering	
sinuvertebral nerves	
sixth cranial nerve (abducent nerve)	nervus abducens
small deep petrosal nerve	
smallest splanchnic nerve	
small sciatic nerve	
smell, nerve of (olfactory nerve)	nervi olfactorii
somatic nerve	
space nerve	
spinal nerves	nervi spinales
spinal accessory	
splanchnic nerve	nervus splanchnicus
stapedius muscle, nerve to	nervus stapedius
statoacoustic nerve	
subclavian nerve	nervus subclavius
subcostal nerve	nervus subcostalis
sublingual nerve	nervus sublingualis
suboccipital nerve	nervus suboccipitalis
subscapular nerves	nervi subscapulares
sudomotor nerves	
superficial cervical nerve	nervus cervicalis superficialis
superficial fibular nerve	nervus fibularis superficialis
superficial peroneal nerve	nervus fibularis superficialis
superior alveolar nerves	nervi alveolares superiores
superior cervical cardiac nerve	nervus cardiacus cervicalis superior
superior cluneal nerves	nervi clunium superiores
superior dental nerves	

nerve	nervus (pl. nervi)
superior gluteal nerve	nervus gluteus superior
superior laryngeal nerve	nervus laryngeus superior
superior lateral brachial cutaneous nerve	nervus cutaneus brachii lateralis superior
superior maxillary nerve	
supraorbital nerve	nervus supraorbitalis
suprascapular nerve	nervus suprascapularis
supratrochlear nerve	nervus supratrochlearis
sural nerve	nervus suralis
sympathetic nerve	
temporomandibular nerve	
tensor tympani muscle, nerve of	nervus tensoris tympani
tensor veli palatini muscle, nerve of	nervus tensoris veli palatini
tenth cranial nerve (vagus nerve)	nervus vagus
tentorial nerve	ramus tentorii nervi ophthalmici
terminal nerves	nervi terminales
third cranial nerve (oculomotor nerve)	nervus oculomotorius
third occipital nerve	nervus occipitalis tertius
thoracic cardiac nerves	nervi cardiaci thoracici
thoracic spinal nerves	nervi thoracici
thoracic splanchnic nerve	nervus splanchnicus thoracici
thoracoabdominal nerves	nervi thoracoabdominales
thoracodorsal nerve	nervus thoracodorsalis
thyrohyoid muscle, nerve to	ramus thyrohyoideus ansae cervicalis
tibial nerve	nervus tibialis
tibial communicating nerve	
Tiedemann's nerve	
tonsillar nerves	rami tonsillares nervi glossopharyngei
transverse nerve of neck	nervus transversus colli
trifacial nerve (trigeminal nerve)	nervus trigeminus
trigeminal nerve	nervus trigeminus
trochlear nerve	nervus trochlearis
twelfth cranial nerve (hypoglossal)	nervus hypoglossus
tympanic nerve	nervus tympanicus
tympanic membrane, nerve of	
ulnar nerve	nervus ulnaris
unmyelinated nerve	
upper lateral cutaneous nerve of arm	
upper subscapular nerve	

nerve	nervus (pl. nervi)
upper thoracic splanchnic nerves	
utricular nerve	nervus utricularis
utriculoampullar nerve	nervus utriculoampullaris
vaginal nerves	nervi vaginales
vagus nerve	nervus vagus
Valentin's nerve	
vascular nerve	nervus vascularis
vasoconstrictor nerve	
vasodilator nerve	
vasomotor nerve	
vasosensory nerve	
vertebral nerve	nervus vertebralis
vestibular nerve	nervus vestibularis
vestibulocochlear nerve (eighth cranial nerve)	nervus vestibulocochlearis
vidian nerve	nervus canalis pterygoidei
visceral nerve	nervus autonomicus
volar interosseous nerve	
Willis, nerve of	nervus accessorius
Wrisberg's nerve	nervus intermedius
zygomatic nerve	nervus zygomaticus
zygomaticotemporal nerves	ramus zygomaticotemporalis nervi

Table of Veins

vein	vena (pl. venae)
accessory cephalic vein	vena cephalica accessoria
accessory hemiazygos vein	vena hemiazygos accessoria
accessory saphenous vein	vena saphena accessoria
accessory vertebral vein	vena vertebralis accessoria
accompanying vein	vena comitans
accompanying vein of hypoglossal nerve	vena comitans nervi hypoglossi
adrenal veins	venae suprarenales
afferent veins	
anastomotic vein, inferior	vena anastomotica inferior
anastomotic vein, superior	vena anastomotica superior
angular vein	vena angularis
anonymous veins	venae brachiocephalicae
antebrachial vein, median	vena intermedia antebrachii
anterior auricular vein	vena auricularis anterior
anterior cardiac veins	venae cordis anteriores
anterior cardinal veins	
anterior cerebral vein	vena cerebri anterior
anterior facial vein	
anterior intercostal veins	venae intercostales anteriores
anterior jugular vein	vena jugularis anterior
anterior labial veins	venae labiales anteriores
anterior pontomesencephalic vein	vena pontomesencephalica anterior
anterior scrotal veins	venae scrotales anteriores
anterior vein of septum pellucidum	vena septi pellucidi anterior
anterior veins of heart	venae ventriculi dextri anteriores
anterior veins of right ventricle	venae ventriculi dextri anteriores
anterior tibial veins	venae tibiales anteriores
anterior vertebral vein	vena vertebralis anterior
appendicular vein	vena appendicularis
aqueduct of cochlea, vein of	vena aqueductus cochleae
aqueduct of vestibule, vein of	vena aqueductus vestibuli

vein	vena (pl. venae)
aqueous veins	
arciform veins of kidney	
arcuate veins of kidney	venae arcuatae renis
arterial vein	vena arteriosa, truncus pulmonalis
arterial vein of Soemmering	vena portae hepatis
articular veins	venae articulares
ascending veins of Rosenthal	venae inferiores cerebri
ascending lumbar vein	vena lumbalis ascendens
atrial veins of heart, left	venae atriales sinistrae
atrial veins of heart, right	venae atriales dextrae
atrial vein, lateral	vena lateralis atrii
atrial vein, medial	vena medialis atrii
atrioventricular veins of heart	venae atrioventriculares cordis
auditory veins, internal	venae labyrinthinae
auricular veins, anterior	venae auriculares anteriores
auricular veins, posterior	vena auricularis posterior
axillary vein	vena axillaris
azygos vein	vena azygos
basal vein, Rosenthal's	vena basalis
basilic vein	vena basilica
basivertebral vein	vena basivertebralis
Baumgarten's veins	
Boyd communicating perforation veins	
brachial veins	venae brachiales
brachiocephalic veins	venae brachiocephalicae
Breschet's vein	venae diploicae
bronchial veins	venae bronchiales
Browning's vein	
bulb of penis, vein of	vena bulbi penis
Burow's vein	
canaliculus of cochlea, vein of	vena aqueductus cochleae
capillary vein	
cardiac veins	venae cordis
cardiac veins, anterior	venae ventriculi dextri anteriores
cardiac vein, great	vena cardiaca magna
cardiac vein, middle	vena cardiaca media
cardiac vein, small	vena cardiaca parva
cardiac veins, smallest	venae cardiacae minimae
cardinal veins	

vein	vena (pl. venae)
carotid vein, external	vena retromandibularis
caudate nucleus, veins of	venae nuclei caudati
cavernous veins of penis	venae cavernosae penis
central veins of liver	venae centrales hepatis
central vein of retina	vena centralis retinae
central vein of suprarenal gland	vena centralis glandulae suprarenalis
cephalic vein	vena cephalica
cerebellar veins	venae cerebelli
cerebral veins	venae cerebri
cervical vein, deep	vena cervicalis profunda
choroid vein	vena choroidea
choroid veins of eye	
ciliary veins	venae ciliares
circumflex veins	venae circumflexae
cochlear aqueduct, vein of	vena aqueductus cochleae
cochlear canaliculus, vein of	vena aqueductus cochleae
Cockett communicating perforating veins	
colic vein, left	vena colica sinistra
colic vein, middle	vena colica media
colic vein, right	vena colica dextra
common basal vein	vena basalis communis
common cardinal veins (ducts of Cuvier)	
common facial vein	vena facialis communis
common iliac vein	vena iliaca communis
communicating veins (perforating veins)	
companion vein, companion veins	vena comitans, venae comitantes
condylar emissary vein	vena emissaria condylaris
conjunctival veins	venae conjunctivales
coronary vein, left	vena coronaria sinistra
coronary vein, right	vena coronaria dextra
corpus callosum, vein of, dorsal	vena dorsalis corporis callosi
corpus callosum, vein of, posterior	vena posterior corporis callosi
corpus striatum, vein of	
costoaxillary veins	venae costoaxillares
cubital vein, median	vena intermedia cubiti
cutaneous vein	vena cutanea
cutaneous vein, ulnar	vena basilica
Cuvier's veins	
cystic vein	vena cystica

vein	vena (pl. venae)
deep cerebral veins	venae cerebri profundae
deep cervical vein	vena cervicalis profunda
deep circumflex iliac vein	vena circumflexa iliaca profunda
deep veins of clitoris	venae profundae clitoridis
deep dorsal vein of clitoris	vena dorsalis clitoridis profunda
deep dorsal vein of penis	vena dorsalis penis profunda
deep epigastric vein	
deep facial vein	vena faciei profunda
deep femoral vein	vena profunda femoris
deep lingual vein	vena profunda linguae
deep middle cerebral vein	vena cerebri media profunda
deep vein of penis	vena profunda penis
deep temporal veins	venae temporales profundae
digital veins	venae digitales
diploic vein	vena diploica
dorsal callosal vein	vena corporis callosi dorsalis
dorsal veins of clitoris	venae dorsales clitoridis
dorsal vein of corpus callosum	vena corporis callosi dorsalis
dorsal digital veins of foot	venae digitales dorsales pedis
dorsal digital veins of toes	
dorsal lingual vein	venae dorsales linguae
dorsal metacarpal veins	venae metacarpeae dorsales
dorsal metatarsal veins	venae metatarseae dorsales
dorsal veins of penis, deep	vena dorsalis profunda penis
dorsal scapular vein	vena scapularis dorsalis
dorsispinal veins	
emissary vein	vena emissaria
emulgent vein	
epigastric veins, superior	venae epigastricae superiores
episcleral veins	venae episclerales
esophageal veins	venae esophageae
ethmoidal veins	venae ethmoidales
external iliac vein	vena iliaca externa
external jugular vein	vena jugularis externa
external nasal veins	venae nasales externae
external pudendal veins	venae pudendae externae
eyelids, veins of	
facial vein	vena facialis
femoral vein	vena femoralis

vein	vena (pl. venae)
fibular veins	venae fibulares
frontal veins	venae frontales
Galen, veins of	venae internae cerebri
gastric veins	venae gastricae
gastroepiploic vein, left	vena gastro-omentalis sinistra
gastroepiploic vein, right	vena gastro-omentalis dextra
gastro-omental vein, left	vena gastro-omentalis sinistra
gastro-omental vein, right	vena gastro-omentalis dextra
genicular veins	venae geniculares
gluteal veins, inferior	venae gluteae inferiores
gluteal veins, superior	venae gluteae superiores
great cardiac vein	vena cordis magna
great cerebral vein	
great cerebral vein of Galen	vena cerebri magna
great vein of Galen	
great saphenous vein	vena saphena magna
hemiazygos vein	vena hemiazygos
hemorrhoidal veins	venae rectales
hepatic veins	venae hepaticae
hepatic portal vein	
highest intercostal vein	vena intercostalis suprema
hypogastric vein	vena iliaca interna
ileal veins	venae ileales
ileocolic vein	vena ileocolica
iliac vein, common	vena iliaca communis
iliac vein, external	vena iliaca externa
iliac vein, internal	vena iliaca interna
iliolumbar vein	vena iliolumbalis
inferior anastomotic vein	vena anastomotica inferior
inferior basal vein	vena basalis inferior
inferior cardiac vein	
inferior veins of cerebellar hemisphere	venae hemispherii cerebelli inferiores
inferior cerebral veins	venae cerebri inferiores
inferior choroid vein	vena choroidea inferior
inferior epigastric vein	vena epigastrica inferior
inferior eyelid veins	
inferior gluteal veins	venae gluteae inferiores
inferior hemorrhoidal veins	
inferior labial vein	vena labialis inferior

vein	vena (pl. venae)
inferior laryngeal vein	vena laryngea inferior
inferior mesenteric vein	vena mesenterica inferior
inferior ophthalmic vein	vena ophthalmica inferior
inferior palpebral veins	venae palpebrales inferiores
inferior phrenic vein	vena phrenica inferior
inferior rectal veins	venae rectales inferiores
inferior thalamostriate veins	venae thalamostriatae inferiores
inferior thyroid vein	vena thyroidea inferior
inferior ventricular vein	vena ventricularis inferior
inferior vein of vermis	vena vermis inferior
innominate veins	venae brachiocephalicae
innominate cardiac veins (Vieussens' veins)	
insular veins	venae insulares
intercapitular veins	venae intercapitales
intercostal veins	venae intercostales
interlobar veins of kidney	venae interlobares renis
interlobular veins of kidney	venae interlobulares renis
interlobular veins of liver	venae interlobulares hepatis
intermediate antebrachial vein	
intermediate basilic vein	vena intermedia basilica
intermediate cephalic vein	vena intermedia cephalica
intermediate colic vein	vena colica media
intermediate cubital vein	
intermediate vein of forearm	
internal auditory veins	
internal cerebral veins	venae cerebri internae
internal iliac vein	vena iliaca interna
internal jugular vein	vena jugularis interna
internal pudendal vein	vena pudenda interna
internal thoracic vein	vena thoracica interna
interosseous veins	venae interosseae
intersegmental veins	pars intersegmentalis
intervertebral vein	vena intervertebralis
intrasegmental veins	pars intrasegmentalis
jejunal and ileal veins	venae jejunales et ilei
jugular veins	venae jejunales
key vein	
kidney, veins of	venae renis
knee, veins of	venae genus

vein	vena (pl. venae)
Krukenberg's veins	venae centrales hepatis
Labbe's vein (acute e)	vena anastomotica inferior
labial veins	venae labiales
labyrinthine veins	venae labyrinthi
lacrimal vein	vena lacrimalis
large vein	vena magna
large saphenous vein	vena saphena magna
laryngeal vein, superior	vena laryngea superior
Latarget's vein	
lateral atrial vein	vena atrii lateralis
lateral circumflex femoral veins	venae circumflexae femoris laterales
lateral direct veins	venae directae laterales
lateral vein of lateral ventricle	vena atrii lateralis
lateral recess of fourth ventricle, vein of	vena recessus lateralis ventriculi quarti
lateral sacral veins	venae sacrales laterales
lateral thoracic vein	vena thoracica lateralis
left colic vein	vena colica sinistra
left coronary vein	vena coronaria sinistra
left gastric vein	vena gastrica sinistra
left gastroepiploic vein	vena gastro-omentalis sinistra
left gastro-omental vein	vena gastro-omentalis sinistra
left hepatic veins	venae hepaticae sinistrae
left inferior pulmonary vein	vena pulmonalis inferior sinistra
left ovarian vein	vena ovarica sinistra
left superior intercostal vein	vena intercostalis superior sinistra
left superior pulmonary vein	vena pulmonalis superior sinistra
left suprarenal vein	vena suprarenalis sinistra
left testicular vein	vena testicularis sinistra
left umbilical vein	vena umbilicalis sinistra
levoatrio-cardinal vein	
lingual vein	vena lingualis
long saphenous vein	vena saphena longus
long thoracic vein	vena thoracica longus
lumbar veins	venae lumbales
Marshall's oblique vein	
masseteric veins	venae massetericae
mastoid emissary vein	vena emissaria mastoidea
maxillary vein	vena maxillaris
Mayo's vein	

vein	vena (pl. venae)
medial atrial vein	vena atrii medialis
medial circumflex femoral veins	venae circumflexae femoris mediales
medial vein of lateral ventricle	vena atrii medialis
median antebrachial vein	vena intermedia antebrachii
median basilic vein	vena intermedia basilic
median cephalic vein	vena intermedia cephalica
median cubital vein	vena intermedia cubiti
median vein of forearm	vena intermedia antebrachii
median vein of neck	vena mediana colli
median sacral vein	vena sacralis mediana
mediastinal veins	venae mediastinales
median vein	vena intermedia
medulla oblongata, veins of	venae medullae oblongatae
meningeal veins	venae meningeae
mesencephalic veins	venae mesencephalicae
mesenteric vein, inferior	vena mesenterica inferior
mesenteric vein, superior	vena mesenterica superior
metacarpal veins	venae metacarpales
middle cardiac vein	vena cordis media
middle colic vein	vena colica media
middle hemorrhoidal veins	venae rectales mediae
middle hepatic veins	venae hepaticae mediae
middle meningeal veins	venae meningeae mediae
middle rectal veins	venae rectales mediae
middle temporal vein	vena temporalis media
middle thyroid vein	vena thyroidea media
musculophrenic veins	venae musculophrenicae
nasofrontal vein	vena nasofrontalis
oblique vein of left atrium	vena obliqua atrii sinistri
obturator vein	vena obturatoria
occipital vein	vena occipitalis
occipital cerebral veins	venae occipitales
occipital emissary vein	vena emissaria occipitalis
olfactory gyrus, vein of	vena gyri olfactorii
ophthalmic vein, inferior	vena ophthalmica inferior
ophthalmic vein, superior	vena ophthalmica superior
ovarian vein, left	vena ovarica sinistra
ovarian vein, right	vena ovarica dextra
palatine vein	vena palatina

vein	vena (pl. venae)
palmar digital veins	venae digitales palmares
palmar metacarpal veins	venae metacarpeae palmares
palpebral veins	venae palpebrales
pancreatic veins	venae pancreaticae
pancreaticoduodenal veins	venae pancreaticoduodenales
paraumbilical veins	venae paraumbilicales
parietal veins	venae parietales
parietal emissary vein	vena emissaria parietalis
parotid veins	venae parotidea
pectoral veins	venae pectorales
peduncular veins	venae pedunculares
perforating veins	venae perforantes
pericardiac veins	venae pericardiales
pericardiacophrenic veins	venae pericardiacophrenicae
pericardial veins	venae pericardiacae
peroneal veins	venae peroneae
petrosal vein	vena petrosa
pharyngeal veins	venae pharyngeae
phrenic veins	venae phrenicae
plantar digital veins	venae digitales plantares
plantar metatarsal veins	venae metatarseae plantares
pontine veins	venae pontis
popliteal vein	vena poplitea
portal vein	vena portae hepatis
posterior anterior jugular vein	vena jugularis posterior anterior
posterior auricular vein	vena auricularis posterior
posterior cardinal veins	
posterior facial vein	vena retromandibularis
posterior horn, vein of	vena cornus posterioris
posterior intercostal veins	venae intercostales posteriores
posterior labial veins	venae labiales posteriores
posterior vein of left ventricle	vena posterior ventriculi sinistri
posterior marginal vein	vena corporis callosi dorsalis
posterior parotid veins	venae parotideae posterioreae
posterior pericallosal vein	vena corporis callosi dorsalis
posterior scrotal veins	venae scrotales posteriores
posterior vein of left ventricle	vena ventriculi sinistri posterior
posterior vein of septum pellucidum	vena septi pellucidi posterior
posterior tibial veins	venae tibiales posteriores

vein	vena (pl. venae)
precardinal veins	
precentral cerebellar vein	vena precentralis cerebelli
prefrontal veins	venae prefrontales
prepyloric vein	vena prepylorica
pterygoid canal, vein of	vena canalis pterygoidei
pudendal veins	venae pudendae
pulmonary veins	venae pulmonales
pyloric vein	vena gastrica dextra
radial veins	venae radiales
ranine vein	vena sublingualis
rectal veins	venae rectales
renal veins	venae renales
retromandibular vein	vena retromandibularis
Retzius' veins	
right colic vein	vena colica dextra
right gastric vein	vena gastrica dextra
right gastroepiploic vein	vena gastro-omentalis dextra
right gastro-omental vein	vena gastro-omentalis dextra
right hepatic veins	venae hepaticae dextrae
right inferior pulmonary vein	vena pulmonalis inferior dextra
right ovarium vein	vena ovarica dextra
right superior intercostal vein	vena intercostalis superior dextra
right superior pulmonary vein	vena pulmonalis superior dextra
right suprarenal vein	vena suprarenalis dextra
right testicular vein	vena testicularis dextra
Rosenthal's vein	
Ruysch's veins	
sacral veins	venae sacrales
Santorini's vein	
saphenous veins	venae saphenae
Sappey's veins	venae paraumbilicales
scleral veins	venae sclerales
scrotal veins	venae scrotales
septum pellucidum, vein of, anterior	vena anterior septi pellucidi
septum pellucidum, vein of, posterior	vena posterior septi pellucidi
short gastric veins	venae gastricae breves
short saphenous vein	vena saphena breve
sigmoid veins	venae sigmoideae
small vein of heart	vena cardiaca parva

vein	vena (pl. venae)
small cardiac vein	vena cordis parva
smallest cardiac veins	venae cordis minimae
small saphenous vein	vena saphena parva
spermatic vein	vena spermatica
spinal veins	venae spinales
spiral vein of modiolus	vena spiralis modioli
splenic vein	vena splenica
stellate veins of kidney	venulae stellatae renis
Stensen's veins	venae vorticosae
sternocleidomastoid vein	vena sternocleidomastoidea
striate veins	venae thalamostriatae inferiores
stylomastoid vein	vena stylomastoidea
subclavian vein	vena subclavia
subcostal vein	vena subcostalis
subcutaneous veins of abdomen	venae subcutaneae abdominis
sublingual vein	vena sublingualis
sublobular veins	
submental vein	vena submentalis
superficial vein	vena superficialis
superficial cerebral veins	venae cerebri superficiales
superficial circumflex iliac ven	vena circumflexa iliaca superficialis
superficial dorsal veins of clitoris	venae dorsales clitoridis superficiales
superficial dorsal veins of penis	venae dorsales penis superficiales
superficial epigastric vein	vena epigastrica superficialis
superficial middle cerebral vein	vena cerebri media superficialis
superficial temporal veins	venae temporales superficiales
superior anastomotic vein	vena anastomotica superior
superior basal vein	vena basalis superior
superior veins of cerebellar hemisphere	venae hemispherii cerebelli superiores
superior cerebral veins	venae cerebri superiores
superior choroid vein	vena choroidea superior
superior epigastric veins	venae epigastricae superiores
superior eyelid, veins of	
superior gluteal veins	venae gluteae superiores
superior hemorrhoidal vein	vena rectales superior
superior intercostal vein	vena intercostalis superior
superior labial vein	vena labialis superior
superior laryngeal vein	vena laryngea superior
superior mesenteric vein	vena mesenterica superior

vein	vena (pl. venae)
superior ophthalmic vein	vena ophthalmica superior
superior palpebral veins	venae palpebrales superiores
superior phrenic veins	venae phrenicae superiores
superior rectal vein	vena rectalis superior
superior thalamostriate vein	vena thalamostriata superior
superior thyroid vein	vena thyroidea superior
superior vein of vermis	vena vermis superior
supraorbital vein	vena supraorbitalis
suprarenal veins	venae suprarenales
suprascapular vein	vena suprascapularis
supratrochlear veins	venae supratrochleares
supreme intercostal vein	vena intercostalis suprema
sural veins	venae surales
surface thalamic veins	venae directae laterales
sylvian vein, vein of sylvian fossa	vena mediae superficiales cerebri
temporal veins	venae temporales
temporomandibular joint, veins of	venae articulares temporomandibulares
temporomaxillary vein	vena temporomaxillaris
terminal vein	vena thalamostriata superior
testicular veins	venae testiculares
thalamostriate veins	venae thalamostriatae
thebesian veins	venae cordis minimae
thoracic veins	venae thoracicae
thoracoacromial vein	vena thoracoacromialis
thoracoepigastric vein	vena thoracoepigastrica
thymic veins	venae thymicae
thyroid veins	venae thyroideae
tibial veins	venae tibiales
trabecular veins	
tracheal veins	venae tracheales
transverse cervical veins	venae transversae colli
transverse facial vein	vena transversa faciei
transverse veins of neck	venae transversae cervicis
transverse vein of scapula	venae transversae scapulae
Trolard's vein	vena anastomotica superior
tympanic veins	venae tympanicae
ulnar veins	venae ulnares
umbilical vein	vena umbilicalis
uncus, vein of	vena unci

vein	vena (pl. venae)
upper limb, veins of	venae membri superioris
uterine veins	venae uterinae
varicose veins	
vena cava, inferior	vena cava inferior
vena cava, superior	vena cava superior
ventricular veins of heart	venae ventriculares cordis
vermis, inferior vein of	vena inferior vermis
vertebral vein	vena vertebralis
vertebral column, veins of	venae columnae vertebralis
vesalian vein	
Vesalius' vein	
vesical veins	venae vesicales
vestibular veins	venae vestibulares
vestibular aqueduct, vein of	vena aqueductus vestibuli
vestibular bulb, vein of	vena bulbi vestibuli
vidian veins	venae canalis pterygoidei
Vieussens' veins	venae cardiacae anteriores
vitelline vein	vena vitellina
vortex veins (vorticose veins)	venae vorticosae